P9-AFZ-432

THE BRAIN HEALTH KITCHEN

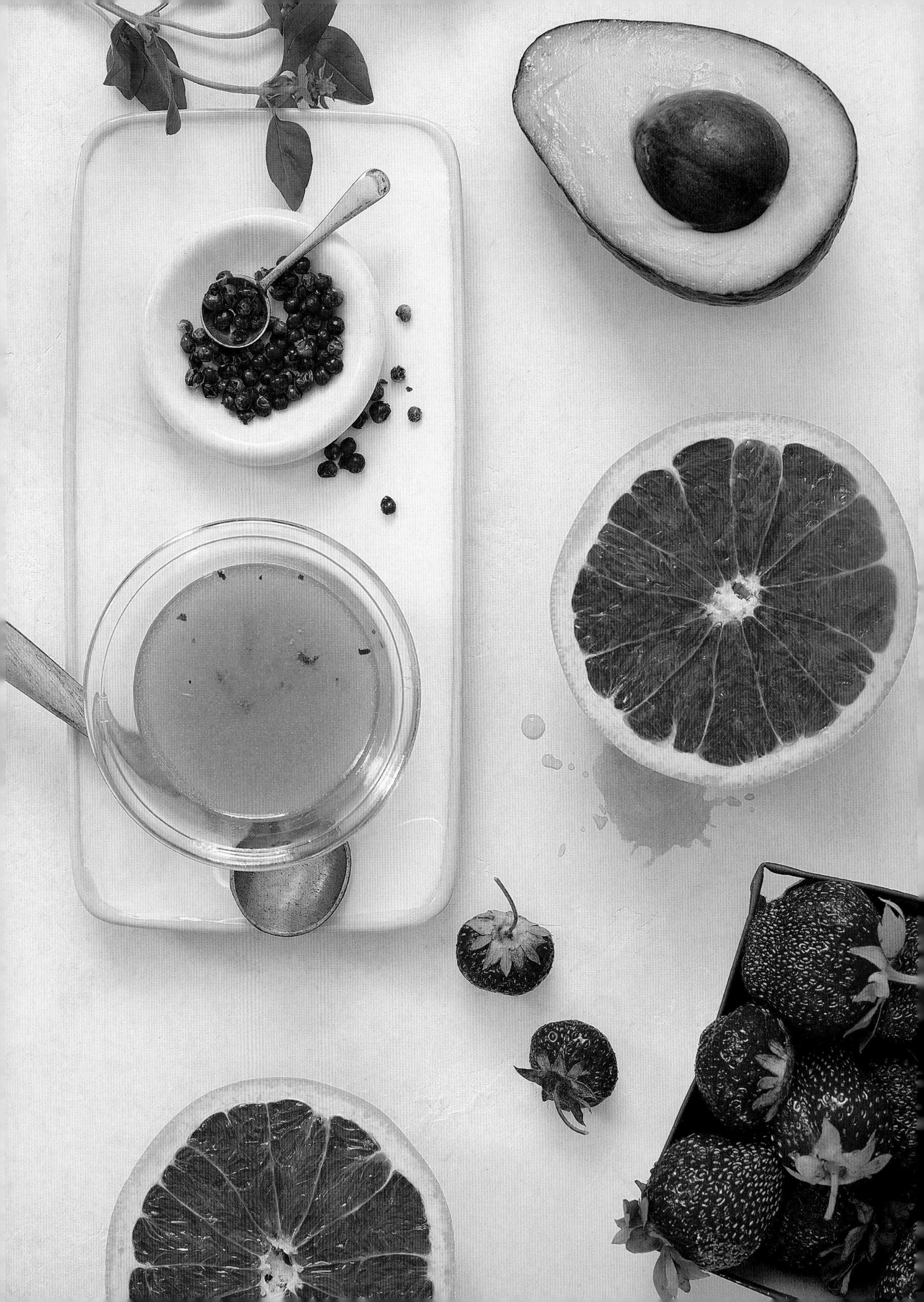

THE BRAIN HEALTH KITCHEN

PREVENTING ALZHEIMER'S THROUGH FOOD WITH 100 RECIPES

ANNIE FENN, MD

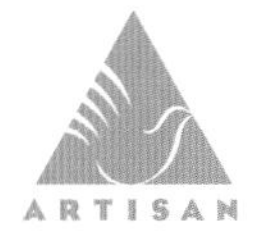

This book is intended as a cookbook, not a medical manual. The information given here is not a substitute for any treatment that may have been prescribed by your doctor. Please seek your doctor's advice before making any decision that may affect your health. The author and publisher are not responsible for any loss, damage, or injury to any person or entity caused directly or indirectly by the information contained in this book.

Library of Congress Cataloging-in-Publication Data.

Fenn, Annie, author.
The brain health kitchen : preventing Alzheimer's through food / Annie Fenn, MD.
New York, NY : Artisan Books, [2023] | Includes index. |
LCCN 2022026462 | ISBN 9781648290367 (hardcover)
LCSH: Alzheimer's disease—Prevention—Popular works. |
Alzheimer's disease—Diet therapy—Recipes. | Memory disorders—Prevention. | Brain—Degeneration—Prevention.
LCC RC523.2 .F46 2023 | DDC 616.8/311—dc23/eng/20220629
LC record available at https://lccn.loc.gov/2022026462
ISBN 978-1-64829-036-7

Design by Renata De Oliveira

Artisan books are available at special discounts when purchased in bulk for premiums and sales promotions as well as for fundraising or educational use. Special editions or book excerpts also can be created to specification. For details, contact specialmarkets@hbgusa.com.

Published by Artisan,
an imprint of Workman Publishing Co., Inc., a
subsidiary of Hachette Book Group, Inc.
1290 Avenue of the Americas
New York, NY 10104
artisanbooks.com

Artisan is a registered trademark of Workman Publishing Co., Inc., a subsidiary of Hachette Book Group, Inc.

Printed in China on responsibly sourced paper

First printing, December 2022
1 3 5 7 9 10 8 6 4 2

TO MY SONS, JACK AND NICK:
MAY YOUR BRAINS THRIVE.

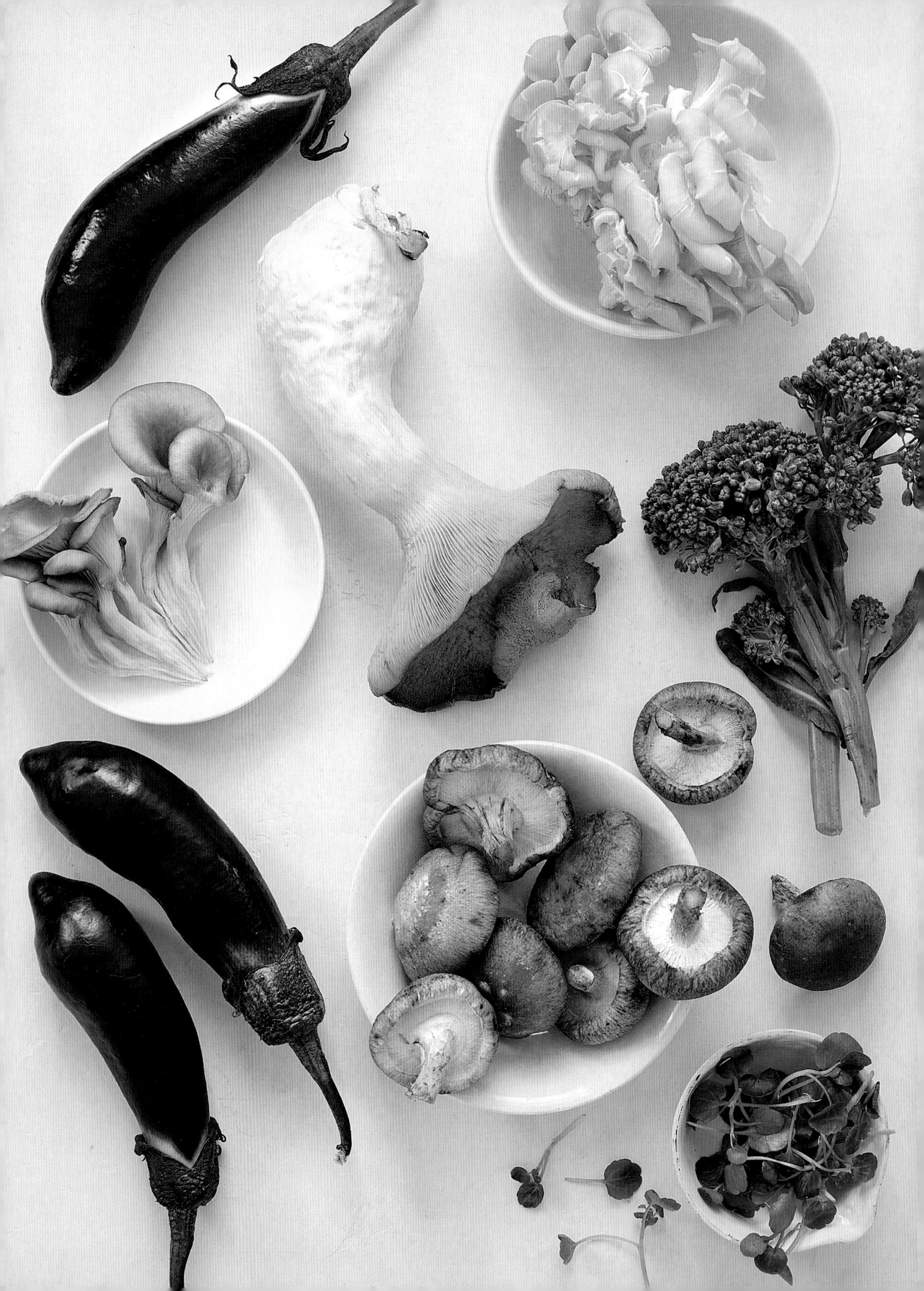

CONTENTS

PREFACE

Hi, I'm Annie: a physician who has always loved food. I didn't choose to become a culinary educator and voice for Alzheimer's prevention. Instead, you could say that Alzheimer's chose me. First, I saw the earliest signs of cognitive decline in my patients, starting in their perimenopausal years. I saw it in my community—in my colleagues, neighbors, book club members, and parents of friends. Then my mother was diagnosed with mild cognitive impairment (MCI)—which turned out to be an early stage of Alzheimer's—in 2015. This devastating development caused me to have an epiphany: all that I had done in my life up to that point—as a physician specializing in menopause, then as a healthy-cooking instructor—gave me a unique set of tools to help others combat this epidemic. That's why I've made it my mission to help *you* take care of your brain while still eating delicious food.

I wrote this book for all of you, whether you've been touched by Alzheimer's or not. As you will see, food choices sit at the core of the Alzheimer's epidemic, but food is also at the heart of the solution. If you are reading and cooking from this book with your sharp and dementia-free brain, I applaud you for being proactive about your brain health. The earlier you begin eating with brain health in mind, the better. In doing so, you will cultivate a brain that is resilient to age-related cognitive decline from all causes, especially Alzheimer's.

If you are experiencing mild cognitive decline, this book will guide you toward action to slow down the aging of your brain. Or if you are witnessing the earliest signs of decline in someone you love, this book will help you help them. Perhaps you have a genetic predisposition to Alzheimer's or another type of dementia. If so, adopting a brain-healthy eating pattern will turn down the volume of your gene variants, lessening their impact on the brain's destiny. Whatever your situation, think of brain-healthy food as your greatest tool to keep thriving through all the seasons of your life.

If you or a loved one has been diagnosed with Alzheimer's (beyond MCI), however, you've entered a different territory of care. Physicians and researchers have not yet discovered how to reverse the disease. Still, a brain-healthy diet is important to support brain function and overall health to reduce symptoms and slow progression. And if you are an Alzheimer's caregiver, you may be at increased risk. I urge you to take extra-special care of your brain by following the guidelines in this book.

The good news is, getting older doesn't necessarily mean you will also experience cognitive decline. There's a myth that dementia is a normal part of aging. It most definitely is not! In the next few decades, however, you will likely see more family and friends diagnosed with Alzheimer's or another type of dementia. That's because the largest population surge in history (hello, baby boomers!) will be entering age groups at high risk for these neurodegenerative diseases. This is happening in my community in Jackson, Wyoming, and—unless you live in a Blue Zone (see page 19)—the numbers show that it's happening in your community, too.

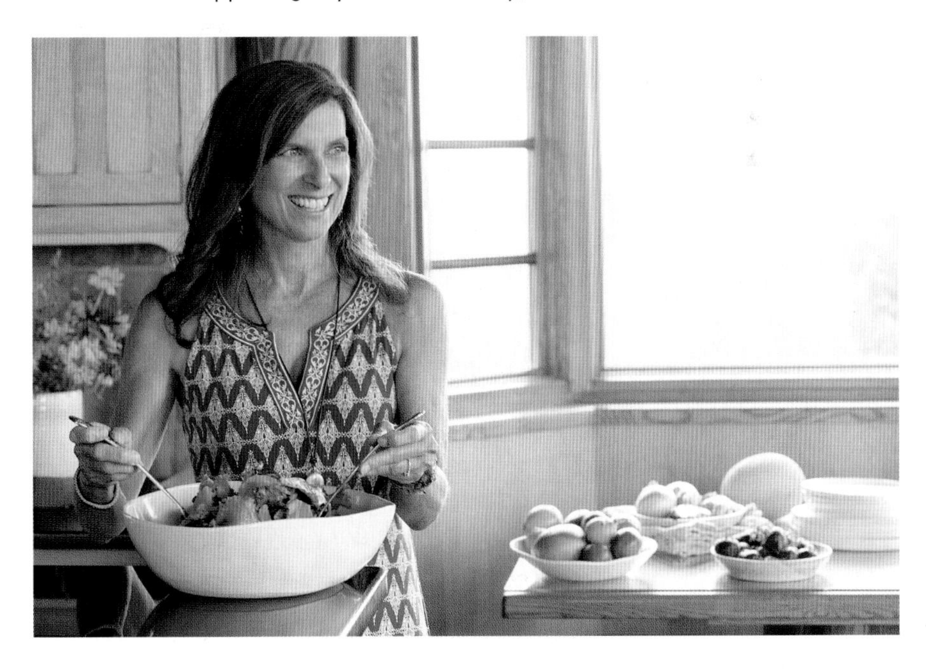

INTRODUCTION

In 2022, more than one in nine people age sixty-five and older have Alzheimer's. One in two over the age of eighty-five has Alzheimer's. That's more than 6.5 million people with Alzheimer's just in the United States, and an estimated fifty million worldwide. With each passing year, the numbers go up.

Lifetime risk is another way to look at estimating how likely you are to get Alzheimer's. This is the probability that someone of a given age will develop the disease during their remaining lifespan. If you are a forty-five-year-old man, for example, your lifetime risk for Alzheimer's is around 1 in 10. If you are a woman, it's closer to 1 in 5. (Yes, women are at greater risk for Alzheimer's than men; I go into some of the reasons on page 25.)

Unless something is done to prevent, slow, or cure Alzheimer's, by 2060 the number of people age 65 and older with this harrowing disease is projected to reach 13.8 million. It's a fate no one would wish on the people they love, but this is the state of the epidemic.

THE POWER OF A BRAIN-HEALTHY DIETARY PATTERN

But there's good news, too. Lifestyle choices—especially what you choose to eat—have a powerful impact on reducing Alzheimer's risk. A 2019 article published in the *Journal of the American Medical Association* found that 60 percent of all Alzheimer's cases could be prevented with dietary and lifestyle behaviors. The Lancet Commission's 2020 update on dementia prevention, intervention, and care identified twelve risk factors for dementia that, if modified, would reduce 40 percent of all cases worldwide. In 2021, a study of more than three hundred thousand dementia-free men and women identified six lifestyle behaviors that reduced age-related cognitive decline by as much as 50 percent later in life. All of these studies found the number one dementia-reducing behavior is a brain-healthy dietary pattern.

How I wish I'd known these numbers and hopeful statistics back when I was practicing medicine or in the decades before my mom was diagnosed with dementia. Back then, the strong link between lifestyle and Alzheimer's risk was just being established through solid scientific studies. As it turns out, the evidence was right in front of me. Unlike most doctors, I always asked my patients about their nutrition history, a general tally of what they ate most days. The women who were more likely to stay mentally sharp with age described a lifetime of eating simple, home-cooked meals—salads, vegetables, beans, grains, and seafood were usually on the menu. Dessert was more likely to be a piece of fruit or a square of dark chocolate than a bowl of ice cream. My patients who complained of cognitive symptoms with age—including my mother—had embraced processed foods: pastries and sweets, processed meat, fried food, and ready-made meals from a box. The difference between these dietary patterns, we now know, can mean the difference between keeping the brain sharp with age and getting Alzheimer's.

MY PATH FROM PHYSICIAN TO ALZHEIMER'S PREVENTIONIST

As a practicing obstetrician-gynecologist, taking care of women was my passion. I became a menopause expert because I sensed that the key to longevity began during the perimenopause stage of life. For years, I listened to patients' frustrations with perimenopausal symptoms. They shared concerns about feeling anxious and overwhelmed, forgetting appointments, and struggling to retrieve a word midsentence—aka "whatchamacallit syndrome"—like they were losing their minds. Along with hot flashes, these minor memory and word-finding problems were a primary reason my patients came to see me. In fact, I heard the same sentence at least once a day: "Annie, I think I have early Alzheimer's."

Meanwhile, each time I visited my mother, I noticed she was more forgetful, confused, and anxious. A few years earlier she had gotten lost going

RACIAL AND ETHNIC DISPARITIES IN ALZHEIMER'S

Twice as many Black Americans and one and a half times more Latinx Americans have Alzheimer's as white Americans. This disparity stems from a complex array of factors—like having more chronic diseases and less access to medical care. Data from the Chicago Health and Aging Project, an ongoing study of the cognitive health of a group of older adults, indicates 19 percent of Black adults and 14 percent of Latinx adults age sixty-five and older have Alzheimer's compared to 10 percent of white older adults. And while the incidence of Alzheimer's may be declining slightly in college-educated white people, rates are going up for non-white people.

Racial disparity in Alzheimer's seems to be rooted in the socioeconomics, health conditions, and life experiences of Black and Latinx populations. Black and Latinx Americans are more likely to suffer from the chronic diseases that increase Alzheimer's risk, such as high blood pressure, diabetes, and obesity—all of which are linked to poor dietary options or choices. They are less likely to have access to good quality education, brain-healthy food, and medical care. Racism influences environmental factors such as where people can live, the quality of schools in their communities, and exposure to environmental pollution, and it likely impacts the brain in ways science is just beginning to understand, such as how childhood segregation can impact mental and cognitive health decades later.

Not only is Alzheimer's more prevalent in non-white communities, existing data represents only a fraction of the number of cases. More studies are necessary to draw conclusions about the true incidence of Alzheimer's in Black and Latinx older adults. Chronic health conditions within these groups may be what's driving Alzheimer's risk. For example, high blood pressure is more common in Black adults than white adults; getting this under control at midlife has been shown to reduce Black dementia rates. Adult-onset diabetes is more common in Latinx adults and a driving risk factor in elevated dementia risk; dietary changes—like the ones in this book—can prevent and treat diabetes (more about diabetes on page 36).

The prevalence of all types of dementia seems to be higher in Indigenous populations than non-Indigenous ones, but high-quality studies are lacking. And while Asian American and Pacific Islander (AAPI) populations are one of the fastest growing groups of older adults, on target to increase in numbers by 145 percent by 2030, there is sparse data to tell us about their incidence of Alzheimer's and dementia. Limited data suggests there are important differences in vulnerability to Alzheimer's in unique subpopulations, such as Vietnamese, Korean, Chinese, Native Hawaiian, and Japanese, but we need more research to understand it. Tackling known risk factors like access to quality medical care, education, and brain-healthy food gives us a clear pathway of how to improve everyone's risk.

to the mall; now she was getting lost in the parking lot of her usual grocery store. She forgot her pin at the ATM and repeated herself frequently in conversation. Since my stepfather had died earlier that year, she had stopped going to church, avoided seeing friends, and mostly stayed home alone. Her longtime hairdresser, Lloyd, would call me to say she wasn't showing up for appointments or that she came on the wrong day.

I took to inspecting her refrigerator first thing each visit—it had become my barometer of how she was doing. When I was a kid, she was particular about keeping a tidy fridge: eggs on the left, milk bottles on the right, vegetables and fruits in separate drawers. Now I saw a half-dozen yogurt containers with spoons sticking out; an open can of Campbell's chicken noodle soup (half eaten, no lid). Often I smelled something fishy wafting from the back of all the cans. Yellow sticky notes plastered the refrigerator door: "Cook the salmon," said one. "Buy Chardonnay," said another.

Even with my medical background, I had missed many of the early signs of age-related cognitive decline in my mother. When Alzheimer's affects someone you love, it's natural to make excuses for the memory lapses rather than face the truth.

I arranged for her to have cognitive testing. She called me right after the appointment, triumphant. "I'm just fine," she would say. "Everyone's a bit forgetful at my age. After all, I'm almost eighty!" Beside the fact that she was actually eighty-three, I was skeptical of her neurological workup. Back then, I didn't know that women are particularly skillful at slipping through the cracks of standard cognitive tests. Because women possess more advanced verbal skills, they can hide their dementia longer from their families and even their doctors. The next time my mom visited me, I took her to see a friend who is a cognitive health specialist.

I left the room while the nurse administered the Montreal Cognitive Assessment (MoCA). MoCA, which includes the clock-drawing test, is an evidence-based screening test for cognitive decline. The simple act of drawing a clock taps into multiple thinking skills. It requires auditory comprehension plus the ability to persist in drawing, remember task instructions, and translate information into a physical act. My mom was asked to draw a clock, fill it with numbers, and draw hands to reflect ten after eleven. She got one point for closing the circle and two points for properly placed numbers, but she was unable to place the hands correctly. An arrow pointed from ten to eleven. Her clock looked like a first grader had drawn it.

It got worse. She missed five out of five words on delayed recall. She knew the month but stated the year to be 1916. The current president? George W. Bush. (This was during the Obama administration.) Her MoCA reflected cognitive decline. The most likely diagnosis: the mild cognitive impairment stage of Alzheimer's disease.

I couldn't get her clock test out of my head. I showed it to my siblings. We all stared at it, astounded. No matter how skilled we had become at making excuses for our mother's memory problems, that clock pretty much said it all. We jumped into action. My brother took over her financial affairs. I took over as her medical power of attorney. While reviewing her records, I was shocked to learn that she had never undergone those cognitive tests I'd asked about before the MoCA, even though I had called her physician to request it. The sad truth is, only about half of all primary care providers have the time and resources to screen patients over 65 for Alzheimer's. It's also possible that Mom had talked her way out of getting tested then lied to us about it later. We were just starting to learn our way around this country of Alzheimer's. Lying, along with confabulation—that is, fabricating stories based on small truths—was part of the terrain.

If my mother was indeed on the road to Alzheimer's, was there a way to slow it down by changing how she ate? What about my patients who already had mild memory problems or worried about developing dementia? I dove into the scientific literature, poring over every study I could find about the impact of food on cognitive function, how our brains age, and the risk of Alzheimer's and other dementias.

Eventually, one of my brothers moved in with her as a temporary solution while we looked into assisted living centers. More than seven years later, he's still taking care of her at home.

My mother is declining, but not as quickly as we had feared. As soon as she was diagnosed, we adapted her meals to closely follow the MIND diet guidelines (page 17). We got rid of the processed food in her diet and watered down her wine until she was no longer drinking at all. Honestly, we are amazed that she's still living at home.

COOKING MY WAY THROUGH LIFE

It wasn't the food I fell in love with while growing up but the ritual of sitting down to eat dinner each night with my family. Sharing food around the table had a magical power over me—one of connection, belonging, and finding my way as the quiet youngest of four kids. Back then, the food was the opposite of brain healthy: a steady American diet of sugary cereals, soda pop, Wonder bread, and frozen dinners. My mother, just like all my friends' mothers, embraced the novel convenience of processed foods. Thankfully, I was lucky to be able to visit my nearby grandparents and delight in home-cooked food. My Sicilian nonna cooked everything from scratch, from an ever-present simmering pot of minestrone soup to handmade pasta topped with bitter greens.

Then, when I was sixteen, I was awarded a scholarship to study in Spain. I traded my junk-food diet for Mediterranean staples like olives, dates, a rainbow of vegetables, strong cheeses, and new-to-me dishes like paella made with four kinds of seafood. I drank wine and sipped coffee. There I learned that what I loved most about food—sharing it around a table with others—was an integral part of an entire culture. As for the food, that was like going from a black-and-white dietary pattern to a technicolor one. With this introduction to the Mediterranean lifestyle, it felt like my life was just beginning.

When I came home from Spain, I started cooking for myself, making my school lunches and dinner at night. At college the next year, I cooked multicourse meals in my dorm room using only a blender and a hot plate. I even kept this love of food alive in medical school. Despite exhausting hours in lectures, laboratories, and hospital rotations, I still made time because food was how I connected with others. My tiny apartment was always full of students sitting on the floor, plates balanced on laps. I collected cookbooks, reading them in bed like novels.

No matter what was going on in my hectic day-to-day life, cooking was my constant companion. Looking back now, I see I had essentially adopted the Mediterranean diet. Eating this way connected me to my family in Sicily, gave me the energy to tackle long hospital days, and punctuated my life with simple moments of pleasure. When my training was over, I moved with my husband to Jackson, Wyoming, then just a community of ten thousand.

After practicing obstetrics and gynecology for more than twenty years, I shifted gears to pursue my love of food. I wanted to learn how thriving communities cooked and ate. I traveled to central Mexico to the mountainous region of Tepoztlán to learn regional vegetable-centric specialties. I learned ancient recipes for salsas and soups at a cooking school in San Miguel de Allende. Another summer, I studied with a woman in Tuscany in her tiny kitchen, learning to braise vegetables, make pasta by hand, and create pesto from just about any combination of nuts, herbs, and cheese. At a boot camp at the Culinary Institute of America, I discovered that professional chefs are not unlike physicians: passionate, detail oriented, and able to work long hours on their feet. Having everything in its place before you start to cook, or mise en place, is not so different from how I'd prepare for surgery. I felt right at home.

Back home, I started teaching cooking classes in my community. First, I joined the staff of my local college as a culinary instructor. My focus: making healthy meals easy and accessible. Then I joined forces with Dr. Martha Stearn, a cognitive health specialist at the local hospital. She created Brain Works, the first-ever community-based dementia prevention course, and I came on to run the culinary program. Soon, news of my brain health–focused cooking classes spread, and my home kitchen became the Brain Health Kitchen.

THE LINK BETWEEN FOOD AND ALZHEIMER'S

Back in 2015, I started systematically researching the different brain-protective dietary patterns—approaches to eating that could prevent or slow down Alzheimer's. Your dietary pattern is more than just the foods you consume consistently throughout your life, it's the how, when, and why of your eating habits. How many meals do you eat each day? How diverse are your food choices? Do you often eat alone or with others? How do you combine different types of food, and what do you drink? Researchers use dietary patterns to evaluate how nutrition affects the risk of Alzheimer's disease. Many of the landmark Alzheimer's studies were done by following the cognitive health of large groups of people over time—prospectively, retrospectively, and in randomized, controlled clinical trials—while having the participants tally the frequency, variety, and specific foods they consume.

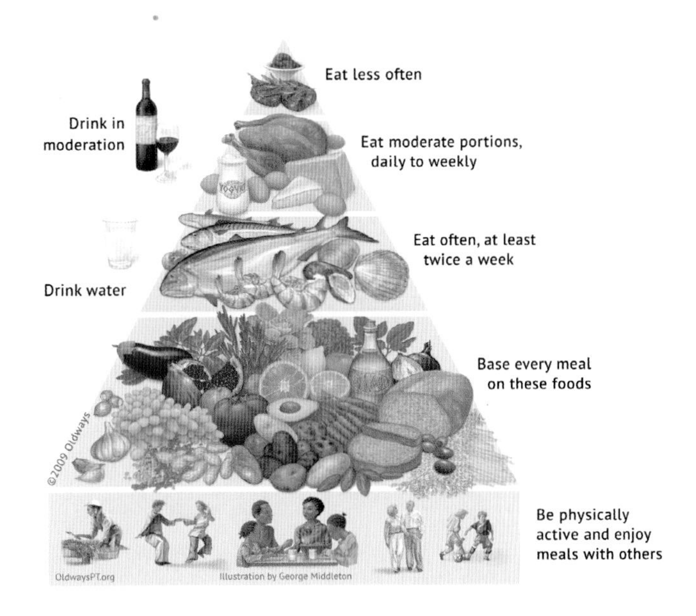

Following the Mediterranean dietary pattern is associated with a lower risk of age-related cognitive decline.

THE MEDITERRANEAN DIET

The Mediterranean diet is characterized by a high consumption of fruits, vegetables, fish and seafood, whole grains, beans and legumes, and olive oil, with a light consumption of red wine. The Mediterranean diet is associated with better overall cognitive health and memory and a lower risk of age-related cognitive decline and Alzheimer's by as much as 40 percent. Brain imaging studies show that people who follow a Mediterranean diet have less brain shrinkage with age, particularly in the hippocampus—the region of the brain first targeted by Alzheimer's disease. More than thirty-five studies support the Mediterranean-style dietary pattern as effective in reducing both cardiovascular disease and Alzheimer's.

THE MIND DIET

MIND stands for the Mediterranean-DASH Intervention for Neurodegenerative Delay. Developed to protect the brain against dementia, this pattern combines the Mediterranean diet and DASH (Dietary Approaches to Stop Hypertension) eating plan with an emphasis on the foods that are most neuroprotective.

The MIND diet guidelines single out ten brain-healthy food groups—berries, leafy greens, vegetables, fish and seafood, whole grains, nuts and seeds, poultry, beans and legumes, olive oil—while also including red wine. The MIND diet minimizes dairy products (like butter and cheese), red meat, and other foods high in saturated fat, like fried and processed foods. When study participants adhered to the MIND guidelines most closely, there were 53 percent fewer cases of Alzheimer's after just four and a half years. Even those participants who followed the diet less rigorously, about half the time, had an astounding risk reduction of 35 percent. Not only that, participants who followed the diet most closely over time actually showed improvement in their cognitive function. Since publication, the MIND diet study has been replicated in other countries, and has been shown to reduce the risks of Parkinson's disease and breast cancer. At the time this book went to print, the MIND Diet Intervention to Prevent Alzheimer's Disease, a placebo-controlled study with one group adhering to the MIND diet compared to another following another healthy diet, was nearing completion.

THE GREEN MED DIET

Like the MIND diet, the Green MED diet is a brain-specific spin on the Mediterranean diet. While it is relatively new, it's already putting up impressive brain-imaging data. Researchers in Israel compared three groups of people given different diets: the standard Mediterranean diet, a reduced-calorie healthy diet, and the Green MED diet—a Mediterranean diet boosted daily with ¼ cup walnuts, 4 to 5 cups of green tea, and a green smoothie made with a protein-rich plant. The Green MED group also cut back even more on meat, especially processed meat. All participants needed to lose weight, were given a free gym pass, and were encouraged to exercise. All had brain scans to determine brain volume at the beginning of the study and after 18 months.

The researchers wanted to learn which dietary pattern would have the most positive impact on brain volume over time.

As you might expect, participants in each arm of the study became healthier, thanks to 18 months of exercise and a healthy diet. They all lost weight, had lower blood pressure, and reduced harmful blood cholesterol. They all had a slower rate of brain shrinkage, too. The group who maintained the most brain volume, however, was the Green MED group. Not only did they hold on to more gray and white matter, they did so in a key area—the hippocampus, aka the memory center of the brain.

THE BLUE ZONES

Another teachable model of what to eat to age without dementia comes from the Blue Zones—the five places on earth where people live the longest: Okinawa, Japan; Sardinia, Italy; Nicoya Peninsula, Costa Rica; Ikaria, Greece; and Loma Linda, California. Identified by *National Geographic* researcher Dan Buettner (author of *The Blue Zones*), these zones are geographically diverse but share common eating habits, such as the leisurely sharing of food with others, and core ingredients, like beans and cruciferous vegetables. The longest-living women, on the Japanese island of Okinawa, enjoyed an abundance of whole soy foods and sea vegetables and were still living active, dementia-free lives way past their nineties. On the Italian island of Sardinia, the world's longest-living men enjoyed a bowl of minestrone soup every day, full of local beans, greens, and vegetables, and still worked and socialized well into their nineties.

VEGETARIAN, VEGAN, AND WHOLE FOOD PLANT-BASED DIETS

Nutrition scientists, such as Dr. T. Colin Campbell (author of *The China Study*), advocate for a diet devoid of animal products, what Campbell calls whole food, plant-based (WFPB; a low-fat vegan diet) for the prevention of cancer and heart disease. Different spins on a vegetarian diet have had excellent support for preventing cardiovascular disease, especially stroke, an important contributing factor to Alzheimer's. A 1993 study of the Seventh-day Adventists in Loma Linda, California (a Blue Zone), looked at plant-rich diets that include dairy and eggs (lacto-ovo vegetarian), eggs (ovo vegetarians), fish (pescatarians), or occasional meat (flexitarians). They found that the more plant-based a person's diet was, the lower their risk of dementia. For instance, strict vegetarians had half the risk of dementia as those who ate animal products sometimes. While updated studies of vegetarian and WFPB diets and Alzheimer's are ongoing, a plant-based diet with very few or no animal products has been proven to reduce the risk of certain types of heart disease and even reverse it, and to reduce stroke risk by as much as 44 percent.

OTHER BRAIN-FRIENDLY DIETARY PATTERNS

There are other neuroprotective dietary patterns, albeit with differing amounts of evidence to back them up. The Nordic Prudent Dietary Pattern, for example, which is similar to the Mediterranean diet but with canola instead of olive oil, has demonstrated improved cognitive function with aging in more than two thousand healthy older adults in Sweden. The Green MED diet, a "greened up" version of the Mediterranean diet, along with exercise, has been shown to slow down the type of brain shrinkage associated with aging. (See page 18 for more.)

Perhaps your dietary pattern aligns with the African, Asian, and Latin American heritage diets. All of these dietary patterns include core brain health lifestyle values like staying active, enjoying food with others, and cooking at home. And crucially, these three patterns are also primarily plant based, drawing from regional foods eaten for centuries. While the scientific literature has been biased toward studying Mediterranean and Asian populations, Latin American and African dietary patterns deserve further evaluation to determine their specific brain health virtues.

THE MEDITERRANEAN AND MIND DIETS RISE TO THE TOP

Throughout my research, the Mediterranean diet and its brain-specific spin-off, the MIND diet, kept rising to the top as the best way to fend off cognitive decline and Alzheimer's. The MIND diet has the most impressive data with a risk reduction of more than 53 percent. Put another way, after following the MIND diet, the subjects' brains performed like someone seven-and-a-half years younger.

All the brain-protective dietary patterns of interest have one thing in common: they are plant rich. Which is to say, they are mostly composed of vegetables, fruits, leafy greens, whole grains, nuts and seeds, and beans and legumes. Further research will determine if a fully plant-based diet is more effective at fending off Alzheimer's than a plant-heavy Mediterranean or MIND diet, which also includes small amounts of animal products, especially fish and seafood.

TURNING THE STANDARD AMERICAN DIET PYRAMID UPSIDE DOWN

The one dietary pattern we know is detrimental to your brain is the standard American diet—aka SAD, the so-called Western diet—which is high in saturated fats, processed foods, and added sugar but low in fiber, nutrients, and brain-friendly fats. In fact, the SAD food pyramid looks like an upside-down version of the Mediterranean one (page 17)—processed foods and animal products fill the base, and plant foods are crowded into the tiny section on top.

It makes perfect sense to me that what you eat has the power to slow down the aging of the brain. After all, I had seen it firsthand in my patients: those who followed a healthy lifestyle, especially a healthful diet, thrived with age. This is what inspired me to find a way to put my longtime love of cooking and food into play to help turn this Alzheimer's epidemic around.

WHAT IS ALZHEIMER'S, EXACTLY?

Dementia is a general term for the loss of brain function targeting memory, reasoning, language, and behavior severe enough to affect daily function. Alzheimer's is the most common type of dementia, accounting for 60 to 80 percent of all cases. The exact cause of Alzheimer's is not known, and as yet, it is irreversible. Even after billions of dollars have been funneled to

WHILE YOU SLEEP, THE BRAIN CLEANS UP

Even while you are sleeping, your brain is hard at work. Short-term memories are sorted, consolidated, and filed away in the long-term storage areas of the brain. With no food metabolites coming in to be dealt with, the brain shifts into cleanup mode. In fact, it has its very own garbage disposal—the glymphatic system—a pressure gradient triggered by sleep that filters out inflammatory particles like beta-amyloid protein. You need multiple cycles of both deep sleep and rapid eye movement (REM) sleep for these filing, restorative, and cleansing functions to happen. Scientists recently discovered that a single night of sleep deprivation increases beta-amyloid load in the brain. Most people aren't getting enough high-quality sleep needed to let the brain do its job. Shoot for seven to nine hours of sleep each night.

develop a treatment, there still isn't a cure. What we do know is this: certain lifestyle choices can slow down brain aging, such as a neuroprotective diet, getting enough good-quality sleep, constantly learning new things, and exercising. Other habits, such as smoking, excessive alcohol use, and a diet of inflammatory foods, can accelerate the path to Alzheimer's.

Your brain is the hungriest, thirstiest organ in the body: it makes up just 2 percent of body weight but requires 20 percent of your body's primary fuel, glucose. Anything that prevents the brain from getting the fuel it needs leads to cognitive decline, whether it be a temporary brain fog or an irreversible dementia.

Think of the healthy brain as a lush, well-nourished landscape with plenty of water and nutrients—a vital, ever-changing ecosystem. Now think of what happens to that landscape during a drought—the ground is parched, the plants lose their source of nourishment, their roots shrivel up, and they wither and die. Even the smallest spark will make the whole place go up in flames.

In the Alzheimer's brain, harmful proteins accumulate over time. Two of these proteins—beta-amyloid and tau—impair how brain cells communicate, repair, grow, and function. Beta-amyloid is continuously cleared from a healthy brain, thanks to your immune system and the glymphatic system (see page 21). However, when it accumulates faster than your body can remove it, the protein sticks together and forms plaques on the surface of cells. In addition, the tau proteins collapse and create tangled bundles of debris that reside inside brain neurons and impair the cell's ability to utilize energy.

When amyloid (the plaques) and tau (the tangles) accumulation reaches a tipping point, even a well-nourished brain becomes starved for fuel. Just like a forest during a drought, the brain becomes vulnerable to a cascade of events set off by inflammation. Chronic inflammation is the brain's worst nightmare—the spark that sets off a smoldering brush fire that grows into a catastrophic forest fire. The amyloid and tau set the scene; inflammation lights the match.

This "amyloid hypothesis" has been the driving theory to explain what happens to the brain as Alzheimer's evolves. Researchers are now questioning whether amyloid is the cause or the result of other factors. Chronic inflammation in the brain may be the overriding factor that makes someone vulnerable to Alzheimer's. Also called neuroinflammation, this comes from many things, including environmental pollution, brain-harming particles in the foods you eat, head trauma, and heavy alcohol use. Having a genetic predisposition to Alzheimer's can make it easier for inflammation to spread. Neuroinflammation becomes a vicious cycle, creating more abnormal protein deposition while hastening the demise of brain cells. The thinking region of the brain (the frontal lobe) becomes disconnected from the primary memory center (the hippocampus). Once-healthy neurons start to shrivel and die and the brain shrinks, a process called atrophy.

Once Alzheimer's becomes symptomatic, short-term memory loss is almost always the first sign. Losing objects of value, as in the proverbial misplaced keys, is secondary to this memory loss. But those suffering from early Alzheimer's also repeatedly mix up dates and appointments (like my mom did with her hair appointments), have trouble coming up with the right word or name, and rapidly forget what they've just read. Apathy and depression are also early signs.

THE OTHER TYPES OF DEMENTIA

Vascular dementia—which is caused by inadequate or obstructed blood flow to the brain—makes up another 20 percent of all dementias. Alzheimer's and vascular dementia often coincide; studies show that up to half of all persons with Alzheimer's also have vascular dementia. That's another reason why researchers and drug developers are shifting their thinking from Alzheimer's being caused by a single factor (such as amyloid protein) to a multifactorial disease model, or one caused by many factors like insulin resistance and faulty cholesterol metabolism. The remaining 10 percent include brain syndromes that can lead to dementia: Lewy body disease (including Parkinson's disease), frontotemporal lobar degeneration, Wernicke's encephalopathy, chronic traumatic encephalopathy (CTE), and others.

IS IT GENETIC?

One of the more prevalent myths about Alzheimer's is that it is always genetic, meaning you get it because you inherited a gene for it from a parent. It's true that about 50 percent of all people with dementia have a genetic risk factor, but less than 2 percent of all people with Alzheimer's got it purely through a genetic mutation. (That's the rare, early-onset Alzheimer's we talk about in the sidebar below.) There are literally dozens of genetic variants associated with an increased or decreased risk of Alzheimer's. The most common variant is apolipoprotein E4, or ApoE4, one that 25 percent of all people carry.

ApoE is a gene that has evolved over time to have three different variants, called alleles: ApoE2, ApoE3, and ApoE4. Everyone inherits two alleles of ApoE. You could have an ApoE2 and an ApoE3, for instance, or a combination of ApoE3 and ApoE4. It's the ApoE4 allele that is considered a risk gene for late-onset Alzheimer's. Possessing one copy of ApoE4

EARLY- AND LATE-ONSET ALZHEIMER'S

In Lisa Genova's book *Still Alice*, a brilliant college professor is diagnosed with Alzheimer's shortly after her fiftieth birthday. This "early-onset" type of Alzheimer's is rare, accounting for fewer than 2 percent of all cases, and is almost always caused by a genetic mutation. People with early-onset Alzheimer's lose cognitive function starting in their thirties, forties, and fifties.

The bulk of the Alzheimer's epidemic—the other 98 percent of all cases—appears after the age of sixty. Note that this "late-onset" Alzheimer's actually begins to attack the brain much earlier, as abnormal proteins build up twenty to thirty years before the first memory lapse. Late-onset Alzheimer's goes through stages based on the severity of symptoms. The earliest stage, however, has no symptoms at all. The updated diagnostic criteria now include this preclinical stage—Stage 0—a decades-long period in which there is evidence of Alzheimer's pathology, like the amyloid and tau, in the brain (based on specialized brain scans) but cognitive function has not yet failed.

Symptomatic late-onset Alzheimer's goes through many stages over decades, starting with mild cognitive impairment (MCI, when memory is impaired but daily function is normal) and progressing to functional impairment, dementia, and on to the final stage in which individuals lose the ability to respond to their environment. Ultimately, people with Alzheimer's have difficulty speaking, swallowing, and walking. In almost every case, Alzheimer's worsens to the point of requiring long-term care. Alzheimer's doesn't just steal memory and function; it kills. One in three seniors dies with Alzheimer's or another dementia.

For the purposes of this book, Alzheimer's refers to the late-onset type, which is mostly preventable, rather than the early-onset type, which, as far as we know, is not.

increases the risk of developing Alzheimer's later in life by three- to fivefold; having two copies increases risk fifteenfold. If you have one or two copies of ApoE2, however, it is actually a good thing—it protects you from Alzheimer's.

While ApoE4 is known as an Alzheimer's risk gene, it exerts its effect on the brain indirectly by how it moves blood cholesterol into cells. A glitch in the gene's structure creates a faulty transport mechanism. The brain cells bear the brunt of the problem, getting too much of the cholesterol known to cause damage to blood vessels (LDL) and not enough docosahexaenoic acid (DHA)—the brain-repairing omega-3 fatty acid.

The crucial thing to understand about ApoE4 is that having one or even two copies of the ApoE4 genetic variant does not mean you are going to get Alzheimer's. It's not like having the gene for sickle cell anemia or cystic fibrosis, which are single-gene defects that give you a 100 percent chance of having the disease. That's why ApoE4 is called a "risk gene"—it modifies risk—but the gene itself is pliable, meaning we can lessen its harmful impact on the brain. A brain-healthy lifestyle has the power to substantially turn down the volume of ApoE4. That's right: this risk gene for Alzheimer's is influenced by your habits.

A FEW REASONS WHY ALZHEIMER'S TARGETS WOMEN

While there are many factors that can increase Alzheimer's risk, being female and aging are the two most common predictors. It has been known for decades, in fact, that women are more likely to develop Alzheimer's than men. At the age of sixty-five, a woman is more likely to be diagnosed with Alzheimer's than breast cancer. Currently, there are 4 million women in the United States in this age group living with Alzheimer's.

Might this be because women live longer than men? It's true, women do outlive men by a slight margin, giving the disease more time to develop. However, the lifespan gap between men and women is narrowing to just a few years and no longer accounts for the discrepancy in case numbers.

To find out why women are more vulnerable, researchers are studying the biological differences between men's and women's brains. The presence of estrogen in a woman's body for much of her life protects the brain by supporting essential brain cell functions, influencing how the brain gets its fuel (glucose), and by fighting off oxidative stress—the inflammatory particles that damage the brain over time.

When estrogen levels decline, as they do in the menopausal transition, it not only triggers the classic symptoms, like hot flashes and memory loss, it leads to vulnerabilities in the actual structure of the brain. Menopause may be a window of opportunity for setting up the pathological changes that lead to Alzheimer's later. Plummeting estrogen triggers an accumulation of beta-amyloid and tau proteins, which further cut off its energy supply. The brain becomes starved for glucose and loses its ability to fend off inflammatory attacks.

It's not surprising, then, that the research suggests the more years of her life a woman has estrogen reaching her brain, the lower her likelihood of developing Alzheimer's. Both early menarche and a later onset of menopause (after the average age of 51.5) bode well for reduced Alzheimer's risk. Conversely, early menopause (defined as loss of ovarian function prior to age forty) increases risk. When researchers looked at women who had undergone surgery that induced early menopause, they were more likely to develop Alzheimer's, especially if they didn't receive hormone replacement therapy. This leads to the question: Should women be taking hormones (usually estrogen with or without progesterone) after menopause to fend off Alzheimer's? The science is still being sorted out, but some studies show a reduced risk of dementia in women who take hormones, but only certain groups and only if taken within a few years of menopause. The decision to take hormones or not must be personalized to your own situation—family history, medical history, age of menopause, and whether or not you have had a hysterectomy that also remove the ovaries.

The good news about menopause, however, is that the female brain is well equipped to emerge from the transition without permanent loss of function. The female brain adapts by changing up its energy sources. However, if a woman is already predisposed to Alzheimer's—because she carries an ApoE4 risk gene (discussed on page 24), for example—proper attention to brain health through the menopause transition is essential to prevent a brain environment that facilitates decline.

Biological differences between male and female carriers of ApoE4 are complex, with a more dramatic impact on women. Female ApoE4 carriers have unique challenges getting enough neuroprotective nutrients to the brain, especially DHA, which may explain their heightened vulnerability to brain aging. Female ApoE4 carriers may benefit from boosting intake of both DHA and EPA with food or supplements. (Read more on page 163.)

Besides biology, there are environmental factors that contribute to a woman's risk. Lack of early childhood education is one of the modifiable risk factors identified by the Lancet Commission, and a common problem in girls throughout the world. Women often suffer from lack of sleep also, when raising small children and going through menopause, and this may have lasting impact on the brain. (This doesn't mean taking sleeping pills is a good idea; it's better to prioritize trying to get adequate natural sleep.) On the plus side, women who work outside the home may be protected from age-related cognitive decline, perhaps because it builds cognitive reserve. Women possess excellent verbal skills, which helps them perform better on standard

WHAT'S GOOD FOR THE HEART IS GOOD FOR THE BRAIN

Keeping your heart and blood vessels healthy is crucial for avoiding Alzheimer's. Besides exercising, not using tobacco, maintaining a healthy weight, and keeping blood pressure under control, this means paying attention to blood cholesterol, especially low-density lipoprotein (LDL). The LDL is the harmful type of blood cholesterol, in contrast to high-density lipoprotein (HDL), which is protective of heart disease. The higher your LDL, the greater your risk of Alzheimer's. That's because LDL creates inflammation inside blood vessels, causing larger vessels to become blocked and smaller ones to collapse, cutting off blood flow to the brain. This could look like a major stroke or a series of small strokes that damages parts of the brain.

Reducing LDL is more about reducing how much saturated fat you consume than watching the dietary cholesterol, which is no longer thought to be a big player (see Eggs, page 281). The brain-healthy dietary pattern is strategically low in total saturated fat, ideally less than 5 percent, which targets achieving an optimal, low LDL. In practical terms, this means limiting foods like red meat, dairy products, and fried and processed food. Instead, choose brain-friendly fats like those in nuts, seeds, avocados, olive oil, and fish.

cognitive tests. When it comes to early detection of dementia, however, this is not a good thing—it masks early signs, and women often go undiagnosed for years (like my mom did). As gender-specific cognitive tests come into use, fewer women will fall through the cracks of early detection, important so that they don't miss out on interventions to slow the course of the disease, if caught early.

PREVENTION IS THE CURE

While Alzheimer's used to be viewed as a disease that happens when you get older, now it is recognized as a process that begins in the brain about twenty years before symptoms appear. This makes early adulthood (the years between thirty and forty-five) and midlife (between forty-five and sixty-five) the time to get your brain on a healthy aging track. This is the golden time to fortify your brain. Your lifestyle, especially what you eat, will have a huge impact on whether you develop Alzheimer's later. Numerous studies now show that at least 60 percent of all Alzheimer's cases can be prevented with healthy lifestyle choices, including a brain-friendly diet. And these same lifestyle choices will reduce the risk of those with a genetic predisposition for Alzheimer's.

To be honest, no one really knows if we can actually "prevent" Alzheimer's. What we do know is this: you can push off cognitive decline further into the future. Slowing down the aging of your brain means expanding your brainspan—the number of years the brain is active and healthy. People who eat a serving of leafy greens each day, for example, have been found to have younger-performing brains—eleven years younger!—than those who don't.

THE FUTURE

Imagine a day when your physician offers you a screening test for Alzheimer's at your annual exam. Detecting sticky proteins that accumulate and damage the brain will be as easy as checking your cholesterol. The test alerts you and your doctor that these are building up in your brain faster than your body can clear them, even though you have no symptoms of dementia or memory loss at all. In other words, you have the preclinical stage of Alzheimer's—Stage 0.

Together, you come up with a plan for cultivating a more Alzheimer's-resistant brain: a brain-healthy diet, sleep, exercise, stress management, and staying socially and cognitively active. The physician offers you a cocktail of drugs to help clear out the abnormal proteins from the brain. This prevents you from getting Alzheimer's. She may even offer you a vaccine that stimulates the immune system to fend off Alzheimer's.

Advancements in early detection and treatment of Alzheimer's are bringing this futuristic view within grasp. After nearly twenty years of research, the first human clinical trial of a nasal vaccine against Alzheimer's has just begun. A blood test now being used in research settings accurately predicts the amyloid protein visualized on a PET scan for those with cognitive impairment. As researchers target disease pathways beyond amyloid—like impaired omega-3 uptake by the brain and female-specific metabolic problems—it opens the door to novel treatments.

Despite the promise of future treatments, prevention should always be our primary strategy. This book is your guide to choosing neuroprotective foods, following a brain-friendly lifestyle, and thriving for many decades. The importance of eating a brain-healthy diet will never go away. It is your first line of defense against this heartbreaking disease, and something you can start as a young adult. As the science evolves, there will hopefully be numerous options for fending off Alzheimer's, but none are likely to be as fundamental as nourishing your brain with neuroprotective foods.

These recipes are both healthful and comforting. You'll learn how to use modern, plant-rich techniques and choose each ingredient strategically for its neuroprotective potential. I obsessed over the recipes so that each one is approachable, beautiful, deeply satisfying, and undeniably delicious. My dedicated tribe of recipe testers (more than fifty home cooks, just like you) have ensured that each recipe will be successful in your own kitchen.

There is much hope that this tsunami of Alzheimer's will be curtailed. Advances in the treatment and prevention aside, wiping out this dreadful disease will never be as easy as taking a pill. The proper care of your complex and precious brain requires a comprehensive approach through all stages of life. Fortunately, it's never too early—or too late—to start taking care of your brain. Your brain health journey begins right now, in your own kitchen, with the foods that will nourish and protect your brain for life.

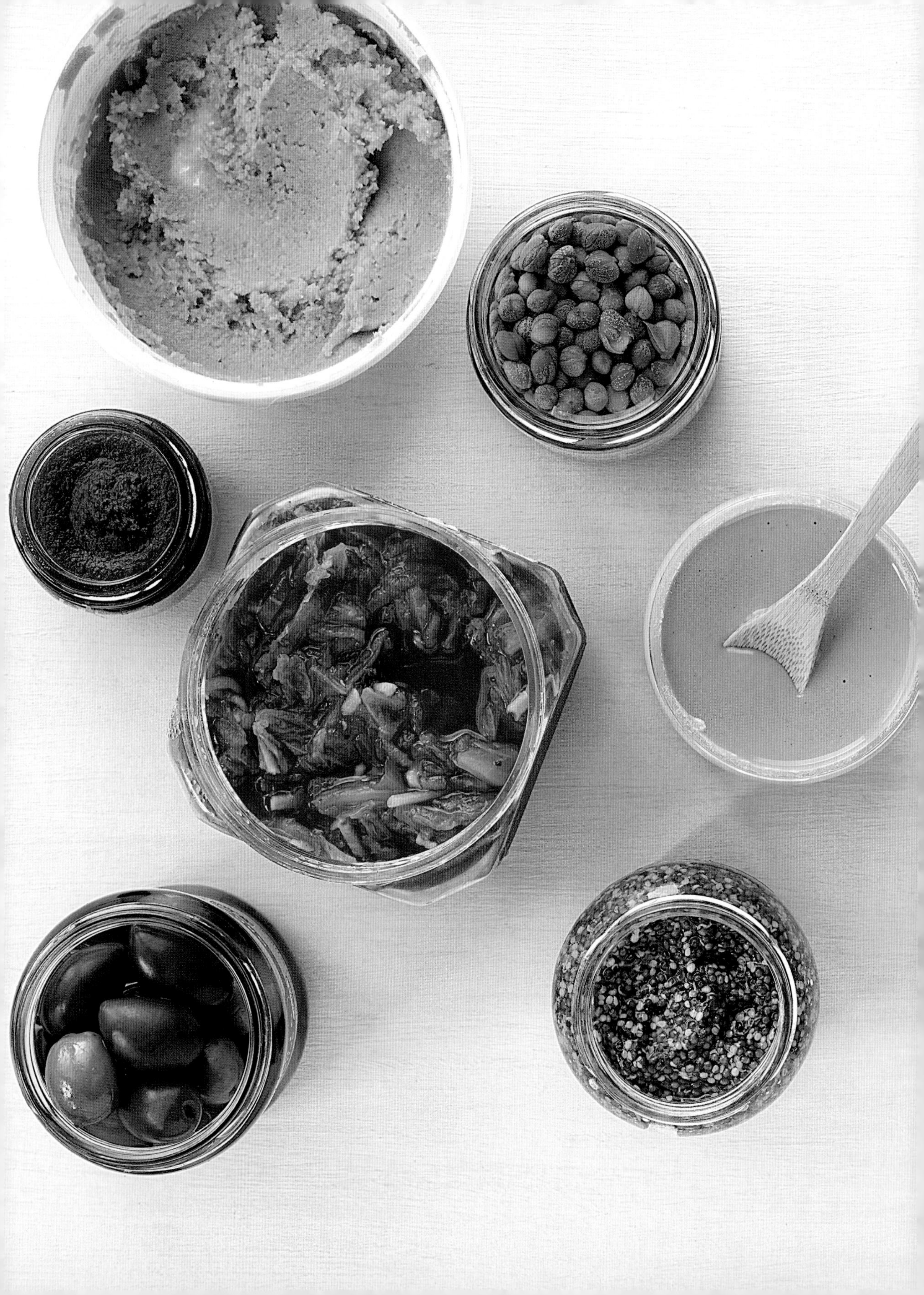

BRAIN HEALTH BEGINS IN THE KITCHEN

Food is your most powerful tool to resist cognitive decline with age. The food you choose to eat can either protect the brain or spur inflammation that accelerates decline. The great news is that neuroprotective food is delicious and building a brain-healthy kitchen is doable and satisfying. It's easy to get started: I'll walk you through what brain-healthy eating means practically, and how to stock up on the best ingredients.

Unlike many health-centric cookbooks, my approach isn't about following a strict plan. Thankfully, brain-healthy eating doesn't require going on a "diet"—aka restricting your eating to lose weight—nor doing a thirty-day "detox" or a cleanse. That's because studies show that these types of dietary approaches aren't sustainable, and brain-healthy eating is about making food choices that will have staying power for the rest of your life.

At its core, brain-healthy eating is a lifestyle founded on a set of attitudes about aging with intention and grace. It's not about counting calories or obsessing about your weight. That being said, don't be surprised if you become leaner and trimmer as you embrace the brain-healthy lifestyle, thanks to an abundance of high-fiber plant foods and an absence of foods laden with empty calories (since those aren't good for the brain). Whether you are thirty-five or seventy-five, this brain health lifestyle is a proactive way to approach aging.

THE BRAIN HEALTH KITCHEN FOOD GUIDELINES

The BHK guidelines are organized around ten brain-healthy food groups—the ones backed by scientific evidence—and the recipes, tips, and sidebars throughout the book will help you incorporate them into your daily life. These ten food groups provide everything an aging brain needs to thrive. The BHK Food Pyramid shows you at a glance what a brain-healthy diet looks like: plant foods fill the base; animal products are optional and, if included, are enjoyed in small amounts; and the foods to limit make up the triangle's smallest tip.

There's room here to adjust this brain-healthy food pyramid based on your personal dietary pattern. If you don't eat meat, for example, just omit that food group. If you are allergic to nuts, get the benefits from that group by eating seeds. The first step toward protecting your brain from Alzheimer's is to find the foods you already love to eat that are also neuroprotective. This is your foundation, the base of your very own food pyramid.

THE TEN BRAIN HEALTH KITCHEN FOOD GROUPS

The BHK food groups reflect a plant-heavy version of the MIND and Mediterranean diets, with more servings of leafy greens and vegetables and fewer servings of food from animals. I based this on the vast amount of data that points to the brain health benefits of eating plants in reducing heart disease, especially stroke. (See What's Good for the Heart Is Good for the Brain, page 27.) In addition, alcohol moves down a notch from its prominence in the MIND and Mediterranean diets based on the latest data (page 356) and the fact that most people don't consume alcohol as the Mediterranean diet intends.

BERRIES

Eat at least one ½ cup (95 g) serving daily.

Regularly eating berries will protect your memory and may slow down the aging of your brain by at least two and a half years. While the Nurses' Health Study showed brain health benefits with just one serving of blueberries or two servings of strawberries each week, which became the basis for the MIND diet guidelines, other studies showed improved memory in older adults with mild cognitive impairment if berries are enjoyed daily. That's why I recommend

THE BRAIN HEALTH KITCHEN PYRAMID

A week of brain-healthy eating looks like this: a strong base of plant foods, one or more servings of fish and seafood, and few (if any) servings of animal products. Drink mostly water. Enjoy coffee and tea daily, if you like. Use extra-virgin olive oil as your primary cooking oil. Reach for at least one serving of fermented foods most days. Treat yourself with a brain-healthy sweet some days.

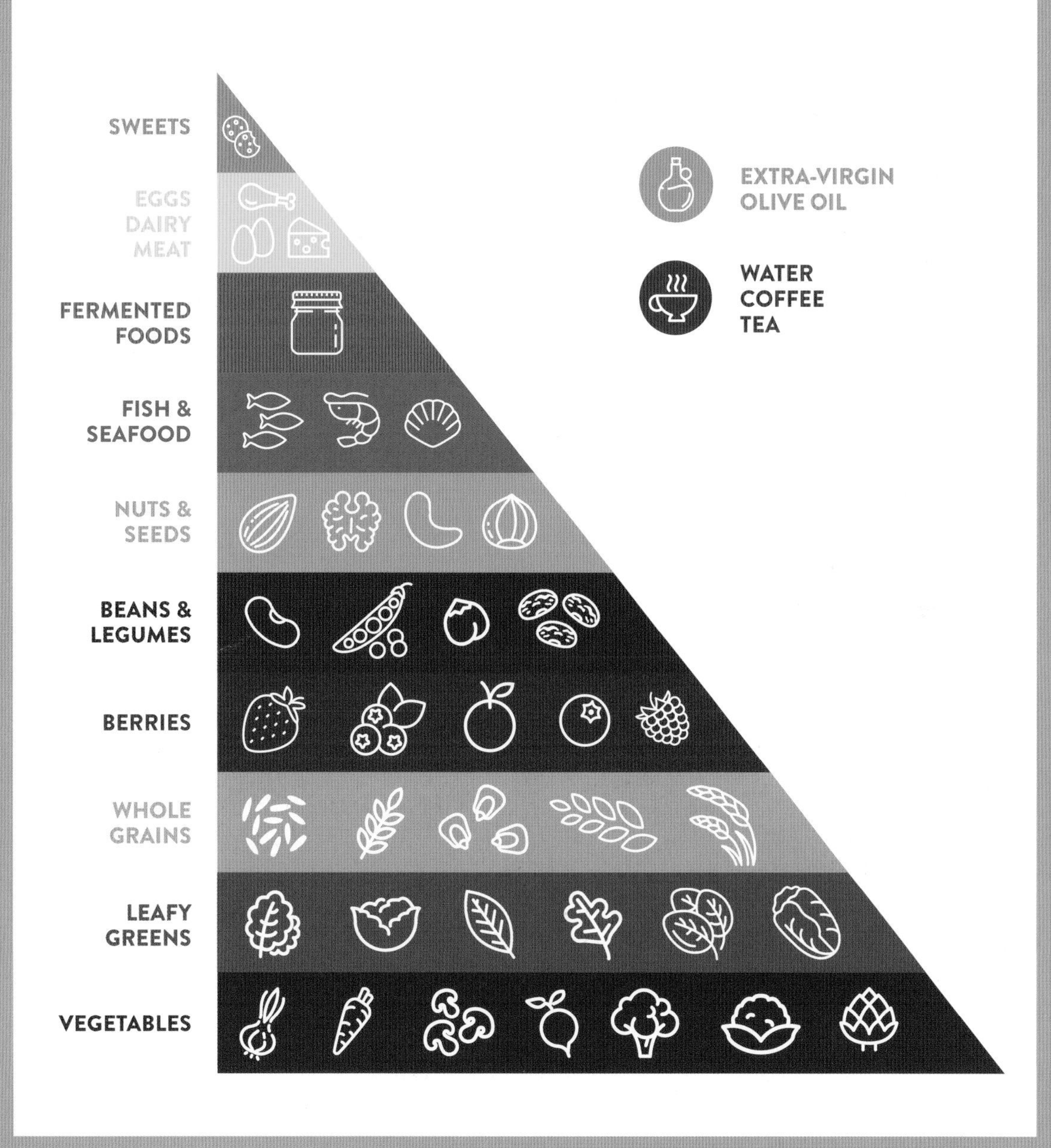

eating a serving of berries every day, if possible. Berries provide a unique package of brain-specific nutrients in a tiny, tasty, fiber-rich matrix. Plus, berries have a low glycemic index, meaning their natural sugars are slowly absorbed and are less likely to elevate blood sugar or stimulate a surge in blood insulin.

LEAFY GREENS

Eat at least 2 cups (80 g) raw or 1 cup (200 g) cooked every day.

Cooked or raw, in a salad or pulverized into a pesto, eating leafy greens daily has a powerful impact on your brain. They are the most nutrient-dense of all the vegetables. The darker the leafy green, the more nutrient-dense.

OTHER VEGETABLES

Eat at least 3 cups (480 g) raw or 1½ cups (240 g) cooked every day.

Eating a wide variety of different-colored vegetables throughout the week is imperative for your brain health (and overall health). That's because vegetables provide many brain-specific nutrients all in one fiber-rich package. Vegetables are a great source of different types of flavonoids, for instance, a family of plant nutrients found in Alzheimer's-resistant diets. Diversity is key. Aim to eat thirty or more different types of plants, mostly vegetables, each week.

- One-third of your vegetables should be cruciferous—broccoli, cauliflower, cabbage, Brussels sprouts, and bok choy—which provides sulforaphane, a key antioxidant that mops up free radicals in the brain.
- Eat at least one serving of colorful vegetables daily, such as carrots, sweet potatoes, and beets.
- Include alliums (garlic, onions, scallions, leeks) frequently in your cooking.
- Enjoy one serving (½ cup/50 g cooked) of mushrooms at least twice a week. (Though technically fungi, we will consider them honorary vegetables throughout the book.)

SEAFOOD

Eat one or more 3-ounce (85 g) servings of seafood each week.

Eating seafood is crucial for your brain health. Choosing the best seafood, however, can be overwhelming given the need to watch out for potential exposure to environmental toxins. Just one serving of high-quality, strategically chosen seafood (see page 152 for tips) provides sufficient DHA, EPA, and a whole host of brain nutrients without exposing yourself to harmful levels of environmental toxins. (Read about supplementing for DHA and EPA on page 163.)

SIX FOOD GROUPS TO LIMIT OR AVOID

While some foods are neuroprotective, others can actually accelerate brain aging. That's why it is just as important to avoid certain foods in your brain-healthy dietary pattern. Some of these brain-harming foods, like butter and cheese, should be limited because they provide too much saturated fat. Others, like ultraprocessed food, should be avoided entirely.

FAST AND FRIED FOOD. Avoid traditional American fast food; its combination of sugar, saturated and trans fats, and salt is especially harmful to the brain. Limit fried food to less than one serving per week, if at all, ideally prepared at home with extra-virgin olive or avocado oil.

PASTRIES AND SWEETS. Limit treats to no more than five servings per week. Avoid all processed and packaged baked goods, which are high in sugar, refined grains, and brain-harming fats. A good rule of thumb: If you want something sweet, make it yourself using the guidelines in this book.

DAIRY. Use small amounts of flavorful cheeses, like Parmesan, feta, and pecorino, sparingly. Reserve full-fat cheese, like cheddar and Brie, for occasional treats. Limit butter intake to less than 1 tablespoon (14 g) per day and choose grass-fed whenever possible. Avoid processed margarine- and butter-like spreads, which harbor brain-harming fats.

ULTRAPROCESSED FOOD. Avoid foods with long ingredient lists and additives such as artificial flavors, added sugars, stabilizers, preservatives, and words that sound more like chemicals than food. These foods include packaged baked goods, chips, candy, store-bought ice cream, boxed cake mixes, conventional pizza, instant noodles, sugary breakfast cereals, flavored yogurt, most energy bars, and processed dairy and meat.

SUGAR- AND ARTIFICIALLY SWEETENED DRINKS. Avoid sports drinks, energy drinks, soda, sweetened coffee and tea, flavored water, milk with added sugar, and fruit juice.

ALCOHOLIC BEVERAGES. If you include alcoholic beverages in your brain-protective diet, do so cautiously and within the context of the light drinking guidelines on page 356: one to six drinks per week. If you don't drink alcohol, there's no reason to start from a brain health perspective.

NUTS AND SEEDS

Eat about ¼ cup (40 g) at least four times each week.

A handful of nuts most days, as a snack or as part of a meal, is proven to reduce your risk of having a heart attack or stroke and also keeps your memory sharp. Regular nut eaters perform better on cognitive tests, with those who eat nuts four times weekly outperforming those who eat nuts just a few times a month. Seeds, while not as extensively studied, are like a bonus brain-healthy food group. If you are allergic to nuts, they are an important source of a similar bounty of nutrients.

WHY TOO MUCH SUGAR IS BAD FOR THE BRAIN

Sugar is both the brain's best friend and worst enemy. That's because a thriving brain requires a constant infusion of sugar—specifically glucose—to perform all of is jobs, even when you sleep. But while the brain is fastidious in its need for glucose, it requires only a small amount each day—62 grams, or about 250 calories, the amount in a few spoonfuls of honey.

Overconsumption of sugar can lead to a condition called insulin resistance in which the pancreas stops responding to every influx of sugar. Insulin resistance in the body leads to metabolic syndrome, prediabetes, and adult-onset diabetes.

Your brain can become resistant to insulin, too. The hippocampus, the primary memory center of the brain, takes the biggest hit of all the brain structures. When the hippocampus can no longer respond to the glucose it needs, it fails, and so does your memory.

It's not surprising, then, that there is a direct correlation between chronically elevated blood sugar levels and the risk of Alzheimer's. Having adult onset diabetes more than doubles the risk. Even having blood sugar readings that are consistently high in the normal range—prediabetes—has been proven to impair thinking and memory functions, and substantially increase dementia risk. Sugar goes by many names in processed foods, such as fructose, sucrose, lactose, maltose, corn syrup, high-fructose corn syrup, and dextrose. Some of the worst culprits for added sugar are boxed cereals, tomato sauce, and yogurt.

The glycemic index—a rating of carbohydrate-containing foods based on how quickly they get broken down into simple sugars—is another way to view food through the lens of brain health. Food that has a low glycemic index and is high in fiber (think carrots, berries, beans, and whole grains) will be kinder to your body and brain than high glycemic index foods like white rice and orange juice.

BEANS AND LENTILS

Eat four or more ½-cup (30 g) cooked servings each week.

All the traditional cultures who enjoy dementia-free longevity include beans and lentils as part of their dietary patterns. Not only are these affordable staples versatile, satiating, and delicious, they stabilize blood sugar and lower harmful blood cholesterol. They also provide the type of fiber health-promoting gut microbiota need to flourish. Beans and lentils boast a wide array of brain-specific phytonutrients, especially the flavonoids that make them speckled and deeply hued.

WHOLE GRAINS

Eat one ½-cup (100 g) cooked serving three times every day.

Three servings a day of whole grains—meaning intact, minimally processed grains—may seem like a lot, but they're worth prioritizing for their dynamic combination of fiber and flavonoids, a key brain health connection. Whole grains provide the added benefit of amplifying the nutrition of the foods with which they're consumed.

MEAT, POULTRY, AND EGGS

Eat small portions (3 ounces/85 g) of chicken or meat up to four times each week; limit eggs based on your personal health factors.

If you choose to include animal products in your brain-protective dietary pattern, do so strategically. At best, things like pastured eggs and grass-fed beef can provide key brain health nutrients like vitamin B12, lutein, choline, iron, and a source of lean protein, not to mention a sense of familiarity to your meals. Eat too much, however, or eat pro-inflammatory foods like hot dogs and other processed meats, and they can contribute to brain aging. If you skip this food group entirely, your brain will still thrive.

OLIVES AND OLIVE OIL

Use olive oil as your primary cooking oil and enjoy olives frequently.

When you make the switch to using mostly olive oil in your cooking, you provide your brain with the brain-friendly ratio of more monounsaturated fats and less saturated ones. Plus, high-quality olive oil provides polyphenols (page 48), potent antioxidants that are part of the reason numerous studies report olive oil consumers suffer fewer heart attacks, strokes, and have lower overall rates of death from any cause. If your dietary pattern precludes the use of cooking oils, get the same brain health virtues from eating olives.

COFFEE, TEA, AND OTHER DRINKS

Drink mostly water, enjoy coffee and tea, and limit alcoholic beverages. While water is the brain-healthiest drink of all, other choices can be a welcome part of your dietary pattern. A substantial body of science says drinking coffee (up to five cups per day) and tea is advantageous for a healthy brain and for fending off Alzheimer's and age-related cognitive decline.

THE FOUR Fs OF BRAIN-HEALTHY FOOD

Cooking from this book will keep you on the brain-healthy track while at home. But what about when you are traveling, grabbing a quick bite at work, eating out, or at a dinner party? You'll need a strategy that's flexible and realistic. That's where the 4Fs come in, an easy-to-remember list of brain-boosting characteristics. Each of the 4Fs—fats, fiber, flavonoids, and fit—provide something your brain needs to thrive. A brain-healthy food will possess at least two of these four properties.

1. **Fats.** Foods rich in brain-friendly unsaturated fats (the MUFAs and PUFAs, page 40, not the saturated ones) provide essential building blocks for brain cells while making food satiating and delicious. Choose foods like avocados, anchovies, extra-virgin olive oil, and walnuts.
2. **Fiber.** Fiber slows down the absorption of sugar, binds harmful cholesterol, provides food for beneficial gut microbes, and even acts as a conduit to help deliver nutrients into the bloodstream where they can then travel to the brain. Fiber-rich foods include artichokes, berries, lentils, and whole grains.
3. **Flavonoids.** The pigments in plants that make them colorful are actually nutrients called flavonoids, a key tool for blocking oxidative stress in the brain (read more on page 39). A flavonoid-rich diet has been linked to reduced Alzheimer's risk. Find them in foods like berries, capers, pears, green tea, red onions, and grapes.
4. **Fit.** Part of nourishing your brain is choosing foods that fit realistically into your life. This means figuring out which neuroprotective foods you

SCIENCE BITE:

ALL ABOUT FLAVONOIDS

What is it that makes foods like berries, green tea, leafy greens, oranges, and pears so good for your brain? In short, it's the flavonoids—a family of plant pigments that make these foods colorful while acting as powerful antioxidants. Evidence is building that a diet rich in certain flavonoid-containing foods can significantly reduce the risk of age-related cognitive decline.

When Rush University researchers followed 921 dementia-free adults with detailed dietary questionnaires and annual neurological examinations over 6 years, they found a strong link between certain foods and reduced Alzheimer's risk. Those who ate about 2 apples or pears a week, for example, which are rich in the flavonoid isorhamnetin, had 38 percent fewer cases of Alzheimer's than those who ate these fruits infrequently. Participants who ate an abundance of foods rich in another flavonoid—kaempferol, found in leafy greens, green tea, soy, and broccoli—had 50 percent fewer cases of Alzheimer's.

Harvard researchers studied the link between cognitive function and flavonoids from a different angle. They tracked diet while evaluating participants for subjective cognitive decline—the subtle type of thinking problems noticed decades before dementia is diagnosed. This powerful 20-year-long study of 49,493 women from the Nurses' Health Study and 27,842 men from the Health Professionals Follow-up Study found that the more certain flavonoid-rich foods were included in the diet, the less likely one was to have subjective cognitive decline. They gave especially high marks to citrus fruits (oranges and grapefruit), berries (blueberries and strawberries), vegetables (peppers, celery, cauliflower, Brussels sprouts), leafy greens, and tea.

love to eat, that you enjoy cooking, that fit within your budget and your lifestyle. Brain-healthy food is a good fit if it checks off one or more of these boxes:

- Big on satisfaction and flavor. This is a food you love and will enjoy often.
- Convenient. This food saves you time or otherwise makes life easier (e.g., good-quality instant oatmeal, jarred marinara, or salsa).
- Gives an emotional boost. This food is part of your belief system, connecting you with your heritage, family, friends, or the people who grew or raised the food.

WORKING YOUR WAY TOWARD A BRAIN-FRIENDLIER DIET

Don't be discouraged if your current dietary pattern doesn't look close to this right now. The goal is not to overhaul your diet all in one go but to introduce more brain-healthy foods over time (keeping the 4Fs in mind) while weeding out the inflammatory ones. Until about ten years ago, my personal dietary pattern was only about 50 percent brain healthy. With time (and great recipes!), I have brought it up to about 95 percent brain healthy, 5 percent other. This gives me permission to enjoy my favorite "real" gelato on the streets of Rome when traveling, barbecued chicken at a friend's house, and occasionally drink more than one 5-ounce (150 ml) glass of wine when out with friends.

The portion sizes and frequencies are based on current scientific evidence. Much like an effective dose for certain medicines, foods can have a medicinal dose (such as one serving of seafood each week). But, again, upping the amount of these foods, if needed, should be done over time until it feels like a sustainable way of eating for you.

Finally, remember that "progress over perfection" is the goal. (Read more on page 44.) As long as you are moving toward a way of eating that is more nourishing to your brain, you are doing a great job. Trying to eat perfectly is not realistic, nor is it the goal. Working your way up to following these guidelines 90 percent of the time is a major accomplishment.

THE SCOOP ON FATS AND BRAIN HEALTH

You may have read the erroneous statistic that the brain is 60 percent fat. That means you should feed the brain an excessive amount of fatty foods, right? Wrong! Nor is it a good idea to follow a "low fat" diet, a trend that is credited with a rise in obesity, diabetes, and cardiovascular disease—all risk factors for Alzheimer's and other dementias.

The good news is this: we already know which fats the brain needs and which ones to avoid. The tricky part can be achieving the right balance between what I call brain-friendly fats with all the others.

SATURATED VS. UNSATURATED FATS

A fat is "saturated" if it is jam-packed with double bonds giving it a rigid structure. This fat occurs in nature (in foods like butter, red meat, and coconut) and can be synthesized in a factory into the trans-saturated fats found in many processed foods (such as margarine, canned cream soups, and frozen pizza and chicken pot pie).

The impact of too much saturated fat in the diet—especially trans fat—is detrimental to the brain in many ways, both directly and indirectly. The rigid structure is directly inflammatory to blood vessels, especially the delicate ones that supply the brain. These fats incite damage to the cells in the pancreas, too, leading to impaired insulin secretion and adult onset diabetes, a major risk factor for Alzheimer's. In addition, a diet laden with saturated fats leads to more harmful blood cholesterol, especially low density lipoprotein (LDL), also a risk factor for Alzheimer's. Consuming saturated fats in the presence of refined sugars, like most standard American diet eaters do, is a recipe for even worse inflammation. Further study is needed to tease out the impact of saturated fat in the diet without all the other brain-harming foods along with it, but the research now suggests: the more saturated fat in the diet, the higher the risk of Alzheimer's and other dementias.

Then there are the "unsaturated" fats—the monounsaturated fatty acids (MUFAs) and the polyunsaturated fatty acids (PUFAs). These fats contain just one or a few double bonds, which makes them pliable as they travel through the body. I call these the brain-friendly fats because they are not only beneficial for health, they are downright essential for thriving brain function. And most people don't get enough.

BRAIN-FRIENDLY FATS

Avocados, olive oil, nuts, and seeds are rich in MUFAs. You get PUFAs from fish and seafood, whole grains, and olive oil. That's the Mediterranean diet in a nutshell. But the Mediterranean diet is not a "low fat" diet; as much as 40 percent of the calories come from fats. Fewer than 5 percent of these are saturated fats, though, which keeps the ratio of unsaturated to saturated fats high. In the MIND diet, the more brain-specific spin-off of the Mediterranean diet, saturated fat intake is even more austere: 3 to 5 percent of total fat consumption. The MIND diet does this by specifically limiting those foods that are high in saturated fats through its five brain-unhealthy foods list: fried and fast food, red meat, butter, cheese, and pastry and sweets.

ESSENTIAL OMEGA-3 FATS

The only category of fat your brain truly requires from the diet is a type of PUFA—the omega-3 fatty acids. These fats are called the essential fatty acids because they need to come from the diet and are therefore an "essential" aspect of what you eat. Omega-3s may be the most important nutrient to fend off age-related cognitive decline. In fact, a low intake of omega-3s is not only correlated with poor cognitive function with age, it is linked to an increased risk of Alzheimer's. Conversely, a diet rich in omega-3s can slow down cognitive decline and decrease risk. (Read more about this in the Fish and Seafood chapter.)

The most important omega-3s for brain health are eicosapentaenoic acid (EPA) and docosahexaenoic acid (DHA). That's because these fats quell inflammation in the brain, repair the age-related damage to brain cells, and actually become incorporated into the cells' protective sheath. Both are plentiful in fish (salmon, mackerel, anchovies, sardines, herring, and cod) and seafood (oysters, mussels, and clams). Grass-fed animal products, like butter and red meat, also provide small amounts of EPA and DHA.

SALT VS. SODIUM

When you get rid of the packaged and processed foods in your pantry, you are also getting rid of most of the salt in your diet. Salt is the ingredient that provides sodium, a mineral your body needs to keep fluids in balance and perform basic physiologic functions. But too much salt, especially if you are salt sensitive, can lead to chronically elevated blood pressure (aka hypertension), which can damage blood vessels and contribute to heart attack and stroke. Hypertension is a common risk factor for Alzheimer's and other types of dementia. Studies show that keeping your systolic blood pressure (the top number) under 130 mm Hg during midlife can reduce the risk of Alzheimer's decades later.

The daily recommendation for salt is 2,300 milligrams per day. That's about 1 teaspoon of fine table salt or 1½ teaspoons Morton kosher salt. Most Americans get 1,000 milligrams more salt than needed, every day! For most people, cutting back on salt is an important strategy for optimizing brain health. For others, like athletes and those with low blood pressure, it's important to get enough. The good news is that when you cook with whole foods (not packaged food), a little bit of salt goes a long way to bring out the flavor in dishes.

Alpha-linolenic acids (ALA) are the third type of omega-3s. ALA comes from plant sources—walnuts, leafy greens, seeds, and algae. The problem with relying on ALA for all the brain's omega-3 needs is that the brain doesn't absorb it in its active form very well. ALA first must be converted to DHA or EPA, an inefficient process that delivers less than 3 percent to the brain. Read more on page 42 about getting enough omega-3s if you don't eat fish and seafood.

A brain-friendly fat intake provides enough of the essential fatty acids (EPA and DHA), minimal saturated fat, and none, if possible, of the trans ones. It's great that the understanding of fats in the diet is moving away from simplistic labeling of "good fats" and "bad fats." (Except for the trans fats! Those truly are the bad fats.) Fat is essential to not just a healthful diet but much of our enjoyment of what we eat. In the case of fats, when you eat foods rich in the brain-friendly ones, there's little room left on the plate for the others.

EATING WITH A BRAIN HEALTH MINDSET

The Brain Health Mindset approaches aging with proactive steps to nourish and protect the brain. Positive lifestyle changes are more likely to become lifelong brain health habits with a few simple guidelines, borrowed from the field of positive psychology.

START WITH A PURPOSE

What motivates you to take care of your brain? Have you lost loved ones to Alzheimer's and want to do everything you can to prevent it in yourself? Maybe you simply want to enjoy your grandchildren and stay sharp in the last season of your life. Clarify what motivates you on this journey. Write it down, be specific, and revisit your purpose often.

EMBRACE A CLEAN SLATE

There are stages in life that are ripe for a fresh start. Perhaps it's a milestone birthday, like turning forty or sixty, or a brush with serious illness. It could be the start of a new year or finding yourself with an empty nest. Maybe it began when you picked up this book. Find your clean slate and use it to move forward as the brain-healthy person you want to be.

WHAT ABOUT ORGANIC?

In a perfect brain-healthy world, all of our food would be grown organically, meaning without harmful pesticides like glyphosate. That's because pesticide exposure is increasingly being proven harmful to brain cells. While a direct link between pesticides and Alzheimer's has not been proven, pesticides are thought to cause cellular stress that creates chronic inflammation in the brain.

In the real world, choosing organic is not always possible. Avoid pesticide contamination in your foods *whenever you are able* by choosing certified organic foods. Sometimes organic food is just not available, is prohibitively expensive, or doesn't seem as fresh as conventional. Other times, it may be raised organically but not have an official USDA Organic stamp (as is often the case with vendors at farmers' markets). Throughout the book, I point out when it is a priority to choose organic and when buying conventional is fine.

BE A BRAIN HEALTH AMBASSADOR

Define yourself as someone who cares about your brain health and is actively taking steps to protect it. When you take care of your brain or when you share that knowledge with the people in your life, you are advocating for their brain health, too. Remind yourself often that you are a brain health ambassador.

CONTROL YOUR ENVIRONMENT

You may be wondering how you will manage to eat less of certain brain-harmful foods, like butter, cheese, and sugary drinks. Won't that take a lot of willpower? First, your brain is wired for instant gratification. Given the choice, it will always go for the quick fix. That's why the concept of willpower is mostly a myth. Rather than relying on superior self control, take charge of your personal food environment. Make the brain-healthy food choice the easier, more accessible one.

FOCUS ON PROGRESS OVER PERFECTION

No matter where you are on the journey to nourishing your brain with neuroprotective food, don't fall into the trap of trying to do everything perfectly. First of all, one perfect brain-healthy diet doesn't exist. Many dietary patterns are neuroprotective, and the one that's best for you will depend on your belief system and what you like to eat.

While it's tempting to say you will only consume brain-healthy food from here on, the reality is this: good eating habits build slowly over time. Rather than vowing to never eat unhealthy food again, start with one meaningful change. If you are a person who never eats leafy greens, for example, your change could be to buy a box of prewashed lettuce and eat one handful of greens every day for a week. Keep doing that for a month, and you have a brain-healthy habit that is proven to slow down the aging of the brain. Every microchange you make that sticks will build a foundation that becomes part of your Brain Health Mindset.

TRACK YOUR PROGRESS WEEKLY, NOT DAILY

Striving to eat right all the time is stressful and unhealthy in itself. And stress, especially chronic stress, is bad for the brain. Rather than obsessing over each food choice throughout your day, think about what you eat over the course of a week. Studies show that your overall dietary pattern—what you eat most of the time—is what matters for long-term brain health. Start by tallying up how many brain-healthy food groups you eat in a week, along with how many unhealthy ones you avoid. (You can use either the MIND diet or a Mediterranean diet scoring system; see Resources, page 390.) Eventually, choosing these foods will become intuitive.

CELEBRATE POSITIVE CHANGES

Be sure to give yourself a pat on the back whenever you make the brain-healthier choice, whether it be having a glass of water instead of a soda or baking with a whole-grain flour instead of all-purpose white. Also, be kind to yourself on this journey. We are all just doing our best.

ASK YOURSELF THIS ONE QUESTION

When faced with a food choice, ask yourself: Is this food likely to be good for my brain or not? After reading and cooking from this book, you will have all the information you need to make the brain-healthy choice. Keep reminding yourself that you value taking care of your brain.

SHOPPING WITH A BRAIN HEALTH MINDSET

Before you head to the grocery store or farmers' market or order groceries, get into your Brain Health Mindset (page 43). Why is this step useful? The number of brain-harming food choices can be overwhelming, for one. Plus, food companies use clever tactics to get you to buy food because it seems healthy or pushes other emotional buttons. Remind yourself that you know how to make the brain-friendly choice. You may be a casual, everyday shopper, picking up what looks good at the market each day. Or you may be a meal planner, crunched for time and getting all your shopping done once a week. Either way, having an overreaching set of values about the foods you bring home will help you develop your own personal neuroprotective dietary pattern. (See Fit on page 38.)

Pause to take a look at your shopping cart as you are checking out. Does everything look colorful, fresh, and healthy? Are there very few boxes and packages of food? If so, this is proof that you are taking the steps needed to nourish your brain. Your Brain Health Mindset is winning!

PANTRY AND SHELF STAPLES

The food in your kitchen cupboards is the heart of your pantry—ready for you with brain-healthy staples for making meals off the cuff. Fill it with canned goods, jarred foods, spices, oils, vinegars, whole grains, legumes, and more.

Snacks

Stock up on nuts: pistachios, cashews, almonds, walnuts, and pecans are all brain-healthy choices. Have a few different nut butters, too—almond and peanut, but also try cashew, walnut, pecan, and hazelnut. (A spoonful of nut butter stuffed into a Medjool date makes a satisfying, fiber-packed snack.) Some seeds are made for snacking, like sunflower and hulled pumpkin seeds (pepitas). If you want something sweet, a square of dark chocolate (60 percent or more cacao) is a good pick.

Spices

Ounce for ounce, spices are the most potent brain foods in your kitchen. Brain health superstar spices often start with the letter *c*: cardamom, cayenne, chile, cinnamon, cumin, coriander, and those that contain capsaicin, like chiles and paprika. Other spices to have on hand include ground ginger, dried oregano, dried thyme, and crushed red pepper flakes.

When you buy spices whole and grind them yourself, they will always be more flavorful and potent. Look for whole coriander, cumin seeds, and peppercorns (especially the pink peppercorns, which are actually berries; see page 57).

Certain spices are worth seeking out because they provide uniquely vibrant flavors and have specific anti-Alzheimer's potential, including sumac (page 57), saffron (page 258), and high-quality turmeric (page 271).

Spices lose their phytonutrient activity over time, so make sure your spices are fresh. Buy only the amount you will use in six months and toss any spices that are more than one year old.

Salt

All you need is coarse kosher salt for most baking and cooking. Different-size crystals and shapes will all vary in measurements. For instance, 1 teaspoon table salt (fine salt) is equivalent to 1½ teaspoons Morton kosher salt or 2 teaspoons Diamond Crystal kosher salt. Throughout the book, I use Morton kosher salt, a type of sea salt with a coarse texture that keeps it from permeating food like finer table salt. Kosher salt has a brighter taste and helps

STORE-BOUGHT BRAIN HEALTH SUPERSTARS

Certain foods deserve to be called out as brain health superstars because they have specific nutrients of interest in Alzheimer's prevention. Many of these superstars can easily be purchased at the grocery store, like anchovies, oat bran, pistachios, and turmeric. Others—such as caper berries, chickpea (aka garbanzo bean) flour, matcha, nutritional yeast, preserved lemons, spelt flour, and sumac—may require seeking out. You'll find these at a health-focused grocery store (where you may also discover new-to-you brain foods!). Everything, of course, can be found online.

Keep in mind that most extremely nutrient-dense foods are also the most perishable (unless canned like anchovies). Buy only as much as you will use in the next six months, and store in airtight containers away from light in a cool cupboard, the fridge, or the freezer.

Throughout the book, superstar ingredients are highlighted with a Science Bite box explaining why they are special and/or offering a tip on how to find them.

bring out the natural flavors of ingredients. Diamond Crystal salt has even bigger crystals and can be tricky to measure consistently.

It's also nice to have a box of "finishing salt" like Maldon, fleur de sel, or Himalayan pink salt. These coarse and flaky crystals add a pop of texture and bring out flavors in a finished dish.

Oils

All you need in your pantry is a short list of brain-friendly oils (page 315). You'll use extra-virgin olive oil (high-end or everyday) for most of your cooking and avocado oil for neutral flavor and high heat cooking. In addition, you may want a few specialty oils for occasional use to add certain flavors, like nut oils and unrefined sesame oil. Pecan oil has a nutrition profile closest to extra-virgin olive oil—high in monounsaturated fats and polyphenols.

While coconut oil has been marketed as a heart- and brain-healthy oil, it is more than 90 percent saturated fat. It has been shown to raise harmful blood cholesterol if consumed regularly (page 41). You may have read that coconut oil can slow the progression of Alzheimer's. Unfortunately, this claim is not supported by legitimate studies. Use this oil sparingly, if at all, for its flavor profile to season certain foods, like stir-fries and curries and the turmeric granola on page 271.

Vinegars

Good-quality vinegar is a fermented food that can brighten soups and stews, balance a salad dressing, and serve as a brain-healthy marinade for meats (page 299). You only need a few types of vinegar: balsamic, red wine, white wine, rice, and apple cider (page 359).

Food in Cans, Boxes, Cartons, and Jars

Fill your pantry with good-quality canned beans and vegetables (artichokes and tomatoes), good-quality marinara sauce, salsas, and jars and tins of olive oil–packed seafood, like anchovies and sardines. See the shopping notes for stocking up on beans (page 391) and whole grains (page 392).

Baking Ingredients

As you cook through the book, you will notice different types of flour than you may already have on hand. Whole-grain (buckwheat, whole wheat, spelt, teff, cornmeal) flours, chickpea (garbanzo bean) flour, nut flours (hazelnut, almond), and seed flours (quinoa) will hopefully come to replace old standbys. Swapping white whole-wheat flour for all-purpose upgrades the fiber content of baked goods, which slows down the absorption of sugar while feeding your gut microbiota. Unless your diet is restricted to certain alternative flours (because you have celiac disease, a gluten allergy, or sensitivity), try to weed out these refined flours that offer neither flavor nor nutrition: rice, tapioca, and arrowroot flours. Purchase high-quality flours in small quantities (enough for about six months) because they may lose antioxidant power with time. (Store nut and buckwheat flours in the freezer.)

Most baking mixes don't deserve a spot in your brain-healthy pantry since sugar is often the first ingredient. Plus, they are packed with chemicals. This includes brownie, cupcake, cake, cookie, and cornbread mixes. Canned frosting? Toss.

FRIDGE

Envision opening your refrigerator to find it bursting with all sorts of fresh and colorful foods: cilantro and parsley stored in jars like flowers (root side down in an inch/2.5 cm of water), salad-ready leafy greens, bundles of Swiss chard, heads of cauliflower and broccoli, a sturdy supply of root vegetables and alliums, and plenty of baskets of berries and other perishable fruits. This is the ideal brain-healthy fridge, stocked with nutrient-rich produce and mostly free from packaged foods.

Fresh Produce

A well-stocked fridge in any of the brain-healthy dietary patterns is jam-packed with fresh produce. When you get home from the grocery store or farmers' market, a few minutes spent cleaning and organizing your produce will help it last longer and be more convenient. (See tips in each chapter opener for how-tos.) Give these perishables the prime real estate of your fridge so you can see what you have at a moment's glance.

Buy only what you can consume in the next several days. Eating a more plant-rich diet may mean more frequent trips to the grocery store. As you discover new-to-you foods and explore different brain-healthy cooking techniques, though, shopping will become more of a stress-reducing activity than a chore. Remind yourself of the big picture: more frequent trips to the grocery store now mean you'll need fewer visits to the doctor's office in the decades ahead.

Condiments

Toss condiments made with unhealthy fats and added sugars. Common culprits are oyster sauce, hoisin sauce, ketchup, barbecue sauce, and teriyaki sauce. Read the label of your mayonnaise; most are rich in saturated fats. Instead, stock up on the following fridge MVPs: flavor-boosting staples that also provide key brain health nutrients for your meals.

BEWARE OF THE HEALTH HALO EFFECT

When a food is marketed to be good for you when in fact it is not, the food company is exploiting the health halo effect. This shows up in buzzwords like *natural* or *light* that bring attention to certain healthful ingredients. In reality, the number of unhealthy ones—such as sugar or inflammatory oils—far outweigh the good.

Case in point: store-bought granola. Granolas have enjoyed carte blanche as "health food" because of ingredients like oats, nuts, and seeds, which provide fiber, antioxidants, and flavonoids. However, most store-bought granolas rely on inexpensive, unhealthy fats like hydrogenated palm and canola oil as a way to create crispy clusters. Most popular brands list sugar high on the list of ingredients.

The health halo effect spills over into shopping habits, too. Studies show that health-conscious shoppers are more likely to indulge in unhealthy foods, like doughnuts, when shopping at a farmers' market instead of the grocery store. When shoppers use reusable bags, they are more likely to fill those bags with indulgent foods, like candy and chips. Researchers postulate that making one virtuous choice—like shopping at the farmers' market—subconsciously makes shoppers feel more deserving and less guilty about choosing unhealthy foods.

With a little practice, you can easily avoid being influenced by the health halo effect. To discern which foods are truly a brain-healthy choice and which ones are just deploying clever, targeted marketing to seem that way, ignore buzzwords, slogans, and images that make foods appear healthful. Go right to the nutrition label and ingredient list; read before you buy. Be mindful that behaving "virtuously" in one area of your life (like using your own shopping bag) doesn't give a green light to act in a negative or overindulgent way elsewhere.

The bottom line: If a food is being marketed to appear good for you, it probably isn't.

- **Miso paste.** Miso is a fermented, plant-based paste that adds umami and salty flavors to foods. If you are new to miso, start with the milder-tasting white (or shiro) miso made from soybeans. The darker the miso, the deeper the flavor; look for yellow, red, or dark brown miso. Miso keeps indefinitely in the fridge.
- **Good-quality fermented vegetables.** Kimchi, lacto-fermented pickles, and sauerkraut are widely available, but many markets carry other fermented vegetables like carrots and cauliflower in the refrigerated section of the grocery store.
- **Mustard.** Look for high-quality mustard without added sugar; bonus if it contains whole seeds, which provide omega-3 fatty acids, protein, and minerals.
- **Curry paste.** Look for red and green curry paste that is low in sugar and saturated fats. Whisk with stock or coconut milk for a quick curry sauce to go with vegetables, chicken, or fish.
- **Olives.** Look for good-quality olives in jars or the bulk section of the grocery store (page 317). Snack on them, dress them up as marinated olives (page 320), add to salads, and fold into soft scrambled eggs.
- **Capers.** These flavonoid-rich berries (page 57) come packed in vinegar, salt, or olive oil. Stock up on all varieties of capers, including the giant caper berries used on page 64.
- **Tahini.** This sesame seed paste, best stored in the fridge, has dozens of uses in your cooking from replacing the butter in cookies (page 265) to sauces (page 192) to making hummus (page 235).

Drinks

Stock your fridge with water, herbal tea, sparkling water, and unsweetened plant-based milks, store-bought or homemade (page 363). Wean out drinks that are sweetened or artificially sweetened.

FREEZER

Your freezer has the potential to be a treasure trove of homemade brain-healthy meals, but it can also be a brain health disaster because many of the ultraprocessed foods come from the freezer aisle at the grocery store. Make room for the good stuff and weed out these foods: frozen pizza, breakfast pastries, ready-made smoothie packs, onion rings, french fries, breaded chicken and fish, prepared pasta meals, frozen desserts . . . the list goes on and on.

The freezer is the right spot for many key brain-healthy ingredients to help you prepare meals more quickly. Nuts like walnuts and pecans are highly perishable, thanks to their delicate fats and vitamin E content; store them, along with nut and whole-grain flours, here in the freezer.

Many frozen vegetables are just as nutritious as fresh ones, such as peas, edamame, corn, cauliflower rice, and butternut squash. A stockpile of frozen berries (blueberries, blackberries, raspberries) will help you enjoy a serving of berries most days. If you eat seafood and meat, you'll use your freezer to store seasonal seafood, like wild-caught salmon and shrimp, grass-fed meats, and high-quality poultry. Stock batches of homemade stocks, pestos, Walnut "Parm," and marinara sauce.

BRAIN-HEALTHY COOKING TECHNIQUES

How you prepare your food can be just as important as the food itself. Whenever heat is applied to a food, it changes the food's structure. This can be beneficial, like the way simmering tomatoes into marinara sauce encourages the fruit's antioxidant lycopene to seep out (page 120). Or, more often, heat creates inflammatory substances in the foods, specifically AGEs (advanced glycation end products, see page 280). That's why the cooking mantra for brain health is "low and slow." Less heat means fewer AGEs accumulate in the food. Slow cooking builds flavor and helps food retain its nutrients and healthy fats.

Brain-healthy cooking techniques include:

1. **Baking at under 400°F (200°C):** preserves nutrients with lower heat and less browning
2. **Boiling:** best for uncracked eggs, which helps them retain nutrients, but not vegetables, which leaches them
3. **Braising:** aka stewing; cooking over low heat in a covered pot within a small amount of liquid
4. **Cold-smoking:** using low temperature (usually under 200°F/95°C) to impart flavor without cooking
5. **Grilling over indirect heat:** grilling in a low-heat zone adjacent to a hot zone

6. **Microwaving:** cooking briefly (less than eight minutes) in the microwave at half power
7. **Poaching:** simmering food in water or another liquid below its boiling point
8. **Pressure cooking:** applying heat and steam at high pressure in a closed system, like an Instant Pot multicooker or a traditional pressure cooker, for a short period of time
9. **Sautéing:** cooking foods quickly over medium-high heat with a small amount of oil
10. **Slow cooking:** simmering covered at a very low heat in a slow cooker or in a pot in the oven or on the stove
11. **Slow roasting:** cooking for a longer time and at lower temperatures
12. **Steaming:** using steam to cook and often adding the small amount of liquid in the pan back into the finished dish
13. **Sous vide:** immersing food in an airtight plastic bag in a device that circulates water at a low temperature
14. **Stir-frying:** quickly sautéing in a large skillet or wok with a small amount of oil

Avoid these cooking techniques:

1. **Broiling:** cooking foods within 3 to 5 inches (7.5 to 13 cm) of the oven heat source, similar to direct grilling
2. **Deep-frying:** cooking foods at a high temperature and submerged in oil
3. **Searing:** quick cooking in a pan over the stove using high heat
4. **Grilling over direct heat:** grilling with food within 6 inches (15 cm) of the heat source, especially if coated in a sweet sauce
5. **High-heat dry roasting:** cooking food, especially meat and chicken, in a hot (more than 400°F/200°C) oven without a braising liquid

With all methods, anything that serves as a barrier between the food and the heat source will help retain nutrients while minimizing AGE formation. This could be a cedar plank or grill basket used while grilling, a nut or breadcrumb coating for fish or chicken, a parchment paper–lined baking pan, or an acid-based marinade (such as yogurt) on fish, chicken, or meat (see Brain-Healthy Grilling Tips, page 292).

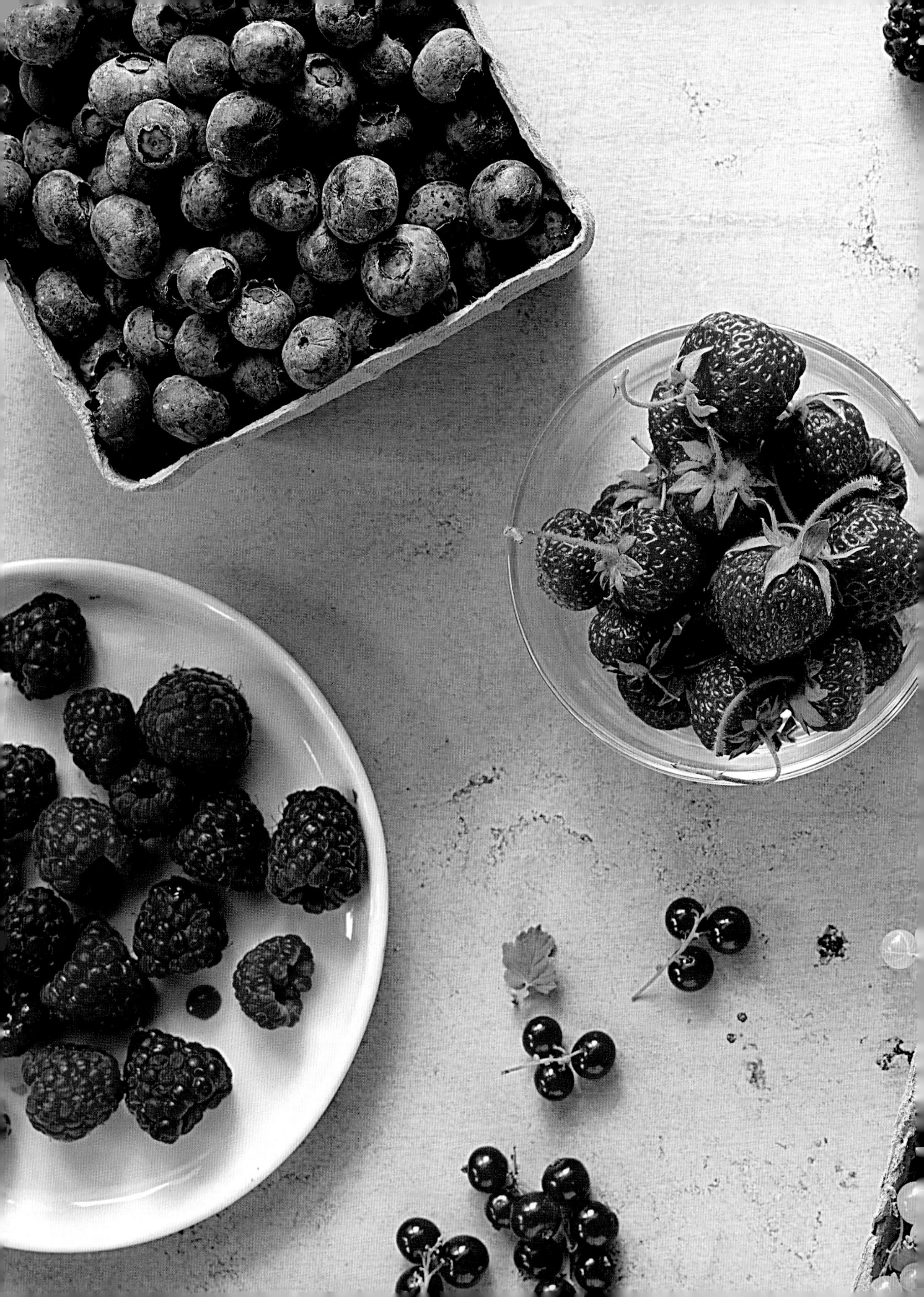

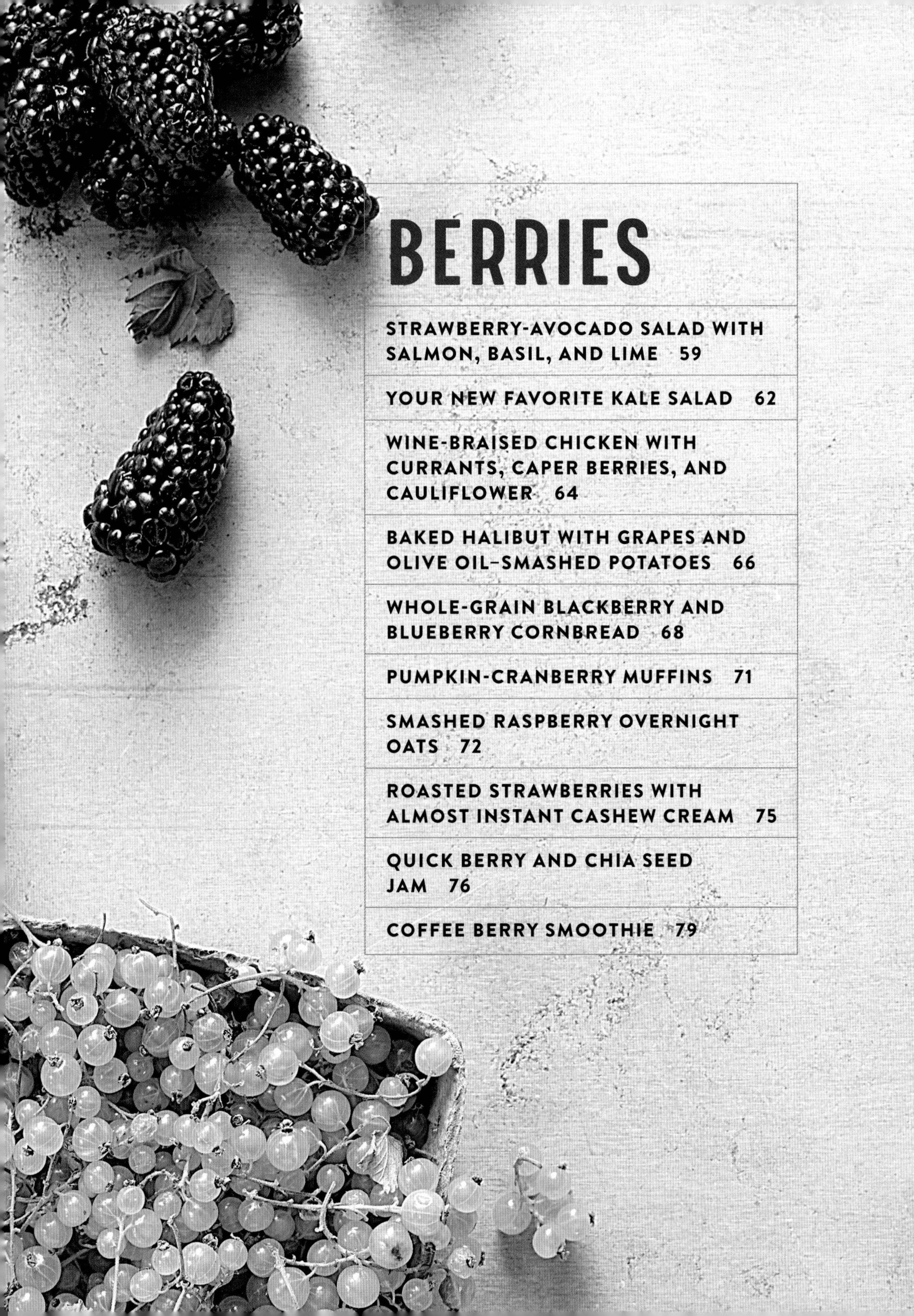

BERRIES

Berries—especially blueberries—have become synonymous with boosting memory and fending off cognitive decline. And for good reason: in both human and animal studies, berries have robust evidence for supporting brain health. Berries are one of the most important foods to help you fend off Alzheimer's and other dementias—thanks to their impressive concentration of polyphenols, all packaged in an irresistibly tasty fiber-rich matrix.

Shoot for eating one ½-cup (95 g) serving of berries every day. If that's not possible, try to get a minimum of two ½-cup servings of berries each week. For most people, it can be tricky to get enough berries without also eating too much sugar. That's because berries are often processed with added sugar and high-heat methods that compromise their beneficial nutrients. Enjoying berries at home doesn't have to mean turning them into a rich dessert. In fact, berries pair well with savory foods, too, like chicken, fish, and salads. And it doesn't mean only fresh berries will do. Think outside the typical bowl of blueberries to try different types of berries and alternatives to fresh, such as frozen, dried, or powdered.

CHOOSING THE BEST BERRIES

Let color be your guide—look for the most vibrant red, purple, blue, or black berries. The darker the berry, the more anthocyanins (see page 60), most of which reside in berry skin. That's why tiny berries with a greater ratio of skin to flesh, like currants and wild blueberries, are rich in antioxidant power, and why whole fruit retains more of these flavonoids than juiced or processed berries.

Plenty of the anthocyanin-rich berries are easy to find at your local grocery store—let's call these everyday berries. Of these, cranberries and blackberries provide the highest antioxidant bang for your buck, followed by raspberries, blueberries, pomegranates, strawberries, and grapes.

Beyond everyday berries, there's a whole world of anthocyanin-rich berry varieties to discover. Some of the harder-to-find berries, what I call the worth-seeking-out berries, boast even more concentrated anthocyanin levels. These include acai, bilberries, black raspberries, boysenberries, goji berries, elderberries, lingonberries, marionberries, mulberries, black and red currants, and white and golden raspberries.

Then there are wild berries, a source of regional pride wherever they grow: dewberries, huckleberries, thimbleberries, cloudberries, olallieberries, aronia berries (aka chokecherries), wild currants, and wild raspberries, to name a few. If you can get your hands on wild berries, they may be the most nutrient-dense fruits of all. Most supermarkets now stock frozen wild blueberries that have been cultivated. Wild blueberries provide 33 percent more anthocyanins than ordinary blueberries.

Not all berries are sweet. Savory berries like capers and caper berries add a vinegary punch to braises and stews. The spices you may not know are berries (allspice, juniper, pink peppercorns, and sumac) offer vibrant pops of flavors and color. All the savory berries are especially rich in flavonoids.

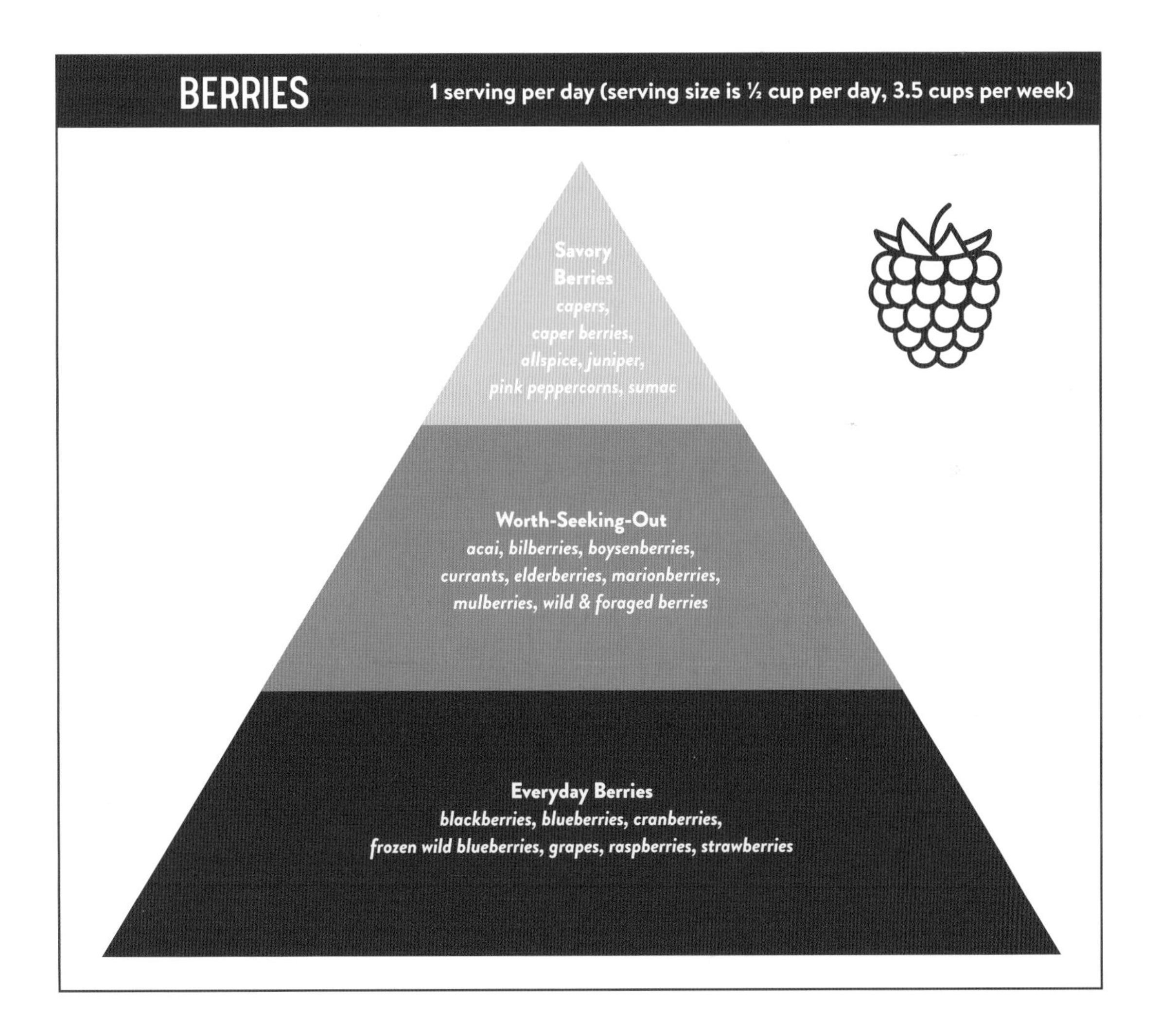

FRESH, FROZEN, AND DRIED

When berries are picked at peak ripeness, they have an alluring, rich hue and irresistible floral aroma. Berries like this don't need much in the way of cooking to make them better. Eat them as is, or if you want to get fancy, add a dollop of Almost Instant Cashew Cream (page 370).

Sometimes the best choice of berries, though, can be found in the frozen food section of the supermarket. When not in season, the "fresh" berries on display in the produce department have traveled halfway around the world, losing nutrient density and flavor as they accrue food miles. Frozen berries can be a higher-quality, more economical choice, with a texture that is well suited to baking. Frozen berries can really shine in many of the recipes in this chapter, especially Whole-Grain Blackberry and Blueberry Cornbread (page 68); as it bakes, the berries collapse into jammy pockets, for a moist cake-like cornbread that's sweet with little added sugar.

Dried berries are another great option to boost your berry intake year-round. These include dried blueberries, cranberries, bilberries, currants, and grapes (aka raisins!). Just be sure to read the nutrition labels of dried berries to avoid those processed with added sugar. Add dried blueberries to grain bowls, salads, breakfast porridges, and fruit crisps.

HOW TO CLEAN, STORE, AND PUT UP BERRIES FOR LATER

Your berries will last longer if they are spread out on a flat surface, such as a rimmed baking sheet or a plate lined with a clean kitchen towel. Store them spread out, barely touching, in the middle of the refrigerator (where they are less likely to freeze). Be sure to eat them as soon as possible. For longer storage, inspect your berries every day, tossing any that are soft, wrinkled, or have visible mold; one bad berry can ruin others touching it. Rinse berries right before eating by placing in a colander and running under cool water.

To freeze, place clean, dry berries in a single layer on a rimmed baking sheet lined with parchment paper; freeze until firm. Transfer to zip-top bags or food-grade containers. These berries will keep for at least six months in the freezer.

STRAWBERRY-AVOCADO SALAD WITH SALMON, BASIL, AND LIME

SERVES 4

¼ cup plus 2 teaspoons (70 ml) extra-virgin olive oil

Four 3- to 4-ounce (85 to 115 g) salmon fillets, about ¾ inch (2 cm) thick

¾ teaspoon kosher salt

1 grapefruit, preferably Ruby Red

2 tablespoons lime juice

1½ teaspoons raw honey

4 loosely packed cups (160 g) mixed baby greens

1 large ripe firm avocado, sliced (see Tip)

1 pound (455 g) strawberries, halved (about 2 cups)

½ cup (10 g) fresh basil leaves, large ones torn into pieces

Flaky salt

Freshly ground pink or black peppercorns

This dinner salad includes three brain-friendly food groups: berries, fish, and leafy greens. I created it to honor the legacy of Dr. Martha Clare Morris, lead researcher of the MIND diet study (see page 17) and author of more than 60 papers on nutrition and brain health. Her research showed that eating an additional ½-cup (95 g) serving of strawberries every week could dramatically reduce Alzheimer's risk.

Besides the strawberries, there's another berry here: pink peppercorns. The fruity flavor of pink peppercorns is a revelation if you've only used black pepper in your cooking. These spicy, dried berries are feisty and floral, adding a pretty finish to many dishes.

Cilantro and mint can be used instead of basil to finish the salad. Tender herbs like cilantro, basil, and mint are leafy greens that are dense with brain-healthy phytonutrients. If you have an abundance of fresh herbs on hand, use all three.

1. Preheat the oven to 350°F (180°C). Coat a ceramic dish or rimmed baking sheet with 1 teaspoon of the oil and place the salmon (skin side down if skin-on) on it. Drizzle the salmon with another teaspoon of the oil and sprinkle with ½ teaspoon of the kosher salt. Bake until the flesh easily flakes with a fork, about 12 minutes for medium-rare or 15 minutes for well done.

2. Meanwhile, zest the grapefruit to yield 1 tablespoon, then cut off the stem ends and use the knife to cut away the peel. Slice between the white pith and the flesh to remove the sections. Squeeze any juice left from the peels into a small measuring cup. Add any juice collected on your cutting board. Discard the peels.

continued

3. In a small bowl, whisk the remaining ¼ cup (60 ml) oil, 1½ tablespoons of the grapefruit juice, the reserved zest, the lime juice, honey, and the remaining ¼ teaspoon kosher salt.

4. Place the greens in a large shallow bowl. Drizzle half the dressing over the greens and toss well. Divide the salad between plates, then top with the avocado, grapefruit segments, and strawberries, dividing evenly. Top each serving with a piece of salmon. Drizzle with the remaining dressing.

5. Garnish each plate with basil leaves, a few pinches of flaky salt, and as much freshly ground pepper as you like.

TIP: *To get beautiful avocado slices, cut each avocado in half from top to bottom and remove the pit. Gently peel back the skin from the flesh and slice each half into six to eight lengthwise slices.*

SCIENCE BITE:

WHY BERRIES ARE AN IMPORTANT BRAIN FOOD

Berries are one of the plant world's best sources of an important brain-boosting flavonoid—anthocyanin. These plant compounds help scrub the brain of inflammatory debris right where your memory needs it the most, in the hippocampus, the brain's primary memory center. Anthocyanins also activate the brain's cleanup crew—groups of cells that work together to clear out plaques and debris, such as the amyloid protein seen in Alzheimer's. It's easy to tell which berries have the most: the darker the berry, the more anthocyanins they provide.

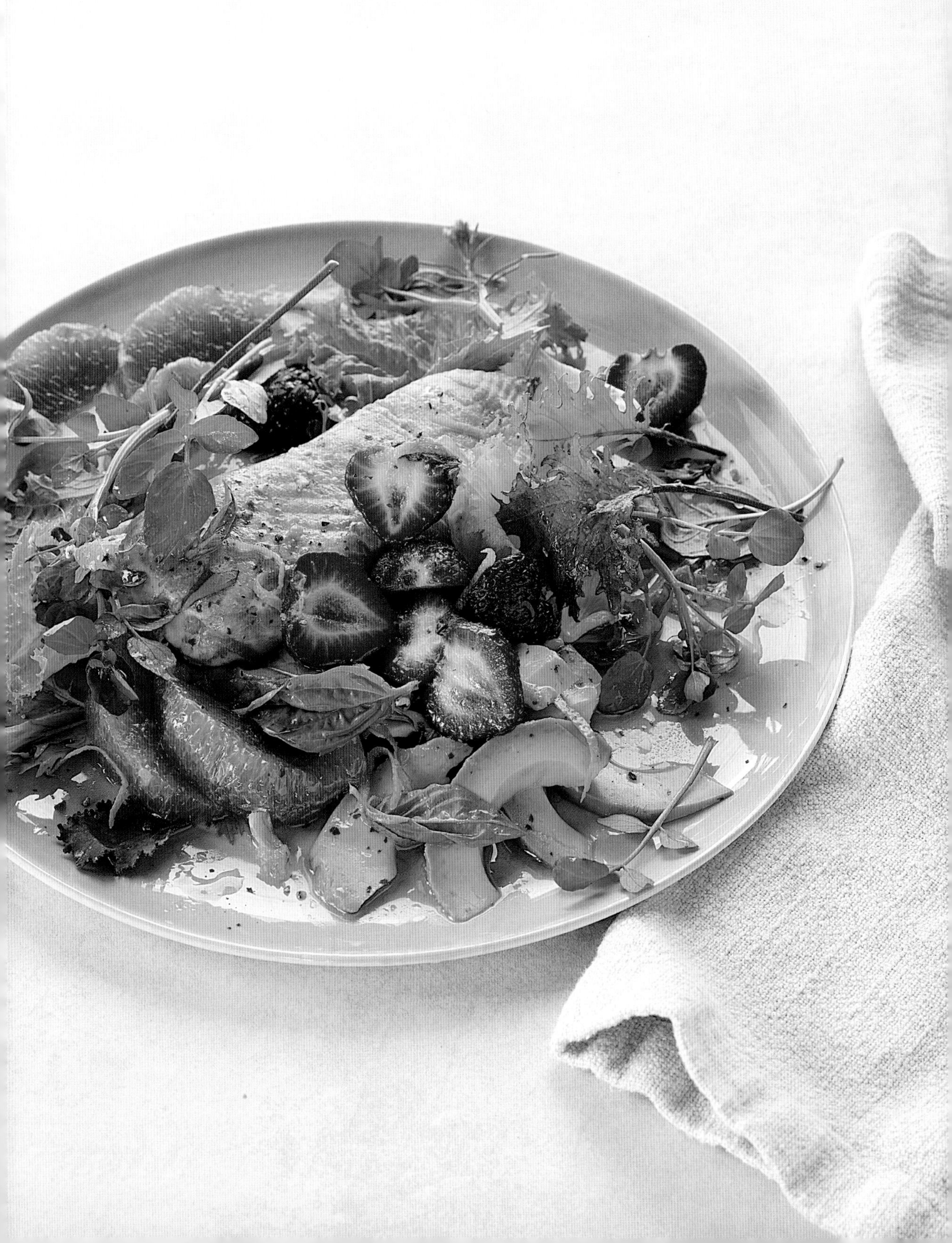

YOUR NEW FAVORITE KALE SALAD

SERVES 4 AS A SIDE

1 bunch lacinato kale (aka Tuscan or dinosaur kale) (6 ounces/170 g)

¼ to ½ cup (60 to 120 ml) Blueberry-Shallot Dressing (recipe follows)

1 large beet (10 ounces/285 g), scrubbed but not peeled, cut into thin rounds

2 tablespoons extra-virgin olive oil

½ teaspoon kosher salt

¼ teaspoon freshly ground black pepper, plus more for serving

1 medium carrot (4 ounces/115 g), scrubbed and shaved into ribbons with a vegetable peeler

½ cup (80 g) golden raisins

½ cup (75 g) toasted almonds, chopped

½ cup (95 g) fresh blueberries

Flaky salt (optional)

You'll avoid too-chewy kale by giving the leaves a short marinade in a warm blueberry dressing, which is a flavorful way to soften the leaves. The combination of raw carrot and beet contrasts the sweet pops of raisin and flecks of toasted almond, making this a crowd-pleasing refresh on the modern classic. Many of my kale-averse family members repeatedly devour this dish.

This is the perfect side salad for simply prepared salmon or shrimp. If you want to eat it as a main course, the recipe doubles easily.

1. Preheat the oven to 400°F (200°C).

2. Strip the kale leaves from the stems; save the stems for another use or compost. Cut the leaves into thin shreds and place in a large salad bowl. Pour ¼ cup (60 ml) of the dressing over the kale, toss well to coat, and let marinate at room temperature for at least 15 minutes and up to 2 hours.

3. Toss the beet rounds on a rimmed baking sheet with the oil, kosher salt, and pepper and separate so they don't touch. Roast for 12 to 14 minutes, until crispy and brown on the edges; set aside.

4. Add the beet, carrot, raisins, and almonds to the bowl of kale. Drizzle with up to ¼ cup (60 ml) dressing, if you like, and toss well. Divide between four plates and top each with the blueberries. Season to taste with flaky salt, if using, and more pepper.

BLUEBERRY-SHALLOT DRESSING

MAKES ½ CUP (120 ML)

¼ cup (60 ml) extra-virgin olive oil

1 medium shallot, (2½ ounces/70 g), finely chopped (about ¼ cup)

¼ teaspoon kosher salt

½ cup (95 g) fresh blueberries

1 tablespoon apple cider vinegar

1 teaspoon fresh tarragon leaves

¼ teaspoon freshly ground black pepper

Up to 1 tablespoon water (optional)

Heat 1 tablespoon of the oil in a small skillet over low heat. Add the shallot and salt and cook, stirring often, until soft and caramelized, 4 to 6 minutes. Add the blueberries and cook until soft, about 2 minutes. Pour the contents of the skillet into a blender with the vinegar, tarragon, pepper, and remaining 3 tablespoons oil. Blend on low speed at first (using a towel to cover the top), then process on high until smooth. Add water by the teaspoonful, if needed, for a pourable consistency.

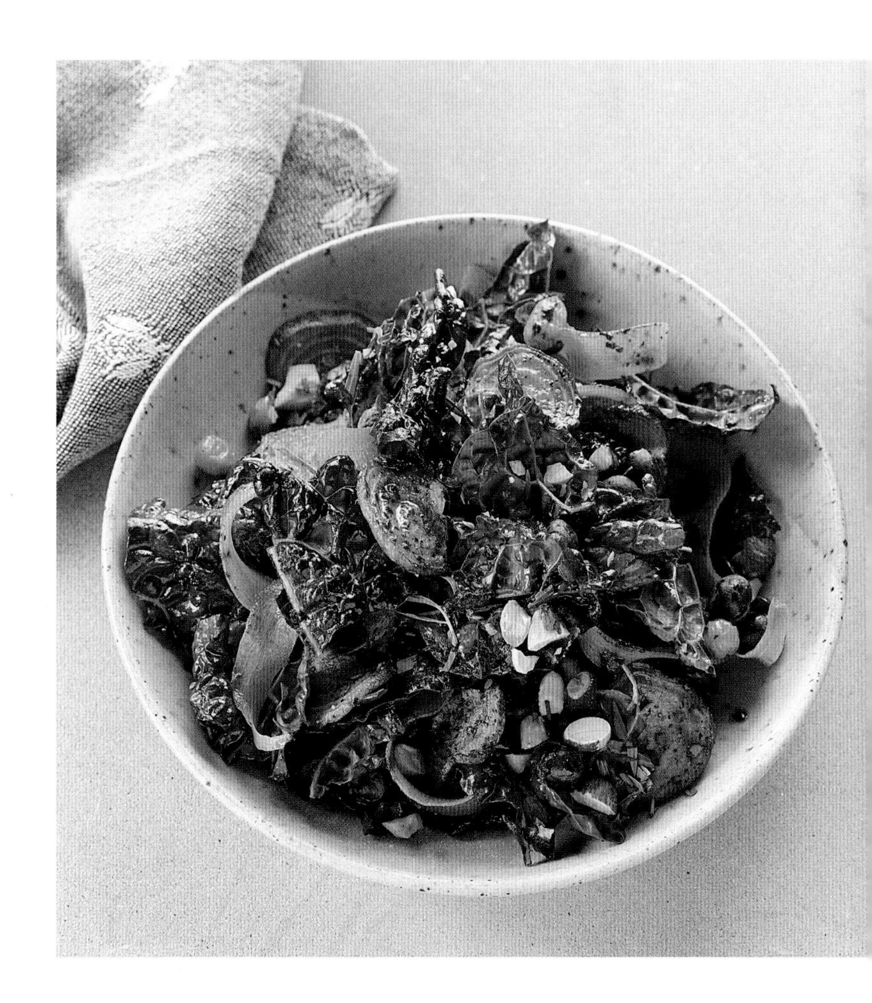

WINE-BRAISED CHICKEN WITH CURRANTS, CAPER BERRIES, AND CAULIFLOWER

SERVES 4 TO 6

½ cup (80 g) dried currants or golden raisins

1 cup (240 ml) boiling water

2 tablespoons extra-virgin olive oil

1 large shallot (5 ounces/ 140 g), thinly sliced (about ½ cup)

8 small boneless, skinless chicken thighs (2 pounds/ 910 g total)

1 teaspoon kosher salt

½ teaspoon freshly ground black pepper

1 cup (240 ml) dry white wine

1 medium head cauliflower (1½ pounds/680 g), cut into 2-inch (5 cm) florets (about 6 cups)

½ cup (60 g) caper berries or ¼ cup (30 g) capers, rinsed

¼ cup (60 ml) white wine vinegar

½ cup (65 g) roasted pistachios

1 loosely packed cup (30 g) fresh flat-leaf parsley leaves, finely chopped

Inspired by Sicilian agrodolce sauce (*agrodolce* means "sour-sweet" in Italian), the sour in this recipe comes from adding vinegar and capers, while fresh or dried berries add sweetness. Currants are traditional in agrodolce dishes, but you could also use raisins, dried blueberries, bilberries, or golden raisins to give the dish its "dolce" component.

Caper berries are the fruit of the caper plant, a shrub that grows wild in Sicily, covering the ancient buildings with vines that bear lavender flowers. Capers are the flower buds of the caper tree, picked just before they bloom. If you can't find caper berries, use a smaller amount of capers instead.

1. Place the currants in a small bowl and pour the boiling water over top. Let sit until soft, about 15 minutes.

2. Warm the oil over low heat in a large skillet with a tight-fitting lid or a Dutch oven. When the oil starts to shimmer, add the shallot and cook, stirring often, until starting to brown, about 5 minutes.

3. Season the chicken with ½ teaspoon of the salt and the pepper. Add the chicken to the shallots and cook over medium heat until the pieces can be easily released from the bottom of the pan, about 5 minutes. Turn the chicken over and add the wine, then the currants and their soaking water. Adjust the heat so the sauce gently bubbles at a low simmer. Add the cauliflower to the pot, and sprinkle with the remaining ½ teaspoon salt. Stir to coat, cover, and cook at a low simmer until you can insert the tip of a knife into the largest piece of cauliflower, 20 to 25 minutes.

4. Stir in the caper berries, vinegar, pistachios, and parsley. Divide between four shallow bowls and serve hot.

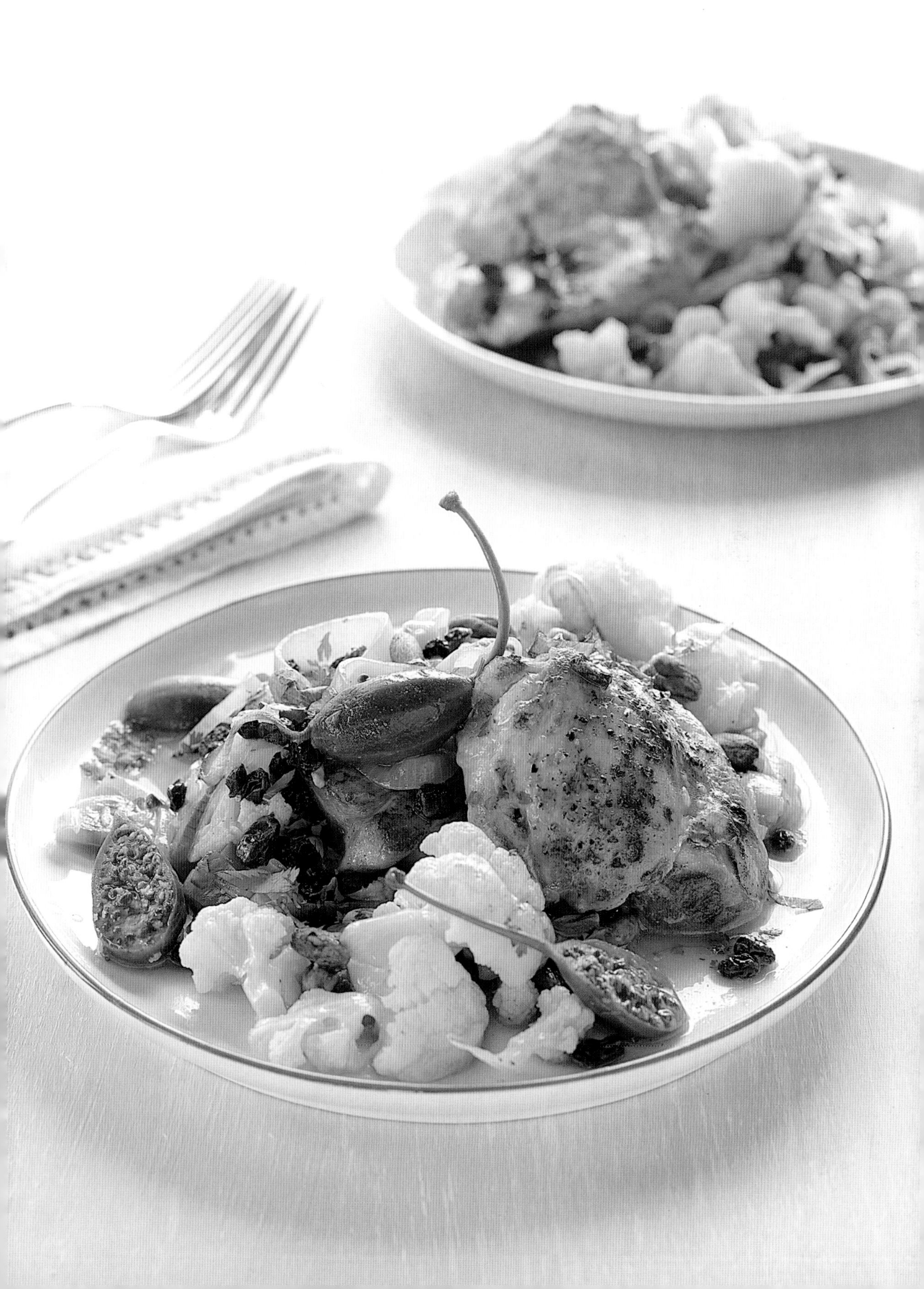

BAKED HALIBUT WITH GRAPES AND OLIVE OIL-SMASHED POTATOES

SERVES 4

1½ pounds (680 g) small potatoes, such as new potatoes or fingerlings

¼ cup (60 ml) extra-virgin olive oil

1½ teaspoons kosher salt

4 ounces (115 g) seedless red or black grapes, halved lengthwise (about 1½ cups)

2 tablespoons apple cider vinegar

½ teaspoon anise seeds or crushed fennel seeds

Four thin 4-ounce (115 g) halibut fillets, skin-on or skin-off

½ teaspoon freshly ground black pepper

1 tablespoon fresh thyme leaves

4 thyme sprigs

Grapes, a type of berry (really!), are famous for their resveratrol content, the same polyphenol found in red wine. In this dish, the grapes collapse into a syrupy sauce as they roast in the oven with apple cider vinegar. Paired with halibut, the sauce adds richness to an otherwise simple baked fish.

Look for different colors and varieties of small potatoes; the purple and red ones are especially rich in flavonoids. Potato skins are nutrient-dense, so small potatoes provide a better skin-to-flesh ratio. Roughly smashed with lots of olive oil (a fruity variety works well here), they turn this simple fish dish into a hearty meal.

1. Set an oven rack in the center position and preheat the oven to 400°F (200°C). Line a rimmed baking sheet with parchment paper.

2. Fit a steamer basket into a large pan with a tight lid and add 2 inches (5 cm) of water. Bring to a boil, add the potatoes, cover, and reduce to a gentle simmer. Cook until very tender, 18 to 24 minutes. Drain off the cooking liquid, if any, and return the potatoes to the pot. While hot, smash the potatoes with a potato masher or wooden spoon. Add 3 tablespoons of the oil and ½ teaspoon of the salt. Mix until the potatoes have a part-chunky, part-smooth consistency. Cover and keep warm on the stove.

3. Meanwhile, toss together the grapes, vinegar, anise seeds, oil, and ½ teaspoon of the salt on the prepared baking sheet. Roast for 18 to 20 minutes, until the grapes are soft and release their juice.

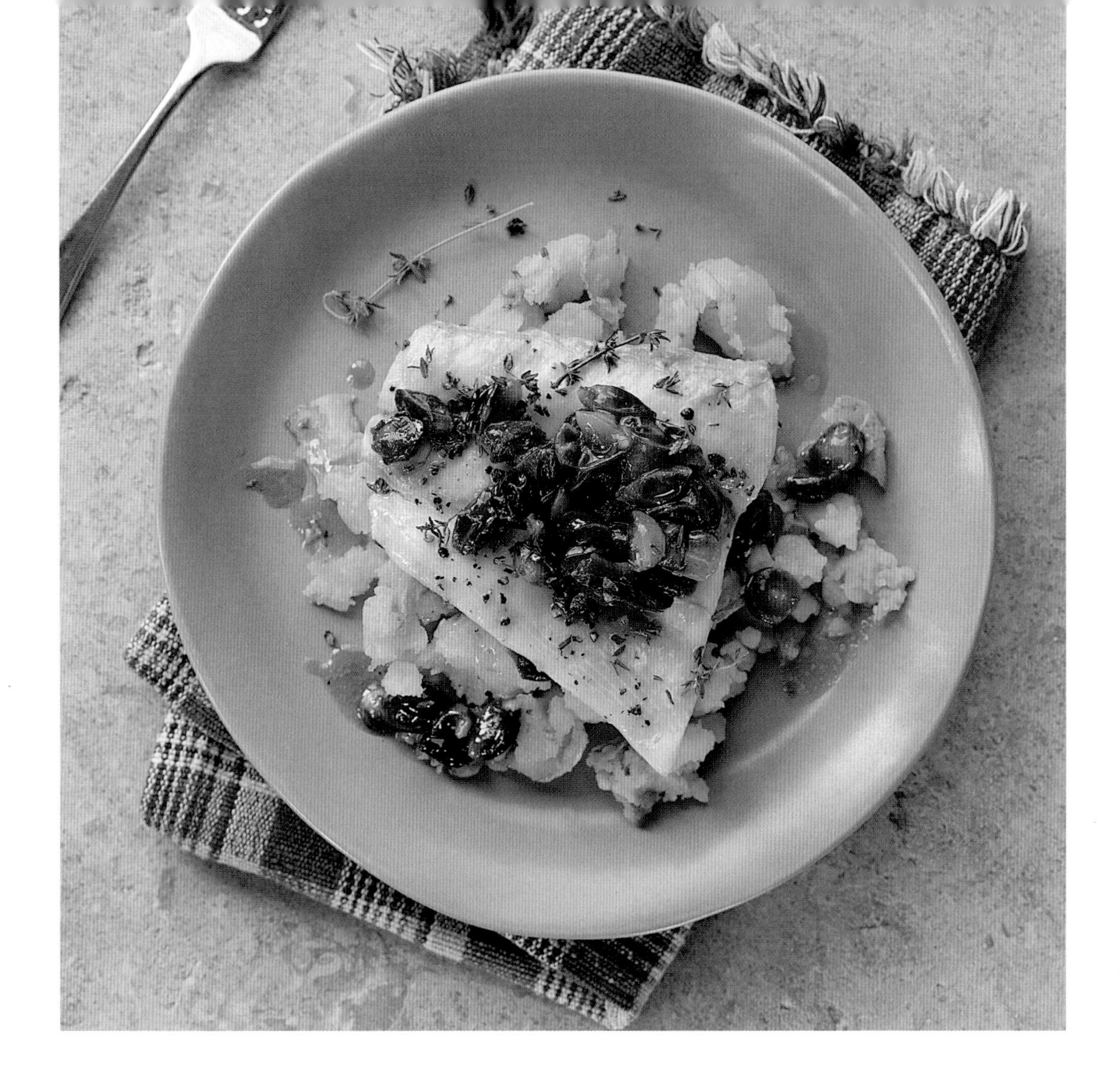

4. Season the fish with the pepper and the remaining ½ teaspoon salt. Remove the pan with the grapes from the oven and reduce the temperature to 350°F (180°C). Nestle the halibut in the sauce (place skin side down, if skin-on), and sprinkle with the thyme leaves. Return the pan to the oven and bake for 15 to 20 minutes, until the flesh is opaque throughout.

5. To serve, divide the smashed potatoes, halibut, and grapes with sauce between four shallow bowls. Garnish with the thyme sprigs and serve hot.

WHOLE-GRAIN BLACKBERRY AND BLUEBERRY CORNBREAD

MAKES ONE 8½-BY-4½-INCH (21 BY 11 CM) LOAF

- **¼ cup (60 ml) extra-virgin olive oil, plus more for the pan**
- **1 cup (140 g) stone-ground cornmeal (medium or finely ground)**
- **1 cup (120 g) almond flour**
- **1 cup (100 g) rolled oats**
- **¼ cup (30 g) flaxseed meal**
- **1 teaspoon baking powder**
- **1 teaspoon kosher salt**
- **½ teaspoon baking soda**
- **2 eggs, at room temperature**
- **1 cup (240 ml) plain, unsweetened whole-milk yogurt**
- **½ cup (120 ml) pure maple syrup**
- **1 tablespoon lemon zest**
- **1 teaspoon pure vanilla extract**
- **3 cups (570 g) blackberries or blueberries, or a mix of both, fresh or frozen (see Tip)**

This brain-healthy remix of cornbread is all about the berries, both swirled into the batter and piled on top, creating jammy pockets in every bite. But it's also about folding in more brain-friendly fats, fiber, and whole grains, with a fraction of the sugar found in typical cornbread. Instead of butter, extra-virgin olive oil creates a crispy crust and a savory, delicate crumb along with more monounsaturated fats.

Using stone-ground cornmeal will upgrade this cornbread in both fiber and nutrition. Machine-milled cornmeal strips the corn kernel of its hull and germ. That's where the brain-healthy vitamins reside, along with its corn-forward flavor and fiber. If a cornmeal product doesn't specify how it's ground, it is probably machine milled.

You can use stone-ground cornmeal that is medium or finely ground with slight differences in textures. For a more cake-like crumb, look for finely ground cornmeal, also sometimes called corn flour.

1. Preheat the oven to 375°F (190°C). Brush an 8½-by-4½-inch (21 by 11 cm) loaf pan with oil, line it with parchment paper so that the edges overhang, and brush the paper with more oil. Set aside.

2. Whisk together the cornmeal, almond flour, oats, flaxseed meal, baking powder, salt, and baking soda in a large bowl.

3. In a separate bowl, whisk the eggs, yogurt, maple syrup, olive oil, lemon zest, and vanilla until combined, then pour over the flour mixture. Fold with a flexible spatula until only a few streaks of dry ingredients remain. Gently fold in half the berries and scrape the mixture into the prepared pan. Top the loaf with the remaining berries.

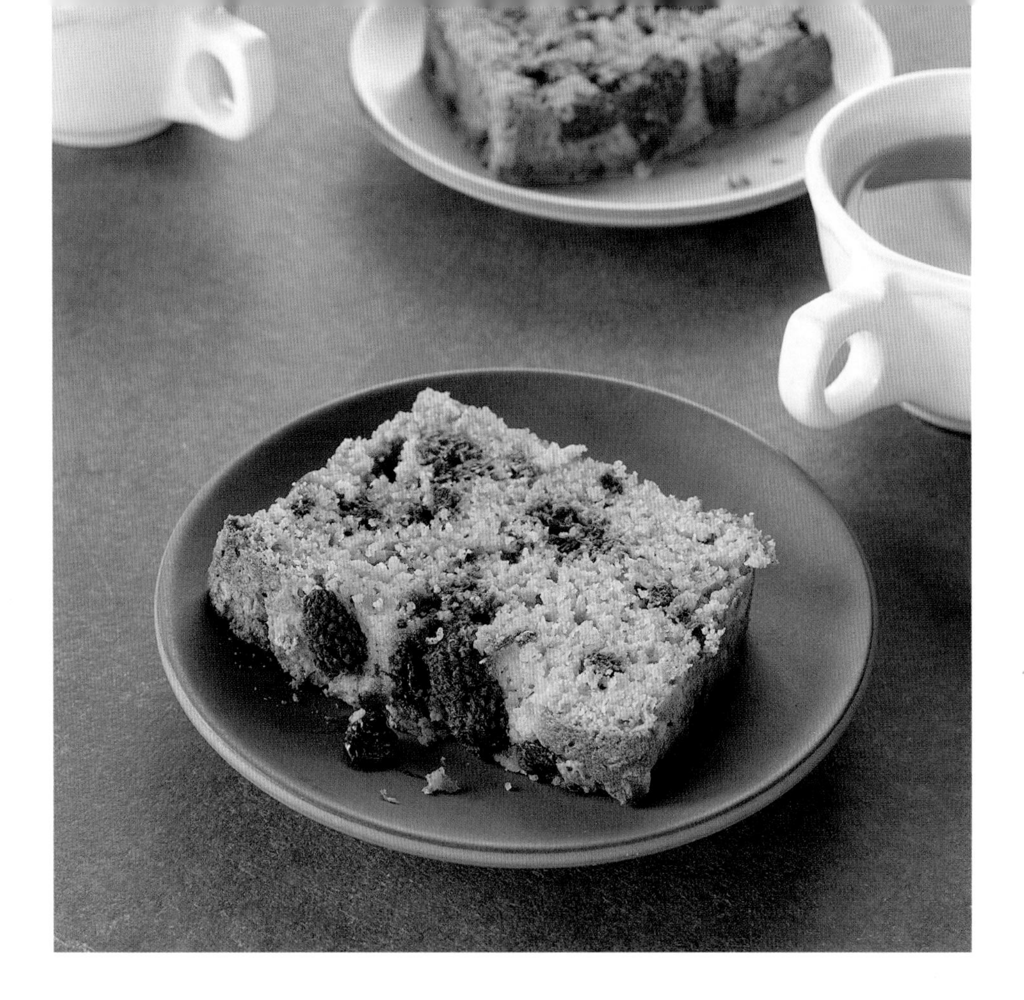

4. Bake for 1 hour 10 minutes to 1 hour 15 minutes, rotating the pan halfway through, until the edges are deeply browned and a knife inserted into the center comes out clean (see Tip). Cool completely, then pull the loaf out of the pan by grasping the parchment overhang on each side. Cut into slices and serve.

5. This cake is best the day it is baked. Because of the large number of berries, store it in the fridge in an airtight container for up to 5 days. The cake can be frozen for up to 6 months. Defrost and warm in the oven at 300°F (150°C) for 10 minutes before serving.

TIP: *If using frozen berries, or a combination of fresh and frozen, the loaf will take about 10 minutes longer to cook. Cover the pan with foil halfway through baking to keep the edges from burning.*

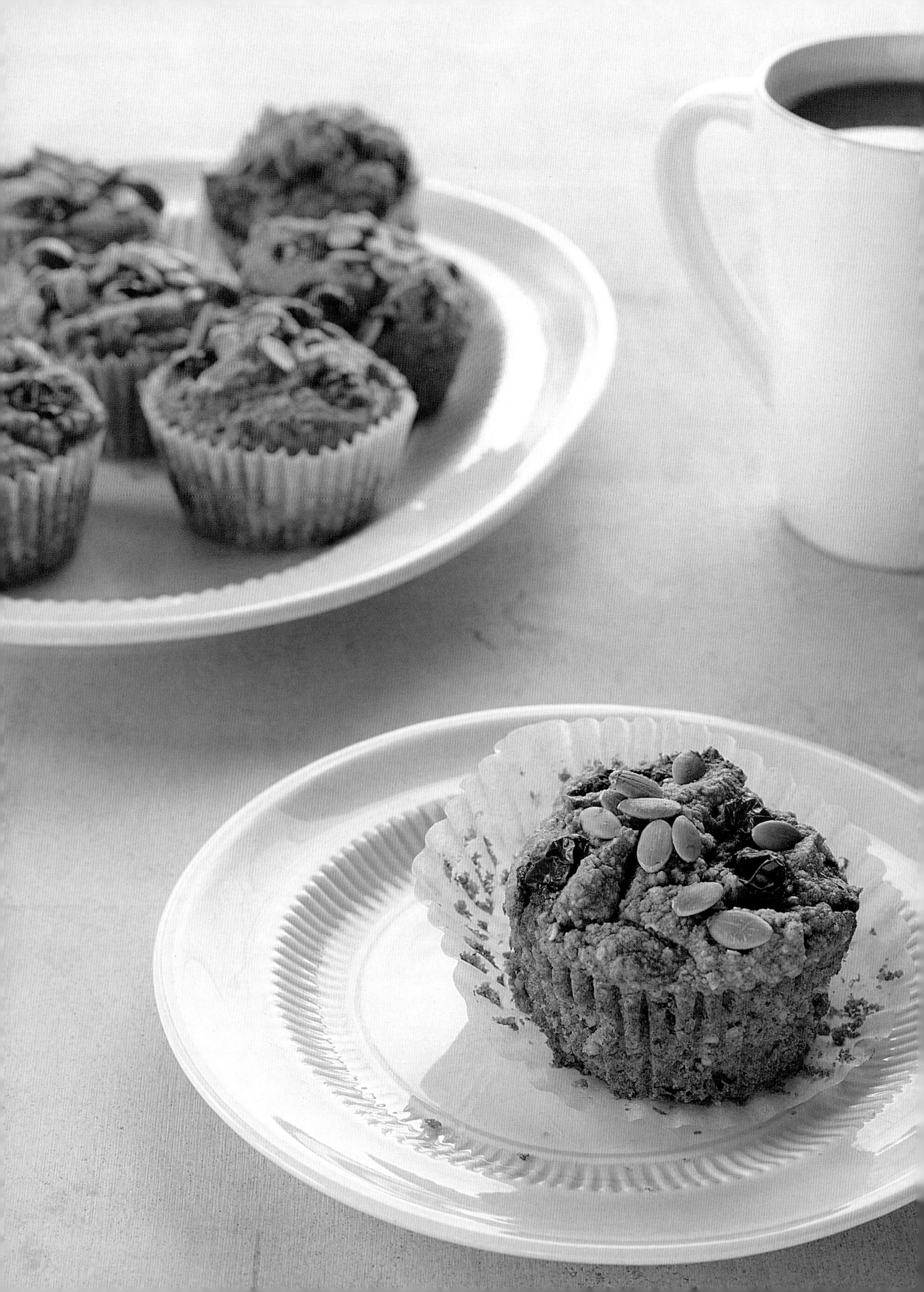

PUMPKIN-CRANBERRY MUFFINS

MAKES 12 MUFFINS

1 cup (115 g) oat flour
1 cup (115 g) almond flour
2 teaspoons baking powder
1 tablespoon ground flaxseed
1 teaspoon ground cinnamon
½ teaspoon kosher salt
1 cup (240 g) canned pumpkin puree
⅔ cup (115 g) coconut palm sugar
½ cup (120 ml) extra-virgin olive oil
1 teaspoon pure vanilla extract
1 teaspoon almond extract
2 eggs
2 cups (220 g) cranberries, fresh or frozen (don't defrost)
¼ cup (30 g) hulled pumpkin seeds (pepitas)

Pleasantly tart and packed with antioxidants, cranberries deserve to be a part of your brain-healthy dietary pattern year-round. It's best to enjoy them as a whole fruit rather than dried or juiced, since those processes add a lot of sugar. For this tender pumpkin muffin, you'll use whole fresh or frozen cranberries, which burst as they bake—adding pockets of jammy fruit. These muffins pack in a nice roster of brain-healthy ingredients, from the almond, oat, and flaxseed batter to the sprinkle of pumpkin seeds on top.

1. Preheat the oven to 350°F (180°C). Line a 12-cup muffin pan with paper liners.

2. Whisk together the oat flour, almond flour, baking powder, flaxseed, cinnamon, and salt in a large bowl.

3. In a separate large bowl, whisk together the pumpkin, sugar, oil, vanilla, and almond extract. Whisk in the eggs one at a time. Fold in the flour mixture until just combined.

4. Gently fold 1⅓ cups (145 g) of the cranberries into the muffin batter. Divide the batter evenly between the muffin cups. Divide the remaining ⅔ cup (75 g) cranberries over the tops of the muffins and gently press them into the batter. Sprinkle with the pumpkin seeds.

5. Bake for 38 to 45 minutes for standard muffins, or until a tester inserted into several muffins comes out clean.

6. These muffins are best the day they are made. Warm day-old muffins in the oven at 300°F (150°C) for 10 minutes. To freeze, wrap in plastic wrap and store in the freezer for up to 6 months.

TIPS: *Save the leftover pumpkin puree and add to oatmeal or a smoothie.*

These muffins work with blueberries (fresh or frozen) or dark chocolate chips instead of cranberries.

SMASHED RASPBERRY OVERNIGHT OATS

SERVES 2

- **1 cup (240 ml) unsweetened plant-based milk, homemade (page 363) or store-bought**
- **¾ cup (75 g) rolled oats**
- **2 tablespoons flaxseed meal**
- **1 teaspoon pure maple syrup (optional)**
- **¼ teaspoon kosher salt**
- **1 cup (180 g) fresh raspberries**
- **¼ cup (40 g) chopped pistachios**

Soaking oats overnight in milk is an easy, make-ahead method for a pudding-like oatmeal. The oats hold their shape as they soak, becoming toothsome yet soft and the base for any number of add-ins. Here you'll swirl in raspberries and flaxseed before topping with pistachios just before eating for a superstar combination of berries, seeds, and whole grains.

Other smashable berries, such as blackberries, would work well, as would mixing up the seeds (chia, hemp, poppy, or sesame) or sprinkling with other nuts (walnuts, pecans, or almonds).

1. Combine the milk, oats, flaxseed, maple syrup (if using), and salt in a medium bowl. Fold ⅔ cup (120 g) of the raspberries into the oat mixture. Using a fork, smash the berries against the side of the bowl and stir into the oats to create swirls.

2. Divide the oat mixture between two 1-cup (240 ml) glass jars, cover tightly, and store in the refrigerator for at least 6 hours and up to overnight.

3. To serve, top with the remaining ⅓ cup berries, dividing evenly, and sprinkle with the pistachios.

4. To store, keep in the refrigerator, tightly covered, for up to 3 days.

TIP: *Use rolled oats (aka old-fashioned oats), not instant or steel-cut ones.*

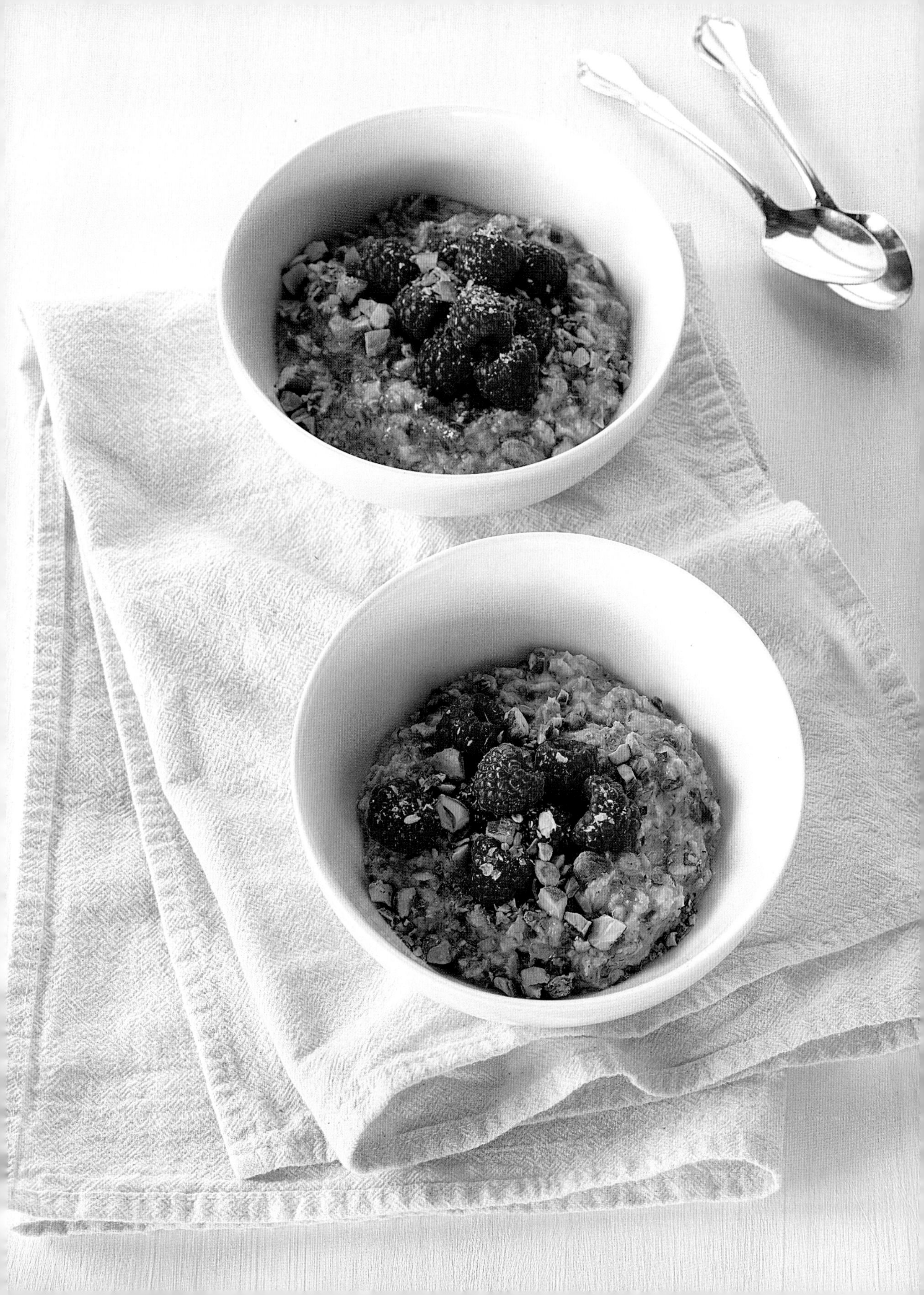

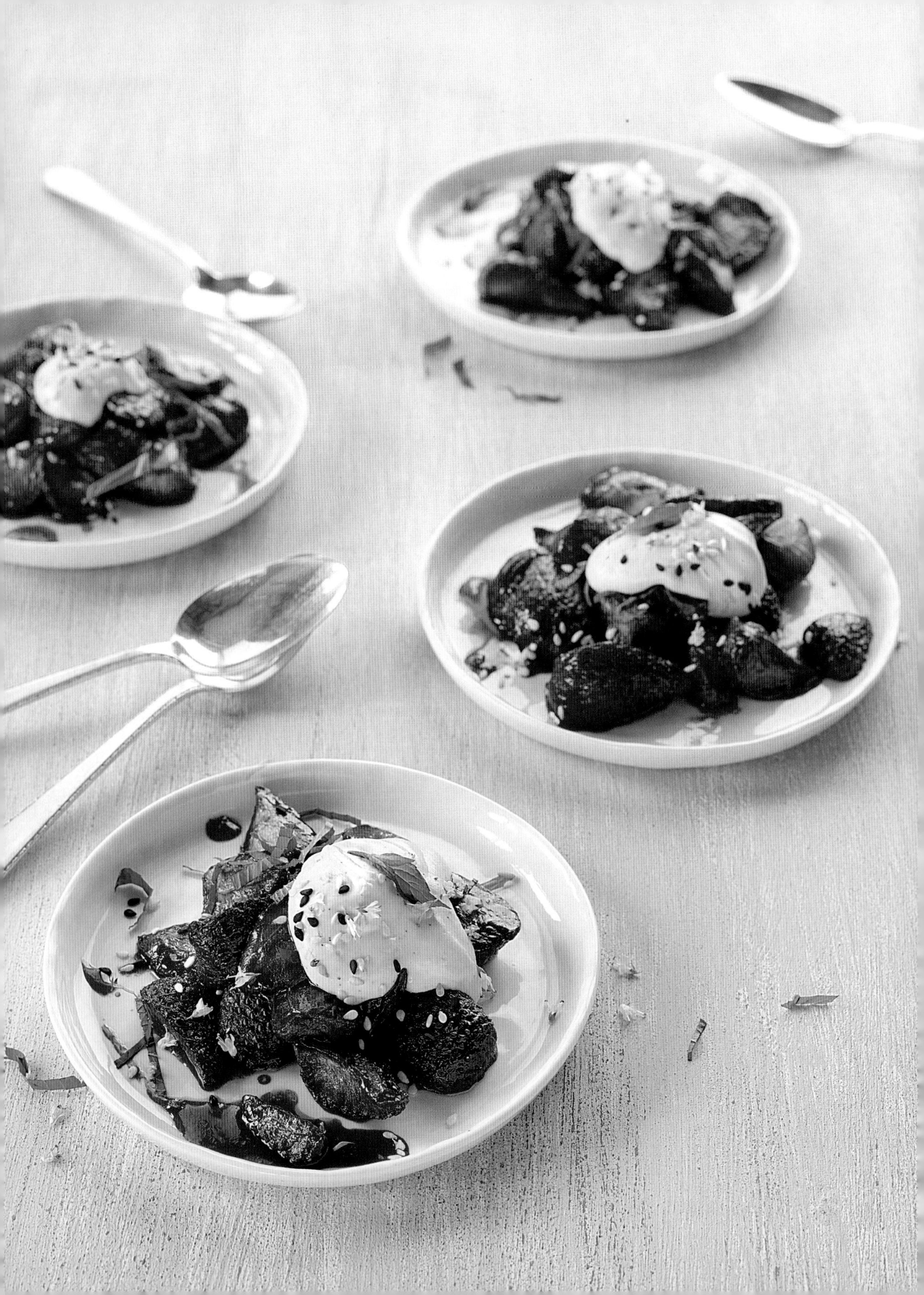

ROASTED STRAWBERRIES WITH ALMOST INSTANT CASHEW CREAM

SERVES 4 TO 6

- **2 pounds (910 g) strawberries, quartered (about 4½ cups)**
- **1 tablespoon extra-virgin olive oil**
- **1 tablespoon balsamic vinegar**
- **½ teaspoon kosher salt**
- **2 teaspoons pure maple syrup**
- **1¼ cups (300 ml) Almost Instant Cashew Cream (page 370)**
- **½ vanilla bean, split and scraped, or 1 teaspoon pure vanilla extract**
- **2 tablespoons unhulled sesame seeds, black, white, or a mix**
- **1 heaping tablespoon slivered fresh mint leaves, plus any flowers from the plant (optional)**

While peak-of-summer strawberries are best simply eaten out of hand, this recipe makes good use of fresh strawberries wherever you can buy them—at the farm stand, your grocery store, or larger big-box stores. Roasting strawberries concentrates their flavor—going from raw to jammy and complex. Paired with vanilla-flecked cashew cream, the strawberries become a fancy dessert thanks to the contrast of sticky fruit with rich cream.

1. Preheat the oven to 350°F (180°C). Line a rimmed baking sheet with parchment paper.

2. Toss the strawberries, oil, vinegar, salt, and 1 teaspoon of the maple syrup in a large bowl. Transfer to the prepared baking sheet and spread in a single layer. Roast for 35 to 40 minutes, until the juices are syrupy and run only slightly when the pan is tilted. While still warm, scrape the roasted strawberries and their juices into a bowl.

3. Meanwhile, stir together the cashew cream, vanilla bean seeds, and the remaining 1 teaspoon maple syrup.

4. To serve, divide the strawberries and cashew cream between shallow bowls. Top with the sesame seeds and mint.

TIP: *The tiny white flowers of a mint plant are not only edible, they are delicious. Use them to garnish the finished dish, if you like.*

QUICK BERRY AND CHIA SEED JAM

MAKES 1¼ TO 1½ CUPS (300 TO 360 ML)

- **3 cups (570 g) fresh or frozen huckleberries, wild blueberries, regular blueberries, blackberries, or a mix**
- **1 tablespoon lemon zest (from 1 large lemon)**
- **¼ cup (60 ml) fresh lemon juice**
- **3 tablespoons pure maple syrup**
- **¼ cup (45 g) chia seeds**

In August, the foothills of the Teton mountains near where I live are thick with huckleberry bushes. The pretty, deep purple berries, a wild cousin of the blueberry, hang in clusters hidden beneath the leaves of waist-high bushes. Huckleberries' thin skin pops pleasantly in your mouth, releasing the tiny seeds encased in their flesh. Wild berries are especially rich in brain-healthy flavonoid compounds—with up to three times more anthocyanins than cultivated blueberries. When I have a glut, I make this quick jam, accented with lemon and a touch of maple syrup.

Making homemade jam means you get the most out of your berries. The high-heat method used to make processed jams inactivates the beneficial antioxidant and polyphenol compounds. Plus, industrially produced jams tend to be low in fiber and high in sugar. This stovetop jam method cooks the berries gently to retain their brain-boosting compounds, fiber, and natural sweetness. The chia seeds give a tapioca-like consistency to the berries while providing omega-3 fatty acids.

1. Combine the berries, lemon zest, lemon juice, and maple syrup in a medium saucepan. Bring to a boil, then reduce the heat to a lively simmer. Cook, stirring occasionally, until reduced by about half and the jam coats the back of a spoon, 12 to 16 minutes for fresh berries and 22 to 26 minutes for frozen ones.

2. Add the chia seeds and cook until the seeds become gelatinous, about 1 minute. Some berries will remain whole after cooking. Remove the jam from the heat and let cool completely. It will thicken as it cools, but you can enjoy it right away as a topping for pancakes, waffles, or toast.

3. To store, transfer to an airtight container and refrigerate for up to 2 weeks or freeze for up to 3 months.

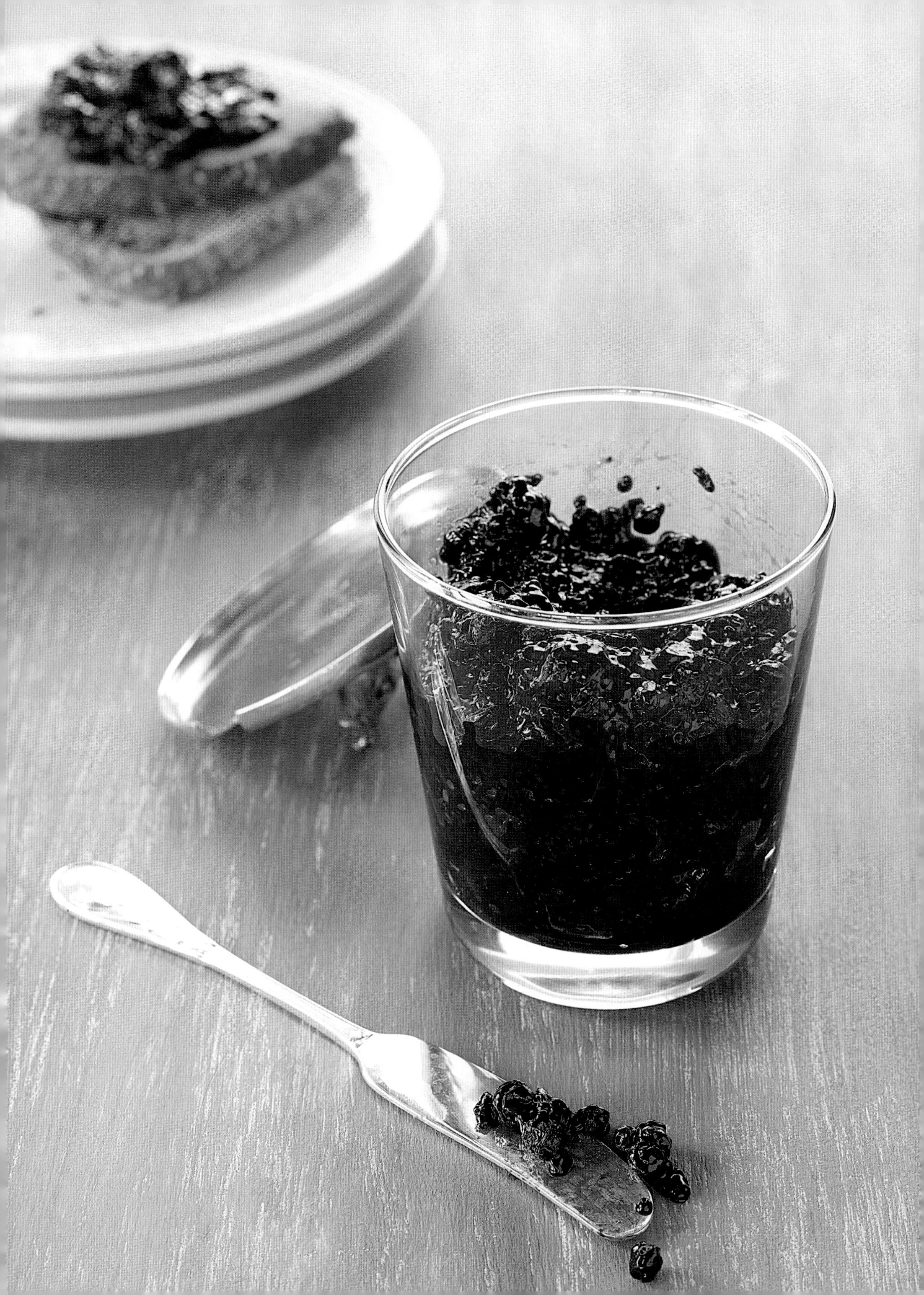

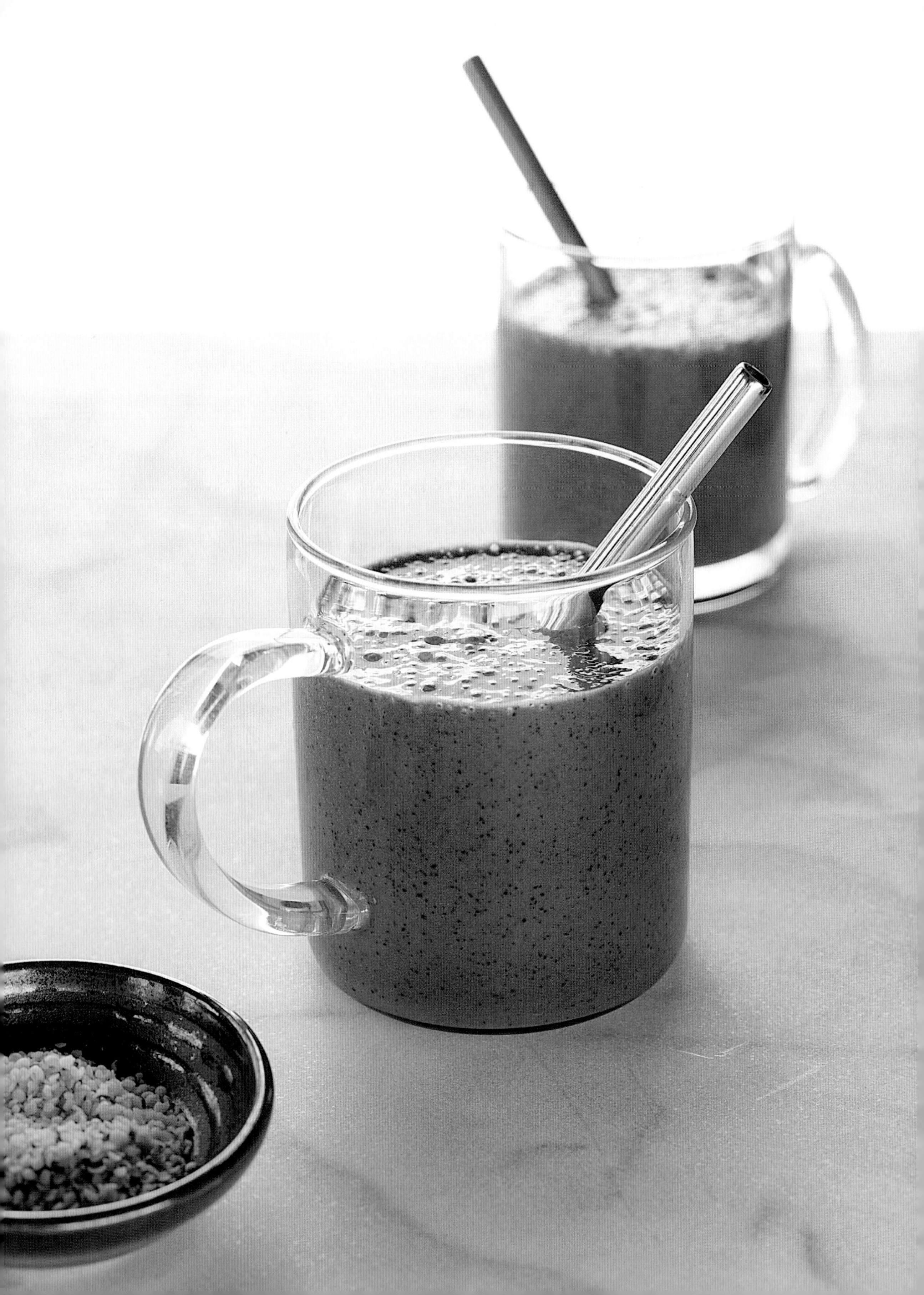

COFFEE BERRY SMOOTHIE

SERVES 2

2 frozen bananas (about 10 ounces/285 g total), broken into pieces

1 cup (190 g) frozen blueberries, blackberries, black raspberries, or a mix

¼ cup (35 g) hemp seeds, plus more for serving

1 cup (240 ml) Basic Nut Milk (page 363) or store-bought nut milk

1 cup (240 ml) freshly brewed coffee, at room temperature or chilled

Coffee and berry flavors work surprisingly well together in this bracing, not-too-sweet smoothie. Some high-quality coffees have fruit-forward flavors. Ethiopian coffee, for example, smells like blueberries! That's because coffee beans are technically a fruit. The beans are actually the pit of a cherry-like fruit now being studied for memory-enhancing properties.

Besides giving you a double dose of berry flavors, there's an abundance of polyphenols from the coffee and the berries, making this a smoothie that quells inflammation and combats oxidative stress in the brain. Hemp seeds blend up creamy and add omega-3 fatty acids and protein.

In the following order, layer the bananas, blueberries, hemp seeds, milk, and coffee in a blender, then blend on high speed until smooth, about 1 minute. Divide between two glasses and top with more hemp seeds, if you like.

TIPS: *To store bananas in the freezer for making smoothies, peel and cut into four pieces each. Store in a zip-top bag or other airtight container for up to 6 months.*

For a thicker smoothie, use ice-cold coffee; for a thinner one, use room-temperature coffee.

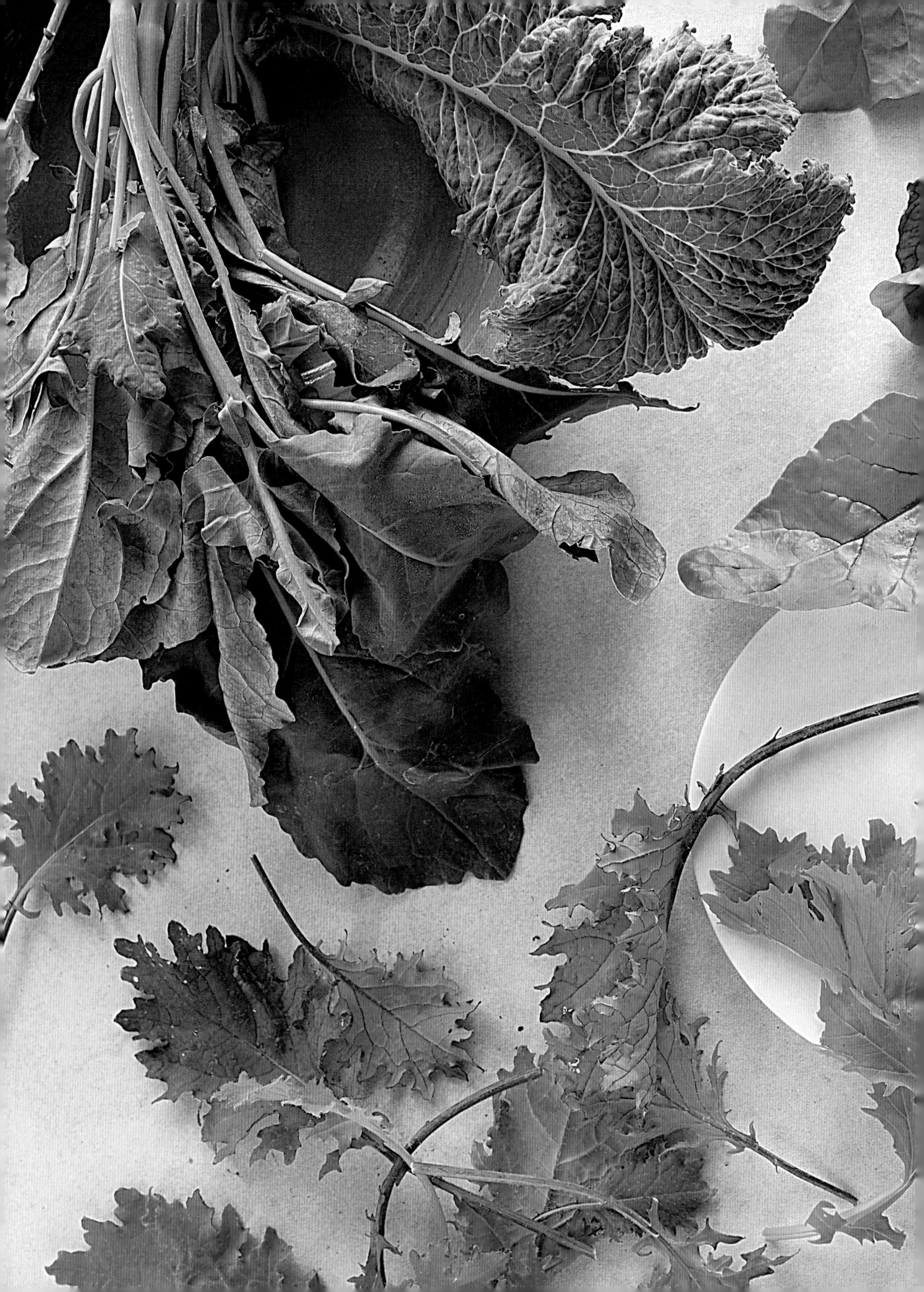

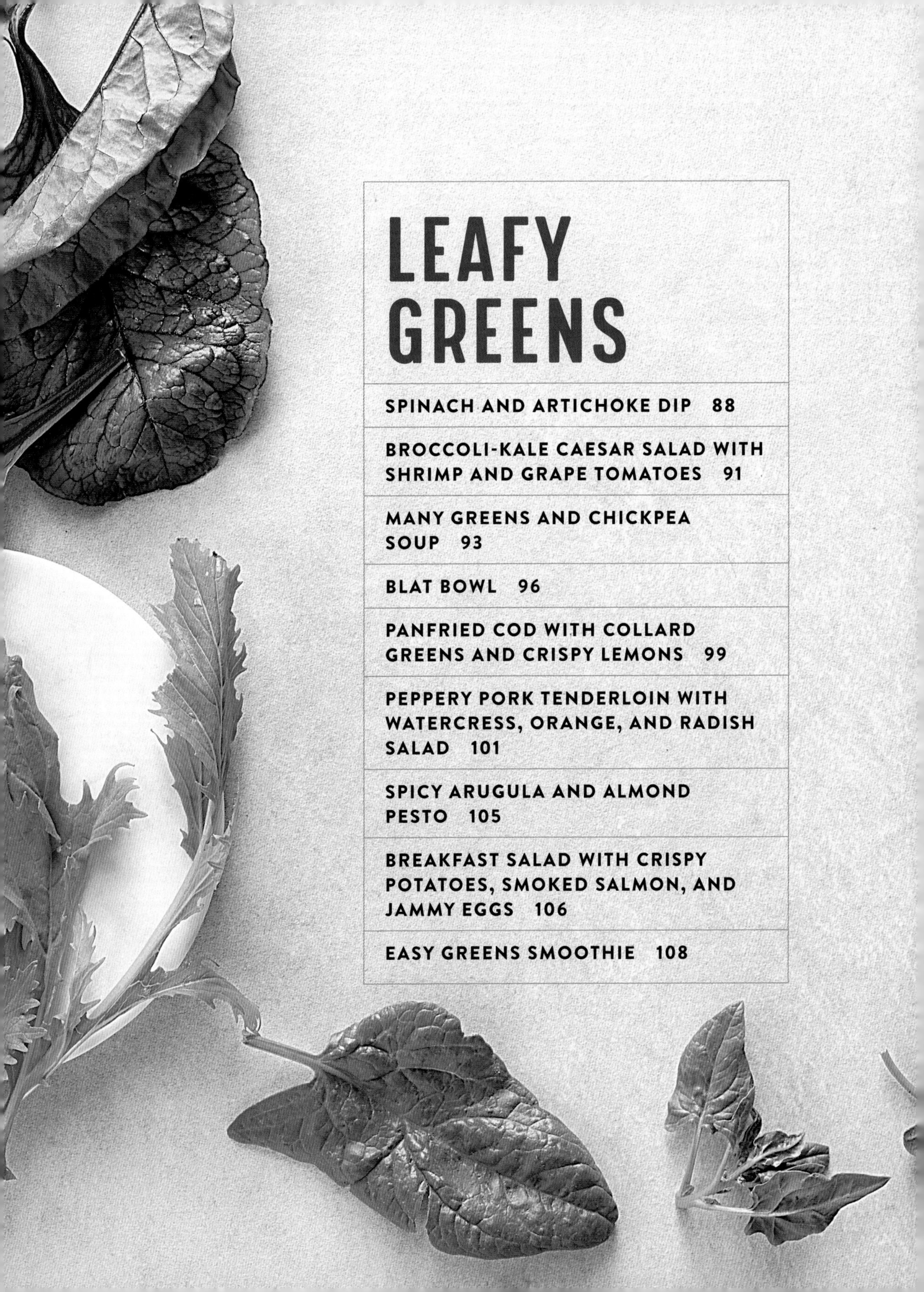

LEAFY GREENS

There's no magic bullet to prevent dementia or Alzheimer's, but please eat more leafy greens. In fact, just one handful of leafy green vegetables every day—cooked or raw—has a powerful impact on your brain.

"Leafy greens" means tender greens like butter lettuce and romaine; hearty greens like kale and collards; fresh herbs like parsley, cilantro, and basil; as well as vegetables like cabbage, beet greens, and carrot tops. It's not just about eating these daily: it's also important to eat a wide variety of leafy greens, from the tender pale lettuces to the sturdy darkest greens.

Be leafy-green curious and try something new at the grocery store or farmers' market—perhaps a bundle of spicy mustard greens, pointy dandelion leaves, or a bag of mizuna (a lacy, peppery lettuce). This might even mean plucking any greens from a stalk of broccoli and including them in your cooking (they are delicious).

Tender greens include mesclun, leaf lettuce, head lettuce, arugula, watercress, and baby versions of spinach and kale. They are what comes to mind when you think "salad." Your salads will be more interesting if you mix up a bunch of different varieties of tender greens and throw in some sturdy greens, too. Mix up the baby lettuces (red romaine, butter, and Bibb) in the Breakfast Salad with Crispy Potatoes, Smoked Salmon, and Jammy Eggs on page 106. (Yes, breakfast is a great time to get in your greens!)

Sturdy greens include kale, collards, Swiss chard, spinach, and chicories like Belgian endive, curly endive aka frisée, radicchio, and escarole. Many of these can be used interchangeably in the recipes. Try swapping in chard for the collard greens in the panfried cod (page 99), baby kale for the spinach in the Spinach and Artichoke Dip (page 88), or watercress for arugula in the BLAT Bowl (page 96). Above all, use what you have or what looks best at the grocery store or farmers' market.

When you find root vegetables that still have their green tops, buy them! This is like getting two vegetables for the price of one. The dark leafy greens of carrots, beets, turnips, and radishes have big, earthy flavors and a high nutrient density. So are the tender stalks and leaves that sprout atop celery root and fennel. In this chapter and throughout the book, fold these bonus stems, stalks, and leaves into your cooking.

Think of tender-stemmed herbs as adding another layer of flavor, color, and antioxidants to your meals. The recipes in this chapter use herbs liberally, both to finish a dish and as the star ingredient. Be sure to include the tender stems of cilantro, dill, and parsley in your meals, too. Not only do they add flavor and nutrient density, they make prep easier.

Microgreens are tiny, edible greens grown from the seeds of vegetables and herbs. They are usually under 3 inches (7.5 cm) long and come in a rainbow of colors. Adding microgreens to a dish is an easy way to punch up flavor and boost nutrient density. In fact, one study measured the lutein, vitamin E, and vitamin C content of microgreens and found that, when compared to their mature vegetable counterpart, they were up to forty times more potent in these nutrients. Add these nutrient-dense sprouts to any dish that could use a splash of color and fresh, crunchy greens. They are particularly good atop the Tuna Burgers with Wasabi Mayo (page 167).

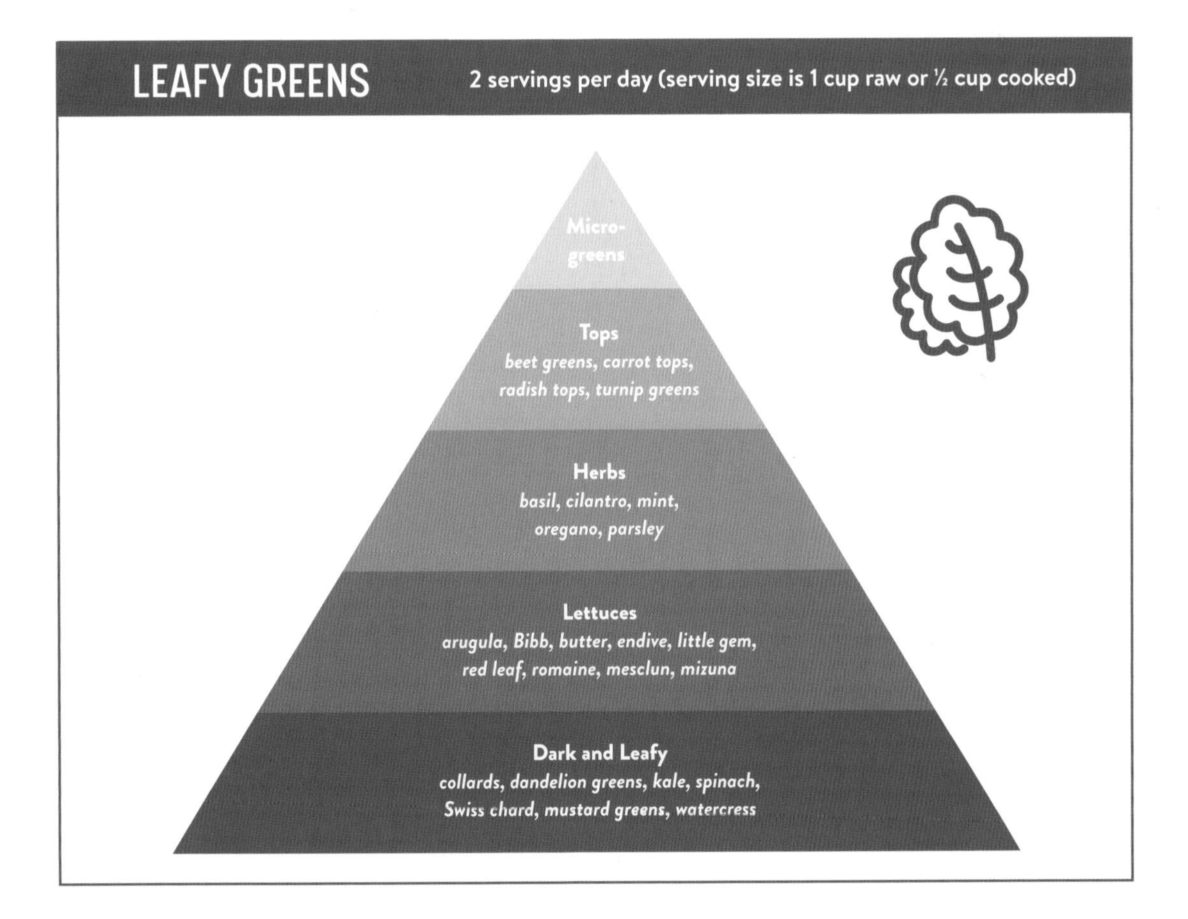

GETTING ENOUGH LEAFY GREENS

Shoot for at least 2 heaping cups (80 g) of raw greens or 1 cup (about 200 g) of cooked ones per day and a variety of greens throughout the week. It's also key to combine leafy greens with the types of foods that enhance their bioavailability—that is, the body's ability to absorb and put their nutrients to work.

The recipes in this chapter are designed to do just that. While you may be accustomed to getting your leafy greens in the form of a salad, this chapter encourages you to start tucking greens into everything from appetizers to soups and even smoothies. Of course, salads are great, and I have two in this chapter that will help you think about them in new ways. Also peppered

EASY WAYS TO EAT YOUR LEAFY GREENS EACH DAY

There are so many easy ways to get leafy green vegetables into your day-to-day diet, and the recipes in this chapter barely scratch the surface. Here are twelve other ways to incorporate these brain health superstars into every meal:

1. Finish a pasta dish with chopped fresh arugula.
2. Add a handful of frozen kale to your fruit smoothie.
3. Make an easy green tahini sauce by blending a handful of flat-leaf (aka Italian) parsley with tahini, lemon juice, and salt.
4. Cook down heaps of chopped kale in a skillet with some water and poach eggs right in the kale.
5. Freeze pesto in ice cube trays and pop out a bright green cube to add to soups and stews.
6. Toss kale and Brussels sprouts leaves with olive oil, paprika, and salt and bake until crispy at 350°F (180°C) to make chips.
7. Create a spicy dipping sauce by pureeing a bunch of fresh herbs with lemon juice, garlic, chiles, and a splash of vinegar.
8. Make fresh spring rolls from tender greens and herbs like mint, basil, and cilantro rolled up along with shrimp, tofu, and avocado.
9. Tuck baby kale or spinach into a sandwich for a nutrient-dense upgrade from iceberg lettuce.
10. Make a green hummus by pureeing spinach, kale, watercress leaves, or arugula along with chickpeas and tahini.
11. Use endive leaves instead of chips for scooping up a dip.
12. Make lettuce wraps by swapping out the sandwich bread and wrap your lunch fixings in butter lettuce cups.

throughout this chapter and the rest of the book are dozens of ideas about how to dress your salads, like the better-for-you take on ranch dressing (using hemp seeds) on page 101.

CHOOSING THE BEST GREENS

Look for bright green, full leaves with no hint of yellow—the latter a sign of poor storage and/or age. Boxes of prewashed greens are undeniably convenient. (Be sure to shake the box before buying to make sure none of the greens are going bad.) But often the best tender greens come in bundles from the grocery store or farmers' market. If you find whole heads of lettuce with their roots and a clod of dirt still attached, like butter lettuce or watercress, they are bound to stay fresh longer.

It's also good to have a stash of frozen greens in your freezer. You can freeze them yourself (see page 87) or purchase kale or spinach in blocks or loose in bags. It's wonderfully convenient to be able to reach for a handful of kale or spinach to add to soups and stews. Not only do they cut down on prep time, but frozen greens also retain nearly all of their beneficial nutrients and, in some cases, may be higher quality than fresh greens.

ORGANIC OR NOT?

Lettuce is one of the most likely vegetables to retain pesticide contamination. If buying conventionally grown lettuces (romaine, red leaf, green leaf), be sure to soak them thoroughly in cold water, which can wash off bacteria from the soil, reduce pesticide residue, and even revive wilted leaves. Don't be concerned by little holes in your organic produce. While these "organic wounds" are a sign that an insect chomped through the leaf, this natural stress may encourage the entire plant to amp up its antioxidant production.

The bottom line: The benefit of boosting your diet with leafy greens far outweighs the potential harm from conventional produce. So if organic greens are too expensive or aren't as high quality as the conventional ones, go for the best greens you can find, organic or not, and wash well.

SCIENCE BITE:

THE POWER OF VITAMIN K

The darker the green—think spinach, kale, arugula, collards, and beet greens—the higher the concentration of vitamin K. Also known as phylloquinone, vitamin K is actually a family of bioactive substances that help maintain strong bones and healthy blood clotting and, research now shows, build resilient brain cell membranes. That may explain why patients with early-stage Alzheimer's have been found to have a much lower dietary intake of vitamin K than cognitively healthy, age-matched adults.

As you get older, your body absorbs less of this fat-soluble vitamin. That's why cooking dark leafy greens with a fat-rich food, like nuts or ricotta, is not only a great food pairing, it helps you absorb more vitamin K, too.

HOW TO CLEAN AND STORE LEAFY GREENS

It takes just a few extra minutes to store your greens properly, ideally as soon as you bring them home. This will pay off later as your greens will stay vibrant and fresh longer, and they'll be partially prepped for a head start on making meals.

To keep tender lettuces, such as mesclun and baby kale, fresh for days, they need to be clean, dry, and surrounded by air. Wash them when you get home from the store by soaking them in cold water, letting the grit fall to the bottom of the bowl. Use a salad spinner to spin them dry and/or pat them dry with clean kitchen towels. Store in the refrigerator right in the salad spinner or wrapped in a folded paper towel and packed loosely into a plastic bag; leave the bag open so some air gets in. Place on the middle shelf of your refrigerator where there's more air circulation, not in the back where it's colder and they could freeze. Your lettuce will stay ready to go for up to five days.

If your lettuces come from the store clean and dry, you can give them a soak and a spin just before using. Farmers' market greens are sometimes already cleaned and dried for you. For boxed greens that have already been washed (or "triple-washed," as some say), store them in their box and wash just before using.

Sturdy greens, such as Swiss chard and collards, last longer if they are kept cold and dry. After you bring them home, release bunches from their rubber bands and ties. Make sure they are dry, then wrap in clean kitchen towels and place in the coldest part of the refrigerator, usually the bottom back shelf. Wash just before use.

You can also freeze sturdy greens for later. Separate the stems from the leaves and reserve the stems for another use. Wash, dry, and coarsely chop. If you don't mind having the greens frozen in one block, pack them tightly into freezer bags or food-safe containers. If you want to be able to grab a handful of greens at a time, for adding to smoothies or chopping later, freeze the leaves individually by spreading them out on baking sheets, then pack into containers.

Separate root vegetables (carrots, beets, radishes, turnips) from their greens as soon as you bring them home. Otherwise, the leaves wilt as the roots continue to draw from their moisture. Plan on using your carrot tops within a few days (make pesto!), and wash and dry the dark leafy greens to add to your stash of lettuces.

Store tender-stemmed herbs—cilantro, parsley, basil—as you would flowers: stems immersed in water, leaves upright in a glass. Store in the refrigerator unless you find a bundle with roots still attached (usually basil); store those in a cool place on the kitchen counter. Refresh the water every few days and they should last for about a week. If you find yourself with an abundance of tender herbs, make pesto (page 105). It freezes beautifully and will brighten up many meals when the weather turns cold.

SPINACH AND ARTICHOKE DIP

SERVES 6 TO 8 AS AN APPETIZER

- **1 tablespoon extra-virgin olive oil, plus more for the baking dish**
- **1 cup (140 g) raw cashews, soaked with water to cover for at least 2 hours and up to overnight**
- **½ cup (120 ml) water**
- **1 large garlic clove, chopped (about 1 teaspoon)**
- **4 cups (535 g) quartered artichoke hearts (from two 14-ounce/400 g cans, or frozen and thawed)**
- **½ cup (120 ml) dry white wine**
- **1 teaspoon kosher salt**
- **3 packed cups (150 g) baby spinach**
- **2 tablespoons fresh lemon juice**
- **⅓ cup (1 ounce/30 g) grated Parmesan cheese (optional; see Tip)**
- **2 tablespoons chopped fresh chives**
- **Freshly ground black pepper**
- **Pita chips, for serving**

Typical spinach artichoke dip wears a health halo that comes from having the word *spinach* in the name. Although it may *sound* good for you, it is all too often loaded with saturated fat and an excessive amount of sodium in a cheesy base that makes it easy to overindulge. Enter this brain-healthy take on the classic dip, which pairs the spinach—and lots of it—with a creamy, cashew-based sauce. If you love artichokes, you'll like this version even better than the standard, since the artichoke flavor really shines, and you still get to dip the crispy chips in the hot, creamy dip.

1. Preheat the oven to 400°F (200°C). Brush a 9-inch (23 cm) square baking dish with olive oil.

2. Drain the cashews and discard the soaking water. Place the cashews in a blender with the fresh water. Blend on high speed until the mixture is creamy and smooth, like the consistency of whipped cream, about 2 minutes. Scrape down the sides of the blender and process for 1 minute longer. Set aside.

3. Heat the oil in a large skillet over medium-low heat. Add the garlic and cook until starting to soften and turn golden, 1 to 2 minutes. Add the artichokes, wine, and salt. Increase the heat until the liquid is gently simmering. Cover and cook, with the lid ajar, until the artichokes are soft and starting to break apart, 7 to 10 minutes. Add the spinach and cook, stirring occasionally, until wilted, 1 to 2 minutes. Stir in the lemon juice.

4. Using a ladle, transfer half of the artichoke and spinach sauce to the blender with the cashew cream. Blend on low speed until smooth, about 1 minute. Scrape back into the pan and stir to combine. Pour into the baking dish, sprinkle with

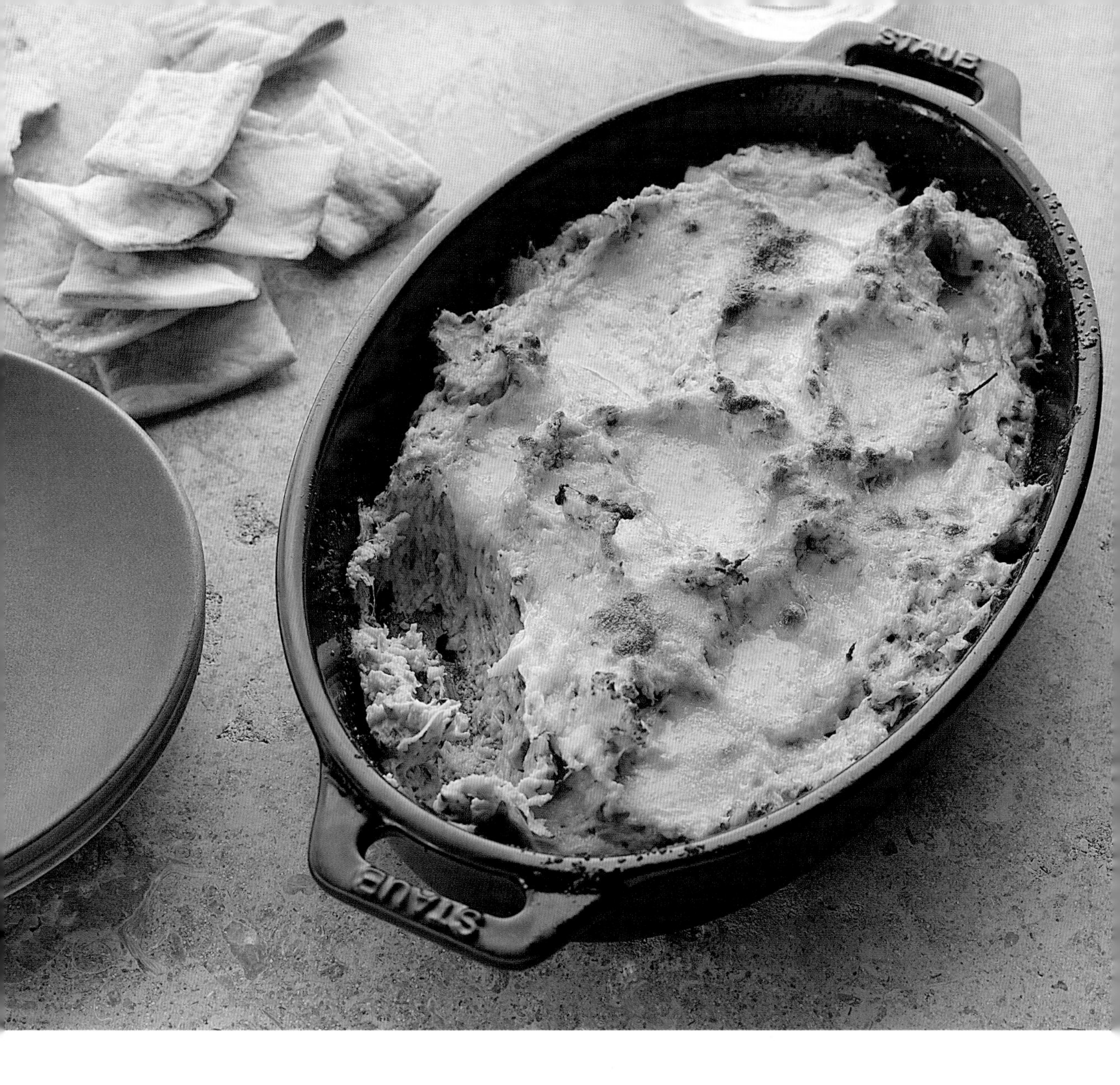

the Parmesan cheese (if using), and bake for 25 to 35 minutes, until the dip is crispy and brown on top and bubbling beneath.

5. Sprinkle with the chives and finish with pepper. Serve the dip hot with pita chips for dipping.

TIP: *To make this dish dairy-free, omit the Parmesan cheese and sprinkle 1 tablespoon of Walnut "Parm" (page 183) or nutritional yeast on top of the finished dip before serving.*

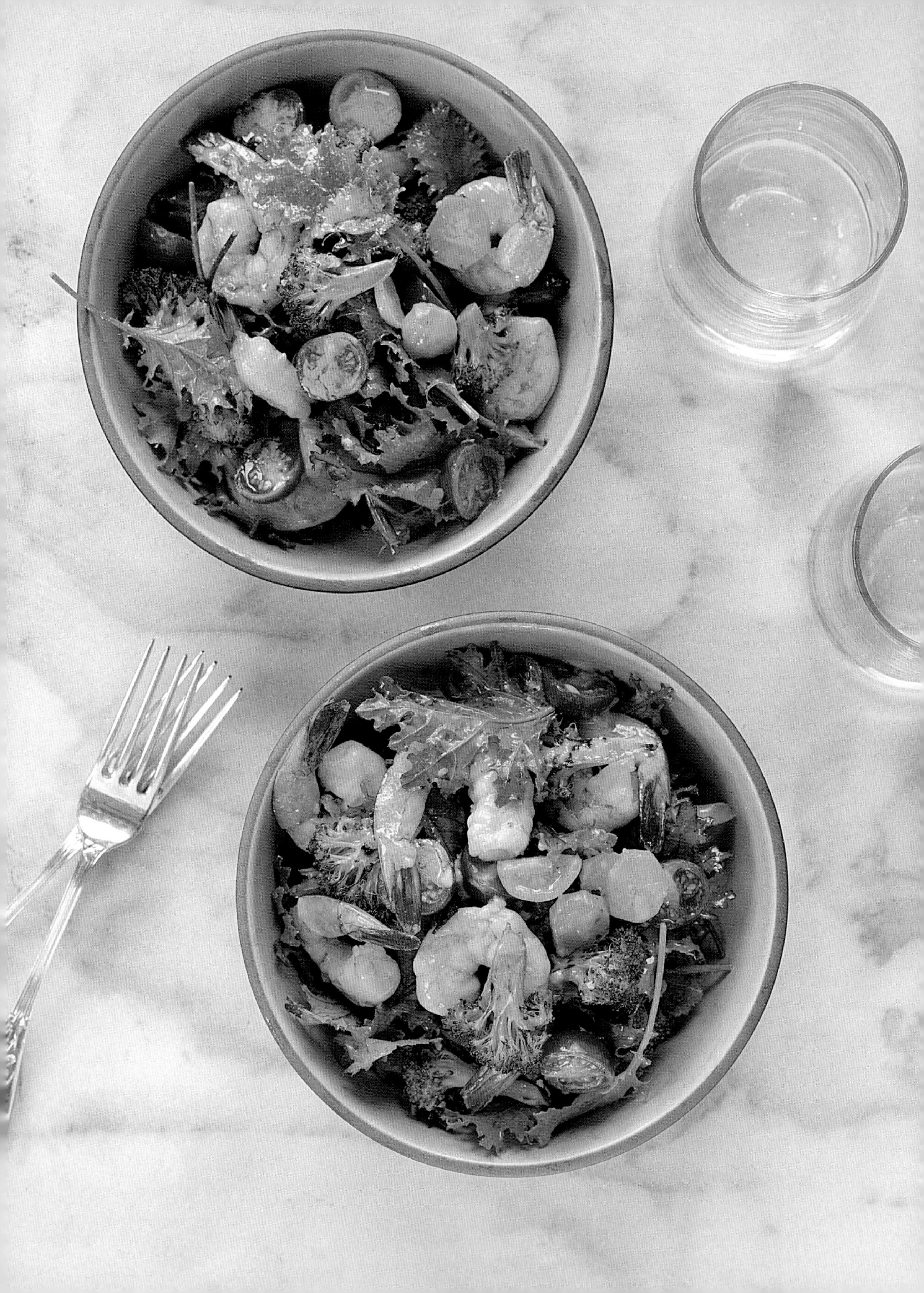

BROCCOLI-KALE CAESAR SALAD WITH SHRIMP AND GRAPE TOMATOES

SERVES 4

4 cups (about 1 pound/ 455 g) broccoli, florets and stem, from 1 large or 2 small heads

¼ cup plus 2 tablespoons (70 ml) extra-virgin olive oil

1 teaspoon kosher salt

¼ teaspoon freshly ground black pepper, plus more for serving

1 pound (455 g) peeled and deveined large shrimp (about 30)

2 oil-packed anchovy fillets

1 large garlic clove, minced (about 1 teaspoon)

¼ cup (60 ml) fresh lemon juice

2 teaspoons Dijon mustard

2 tablespoons vegan mayo or Almost Instant Cashew Cream (page 370)

4 cups (170 g) baby kale

1 cup (150 g) grape tomatoes, sliced lengthwise

Instead of the romaine you'd expect in a Caesar salad, this one includes kale, a powerhouse of folate, calcium, and vitamins C, A, and K. Roasted broccoli florets provide a nice crispy contrast to the creamy Caesar dressing, as well as an abundance of fiber and nutrients, especially anti-inflammatory sulforaphanes.

Between the anchovies in the dressing and the shrimp, this hearty salad is a full meal that packs in DHA and EPA. You'll roast the shrimp along with the broccoli toward the end of its cooking time, all on the same pan.

1. Preheat the oven to 400°F (200°C).

2. Cut the stem from the head of the broccoli, peel it with a knife, trim off the woody end, and slice into ½-inch (1.25 cm) rounds. Separate the crown into florets that are roughly the same size, about 2 inches (5 cm) long.

3. Toss the broccoli, 1 tablespoon of the oil, ¼ teaspoon of the salt, and the pepper on a rimmed baking sheet. Spread the broccoli out so that the pieces are not touching. Roast for 30 minutes, until the broccoli is almost done, then pull the pan from the oven.

4. As soon as the broccoli goes into the oven, rinse the shrimp under cold water and pat dry with paper towels. Toss with 1 tablespoon of the oil and ¼ teaspoon of the salt in a small bowl. When the broccoli is nearly done (after about 30 minutes), nestle the shrimp on the same pan and bake for 6 to 8 minutes, until the shrimp is pink and opaque and the broccoli is brown and crispy around the edges.

continued

5. Meanwhile, make the dressing. Use the flat side of a knife to mash the anchovies and garlic together on a cutting board to make a rough paste. Scrape into a small bowl with the lemon juice, mustard, mayo, and the remaining ½ teaspoon salt and whisk until smooth. Gradually add the remaining ¼ cup (60 ml) oil, whisking constantly until emulsified.

6. Toss the kale, broccoli, shrimp, and tomatoes with half the dressing in a salad bowl and divide between four plates. Drizzle with more dressing, if you like, and season with more pepper. Serve with extra dressing on the side.

7. To store any leftover dressing, keep it in an airtight container in the fridge for up to 5 days.

ANCHOVIES: WHOLE, FILLETS, AND PASTE

Canned anchovies come whole or as a flat fillet, packed in water or in oil. All are salty, so be sure to rinse them well before use if you are watching your sodium intake. To use canned whole anchovies, slip off the skins and remove the tiny spine (although some people eat them bones and all). Look for whole anchovies on ice at the fish counter of your supermarket. The white anchovies, also called alici, are delicious served simply on toast drizzled with extra-virgin olive oil. Anchovy paste varies tremendously, depending on the brand; some taste more assertive than others. It offers a convenient way to add a punch of briny, umami flavor to a dish without opening a can. In any recipe, substitute ½ teaspoon anchovy paste for 1 teaspoon chopped anchovy fillets.

MANY GREENS AND CHICKPEA SOUP

SERVES 4

- **2 tablespoons extra-virgin olive oil, plus more for drizzling**
- **2 large leeks (1¼ pounds/ 570 g), white and tender green parts thinly sliced**
- **1 large fennel bulb (1 pound 5 ounces/595 g), cored and chopped, fronds reserved for another use**
- **1 bunch kale (5½ ounces/ 150 g), leaves coarsely chopped, stems chopped into ½-inch (1.25 cm) dice**
- **2 oil-packed anchovy fillets, finely chopped**
- **2 large garlic cloves, minced (about 2 teaspoons)**
- **1 teaspoon kosher salt**
- **½ teaspoon freshly ground black pepper**
- **6 cups (360 ml) water**
- **1½ cups (250 g) cooked chickpeas (see page 215) or one 15-ounce (425 g) can, liquid reserved (see below)**
- **1 cup (240 ml) bean broth (page 220) or chickpea liquid from the can**
- **1 bunch watercress (7½ ounces/215 g), leaves and tender stems, roughly chopped**
- **1 tablespoon white wine vinegar**

continued

When you want a restorative meal that's hearty and green, this is the soup for you. Inspired by old-school Green Goddess dressing, it includes some ingredients with big personalities, like anchovies and tarragon, which amp the stock with umami. These flavorful ingredients are the key to a filling bowl of soup that doesn't take long to make.

Embrace the flexibility this recipe offers. Omit the anchovies to make it vegetarian. You could use another sturdy green besides kale, like Swiss chard, spinach, escarole, or collard greens. Other herbs, such as cilantro and chives, work here, too, but tarragon is worth seeking out. An assertive, anise-flavored herb with a long tradition of medicinal use, tarragon will keep in your crisper drawer for a long time.

1. Heat the oil in a large pot over medium heat. Add the leeks, fennel, kale stems, anchovies, garlic, ½ teaspoon of the kosher salt, and the pepper. Cook over medium heat, stirring often, until the vegetables are soft and fragrant, about 10 minutes.

2. Stir in the water, chickpeas and their liquid, and the remaining ½ teaspoon kosher salt. Bring to a boil, then reduce to a simmer and stir in the kale leaves. Continue to cook until all the vegetables are very soft, 8 to 10 minutes.

3. Just before serving, stir in the watercress, vinegar, and parsley.

continued

- **1 loosely packed cup (20 g) fresh flat-leaf parsley leaves, chopped**
- **½ cup (120 ml) plain, unsweetened yogurt (coconut, whole milk, or nut-based)**
- **2 tablespoons fresh tarragon**
- **Flaky sea salt (optional)**

4. To serve, ladle the soup into bowls and top each with a dollop of yogurt and a drizzle of extra-virgin olive oil. Tear the tarragon into pieces and sprinkle over the top. Season to taste with flaky salt (if using) and more pepper.

5. To store, refrigerate leftover soup in an airtight container for up to 4 days or freeze for up to 3 months.

SCIENCE BITE:

DO FRESH GREEN HERBS IMPROVE MEMORY?

Of all the green herbs purported to enhance memory, parsley is the most likely candidate. That's because parsley is rich in the flavonoid apigenin, a nutrient shown to protect brain cells from oxidative stress, increase blood flow to the brain, reduce the deposition of amyloid protein, and improve memory tasks in animal studies. Other culinary herbs, such as mint, basil, and cilantro, may also help block oxidative stress in the brain, although a direct impact on memory has not been proven.

Even though it may be difficult to prove the benefit of individual herbs, when used in abundance as part of a dietary pattern, such as the Mediterranean diet, they seem to work in synergy with other plant foods to optimize brain health. Apigenin is also found in celery, oregano, and green tea.

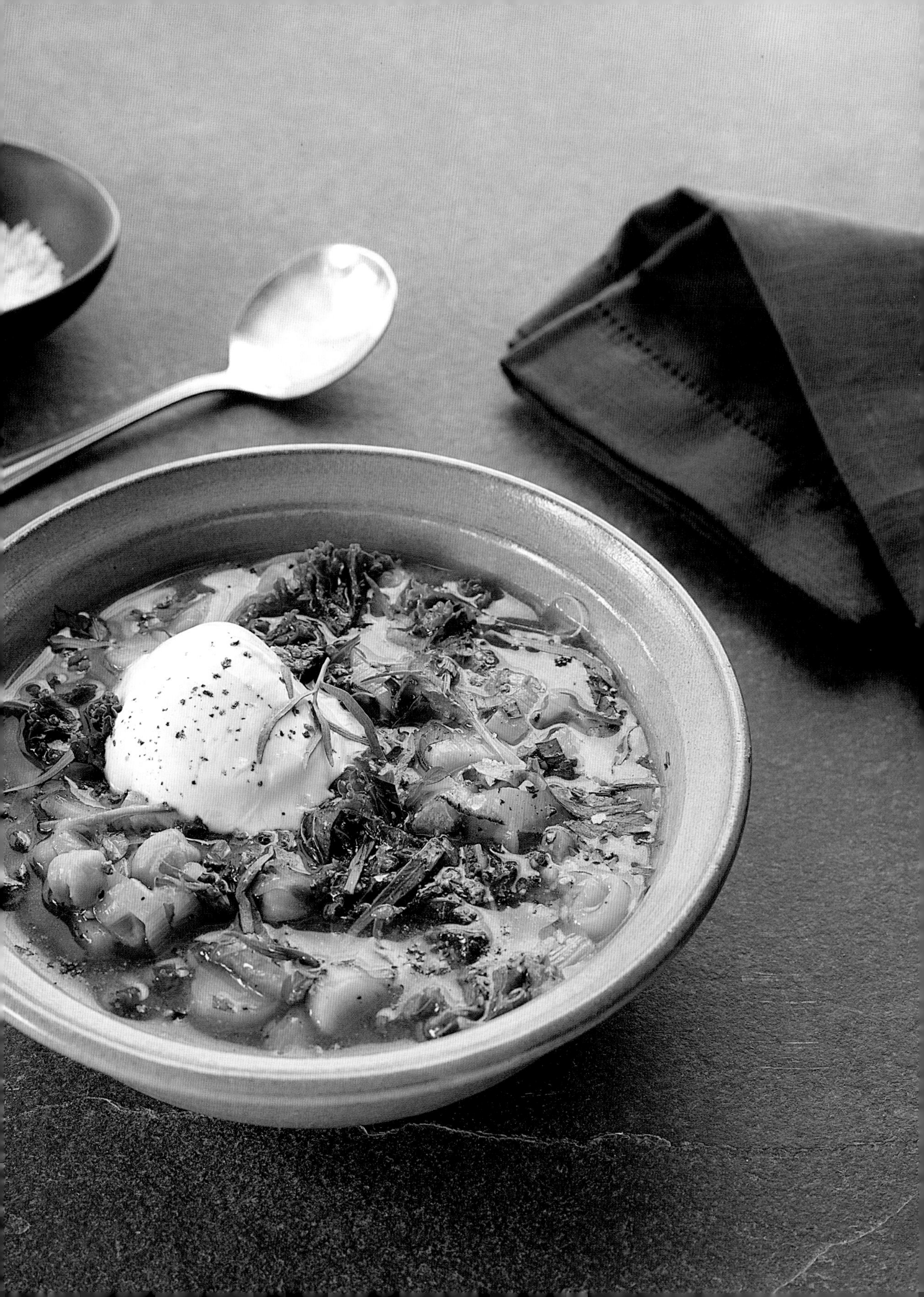

BLAT BOWL

SERVES 4

1½ teaspoons kosher salt

1 cup (190 g) brown rice, rinsed

2 tablespoons extra-virgin olive oil

½ cup (60 g) chopped pancetta

¼ cup (70 g) Spicy Arugula and Almond Pesto (page 105) or store-bought pesto

2 tablespoons white wine vinegar

Up to 2 tablespoons water

1 romaine heart, thinly sliced (115 g)

2 loosely packed cups (80 g) arugula leaves

2 medium avocados, sliced

2 medium or 3 small tomatoes (9 ounces/ 260 g), sliced ½ inch (1.25 cm) thick

¼ cup (2 ounces/60 g) crumbled goat cheese

Freshly ground black pepper

Toasted whole-grain bread, for serving

Everything you love about a BLAT (aka BLT sandwich with avocado) comes together in this simple, whole-grain bowl. Crispy bits of pancetta stand in for the bacon, while arugula and romaine play the part of lettuce. These join up with thick slabs of fresh tomato to top warm brown rice, and the zingy pesto dressing brings bright flavor.

1. Fill a medium pot with water and 1 teaspoon of the salt and bring to a boil. Add the rice and stir. Boil, uncovered, until the rice is chewy and tender, 28 to 35 minutes. Drain in a colander, then return to the pot. Cover the pot and set it away from the heat while you prepare the rest of the salad bowl.

2. Heat 1 tablespoon of the oil in a small skillet over low heat. Add the pancetta and cook, stirring occasionally, until golden brown and crisp, 3 to 5 minutes. Transfer to a paper towel–lined plate; set aside.

3. Whisk together the pesto, vinegar, 1 tablespoon water, and the remaining 1 tablespoon oil in a small bowl. Add up to another tablespoon of water, if needed, to make a pourable dressing.

4. Toss the romaine and arugula in a large bowl with half the dressing. Divide the rice between serving bowls, then top with the dressed greens, avocados, and tomatoes. Drizzle with the remaining dressing and sprinkle with goat cheese and the pancetta crumbles. Season to taste with pepper and serve with warm, toasted bread.

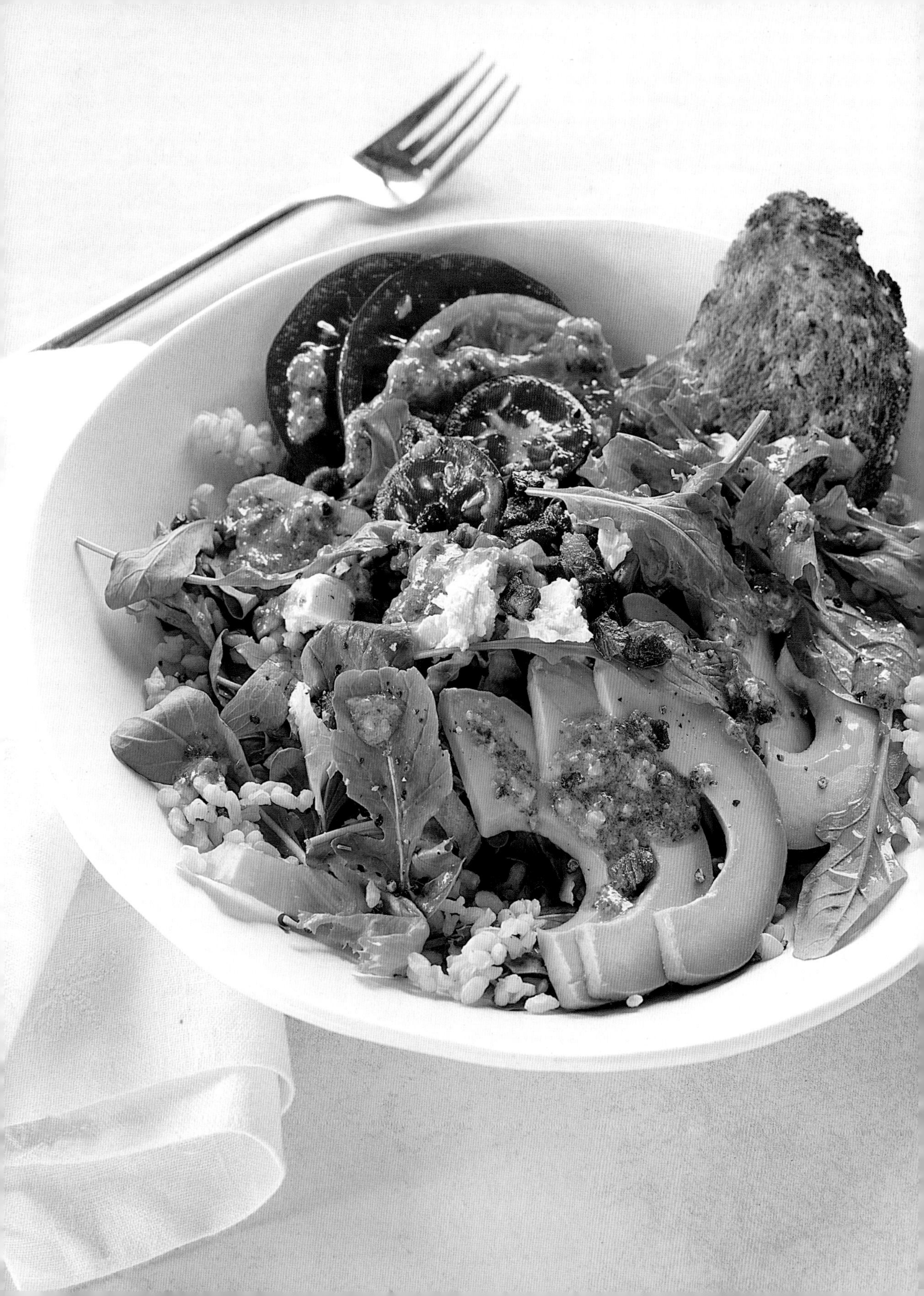

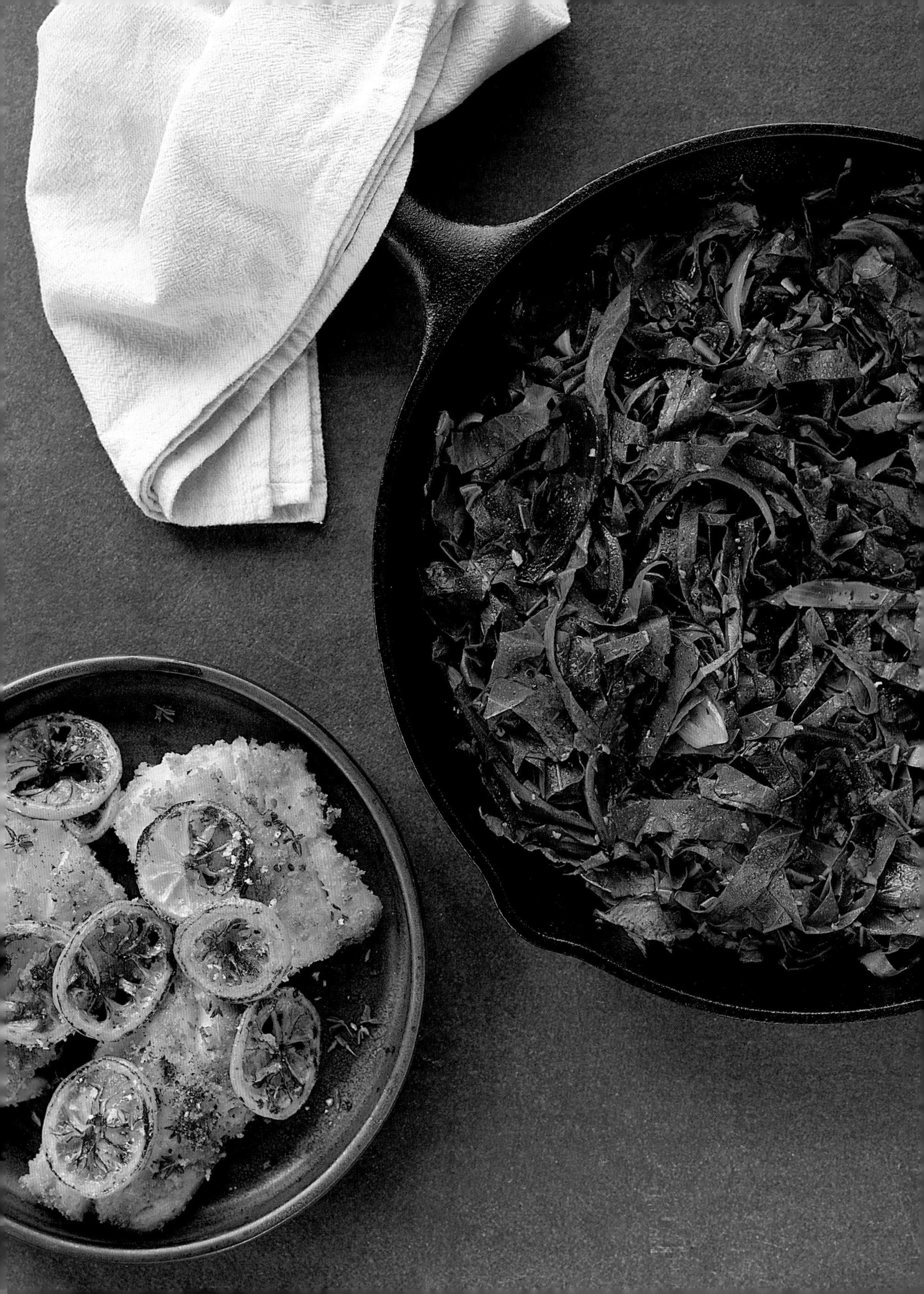

PANFRIED COD WITH COLLARD GREENS AND CRISPY LEMONS

SERVES 4

3 tablespoons avocado oil or olive oil

1 medium red onion (10 ounces/285 g), sliced ½ inch (1.25 cm) thick

1½ teaspoons kosher salt

1 large garlic clove, chopped (about 1 teaspoon)

2 bunches collard greens (about 1 pound/455 g total), leaves thinly sliced, and stems discarded (see Tip)

½ cup (120 ml) dry white wine

Four 4- to 6-ounce (115 to 170 g) skinless cod fillets, about ½ inch (1.25 cm) thick

1½ cups (90 g) whole-wheat panko breadcrumbs

2 teaspoons fresh thyme leaves, plus more for serving

¼ cup (60 ml) Almost Instant Cashew Cream (page 370) or vegan mayo

1 large lemon, thinly sliced, seeds removed

Freshly ground black pepper

Flaky salt (optional)

Although a time-honored way of cooking collards (especially in the American South) is to braise them in a pot for hours, they also taste great cooked quickly in this brain-healthy take on fried fish. A shorter cooking time keeps more of collards' bioactive nutrients from seeping out into the cooking water, preserving their fresh, grassy flavor. Coating the fish with cashew cream and breadcrumbs helps protect the delicate omega-3 fatty acids from the direct heat of the pan.

1. Heat 1 tablespoon of the oil in a large skillet over medium heat. Add the onion and ½ teaspoon of the kosher salt. Cook, stirring often, until soft and golden brown, 10 to 12 minutes.

2. Add the garlic and cook until fragrant, about 1 minute. Add the collard greens and wine and stir to coat evenly in the liquid. Increase the heat until the liquid is gently simmering, then cover the pan with the lid ajar. Cook until the greens are soft, 15 to 20 minutes.

3. Meanwhile, cook the fish. Combine the breadcrumbs, thyme, and ½ teaspoon of the kosher salt on a plate or pie tin. Spread in an even layer. Working with one fillet at a time, brush the fish on both sides with the cashew cream, then roll in the breadcrumb mixture, gently pressing to adhere. Set the coated fillets on a plate.

4. Line a plate with paper towels. Heat the remaining 2 tablespoons oil in a large nonstick skillet over medium heat. Add the lemon slices so that they are not touching and cook, turning once, until golden brown and crispy on both sides, 4 to 6 minutes. Transfer to the paper towel–lined plate, reserving the skillet and oil.

continued

5. Return the skillet to the heat and add the coated fillets. Cook, turning once, until golden brown and crispy on both sides, 5 to 7 minutes per side.

6. To serve, divide the collard greens between four plates. Top each with a piece of fish and a few slices of lemon. Finish with a few thyme leaves, pepper to taste, and flaky salt (if using).

TIP: *To turn a pile of collard greens into ribbons quickly, stack the leaves on top of each other and roll up like a cigar. Cut into ¼-inch-thick (6 mm) slices. Untangle with your hands and chop any that are too long.*

SCIENCE BITE:

THE SYNERGY OF CITRUS AND LEAFY GREENS

The liberal use of citrus in the brain-friendly Mediterranean diet (see page 17) may also be one of its secret powers to help you absorb more nutrients from food. First, the vitamin C in citrus enhances your body's ability to absorb key brain health nutrients in leafy greens: iron, folate, lutein, and phylloquinone (aka vitamin K).

Second, a unique flavonoid called beta-cryptoxanthin is present only in citrus peel, meaning the zest of citrus is a powerful antioxidant on its own. When a population of healthy elders were compared to those with dementia, the amount of beta-cryptoxanthin detected in the body was directly associated with higher scores on cognitive testing. In another study of nearly three thousand middle-aged adults followed for thirteen years, those consuming orange-colored fruits (not just orange juice but the whole fruit) had more of this flavonoid and higher scores on tasks like counting backward, recalling words, and speaking fluently.

The great news is, citrus adds a ping of bright flavor, welcome acidity, and color to vegetables, grains, nuts, and beans—which means what's delicious is also what's brain healthy.

PEPPERY PORK TENDERLOIN WITH WATERCRESS, ORANGE, AND RADISH SALAD

SERVES 4 TO 6

5 tablespoons (55 g) hemp seeds

1 tablespoon plus ¼ teaspoon coarsely crushed pink peppercorns

1 teaspoon kosher salt

1 pound (455 g) pork tenderloin

5 tablespoons (75 ml) extra-virgin olive oil

2 loosely packed cups (340 g) fresh cilantro leaves and tender stems

¼ cup (60 ml) fresh orange juice

Up to 2 tablespoons water (optional)

6 cups (150 g) watercress leaves and tender stems

1 small napa cabbage (about 10 ounces/285 g), thinly sliced (about 4 cups)

2 medium oranges (Cara Cara, navel, or Seville), peeled and sliced into rounds

1 small bunch radishes (about 6 ounces/170 g), thinly sliced lengthwise

Freshly ground black pepper

Flaky salt (optional)

Look out, kale: watercress might be the most nutrient-dense leafy green. While watercress has been around forever, you may be seeing it more now in grocery stores. That's a good thing, because these peppery greens add a spicy dimension to any dish; here it pairs well with oranges, radishes, and peppercorn-coated pork. Watercress is extremely rich in nutrients, with slightly more vitamins A, C, K, lutein, iron, and zeaxanthin than other dark leafy greens.

Serving a big salad with a small amount of meat is a great strategy for brain-healthy eating. Pork tenderloin, lower in saturated fat and calories than beef or lamb, is a particularly good choice. It's also a rich source of thiamine, a B vitamin that supports brain cell function.

The hemp seed dressing is a creamy green version of ranch. Keep the recipe in your back pocket for dressing other greens, especially peppery ones like watercress and arugula.

1. Preheat the oven to 350°F (180°C).

2. Stir together 3 tablespoons of the hemp seeds, 1 tablespoon of the pink peppercorns, and ½ teaspoon of the kosher salt in a small bowl. Rub the tenderloin with 1 tablespoon of the oil and coat with the hemp-peppercorn mixture, pressing with your fingers so it adheres. Place the pork on a rimmed baking sheet and roast for 20 to 30 minutes, until the juices run clear when pierced with a knife or a meat thermometer registers 145°F (63°C). Tent with a piece of foil and set aside to rest.

3. Meanwhile, make the dressing. Place the cilantro and orange juice with the remaining ¼ cup (60 ml) oil, 2 tablespoons hemp

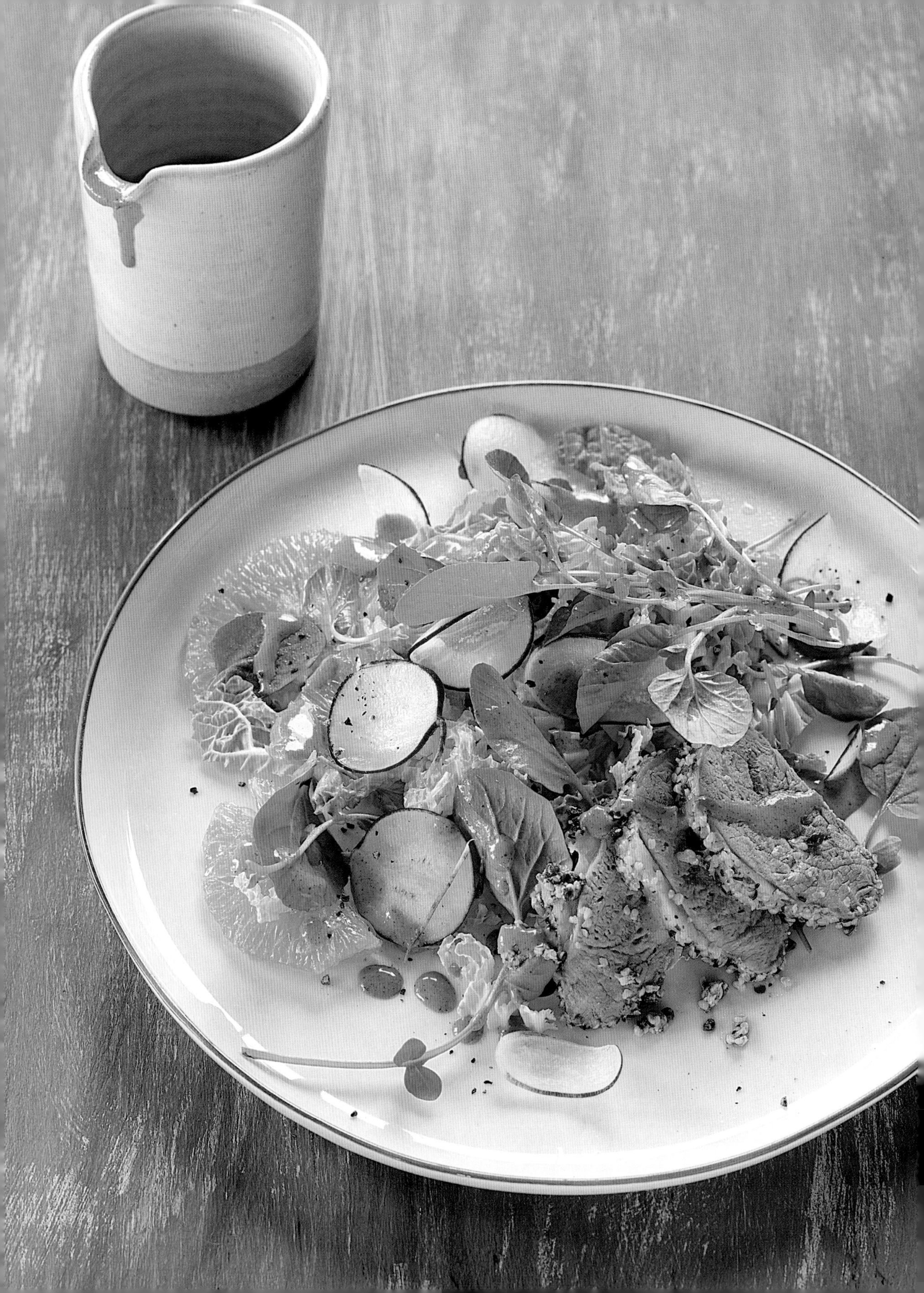

seeds, ½ teaspoon kosher salt, and ¼ teaspoon peppercorns in a blender and blend on high speed until smooth, about 2 minutes. Thin with up to 2 tablespoons water, if you like, for a pourable consistency.

4. Toss the watercress, cabbage, oranges, and radishes, in a large bowl with half the dressing. Divide the salad between serving plates. Top each plate with two ½-inch-thick (1.25 cm) slices of pork and drizzle with the remaining dressing. Garnish with pepper and flaky salt, if using.

SCIENCE BITE:

WATERCRESS IS GOOD FOR YOUR BRAIN AND YOUR EYES

Dark leafy greens like watercress aren't just beneficial for slowing down cognitive decline, they can also contribute to eye health. That's because the leaves are packed with two carotenoids (lutein and zeaxanthin) that actually block blue light from hitting the retina. Less light-induced oxidative stress to the eye means a lower risk of developing macular degeneration with age, a leading cause of vision loss in later years. Getting lutein and zeaxanthin from food has been shown to be especially impactful on those with a genetic predisposition to age-related macular degeneration. Pistachios, eggs, and other dark leafy greens provide a good source of dietary lutein and zeaxanthin.

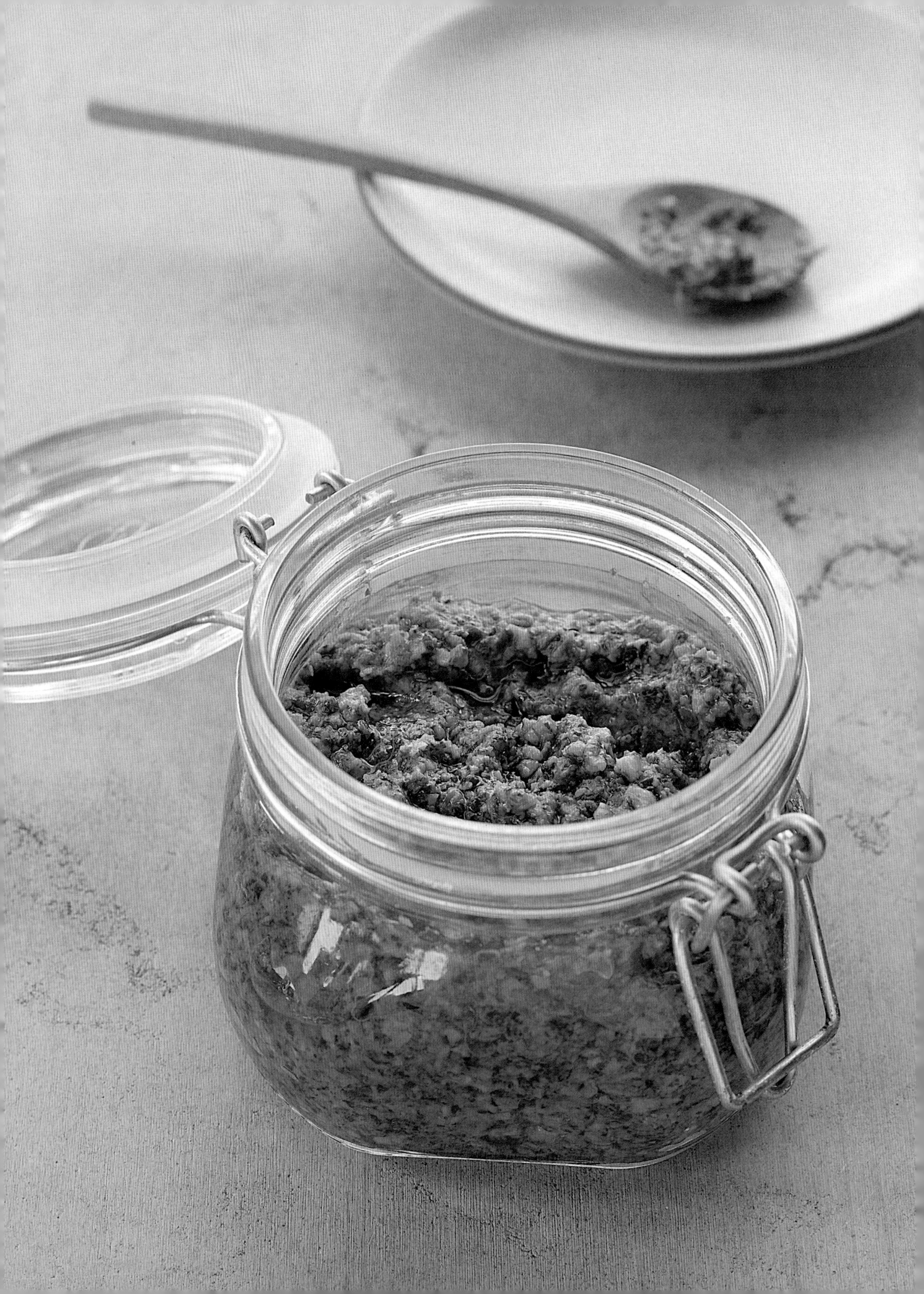

SPICY ARUGULA AND ALMOND PESTO

MAKES 2¼ CUPS (630 G)

4 loosely packed packed cups (160 g) arugula leaves

1 cup (150 g) almonds, toasted (page 190) and cooled

¼ cup (60 ml) fresh lemon juice

2 tablespoons nutritional yeast (see Tip)

1 tablespoon lemon zest

2 large garlic cloves

1 small serrano chile, seeds and stem removed

½ teaspoon kosher salt

⅔ to 1 cup (160 to 240 ml) extra-virgin olive oil

You might be used to tossing pesto with pasta to make an addictively good, comforting dish. Seen through the lens of brain health, pesto can also be a delicious way to eat leafy greens—along with other neuroprotective foods, like nuts, seeds, garlic, and extra-virgin olive oil. Go beyond pasta and enjoy pesto dolloped on soup, folded into scrambled eggs, and stirred into whole grains like quinoa and farro.

An assertive, peppery green like arugula makes a pesto with lots of personality. If you have different types of extra-virgin olive oil in your pantry, choose one with a mellow flavor profile, since a peppery olive oil would compete with the arugula. This pesto is wonderful stirred into cashew cream to use as "mayo" on a roasted vegetable sandwich.

Combine the arugula, almonds, lemon juice, nutritional yeast, lemon zest, garlic, chile, and salt in the bowl of a food processor or blender. Pulse until you have a chunky mixture, 1 to 2 minutes. Scrape down the sides of the bowl. Slowly pour ⅔ cup (160 ml) of the oil over the pesto while pulsing until uniformly green with small bits of nuts visible. Add up to ⅓ cup (80 ml) more oil, if you like, for a thinner, more sauce-like consistency.

TIPS: *Pesto keeps in an airtight container in the refrigerator for up to a week. Because the greens will turn brown when exposed to air, cover the top of the pesto with a thin layer of olive oil. Pesto freezes well, too, for up to 6 months. Make batches of pesto when the greens are abundant and less expensive and freeze single portions in an ice cube tray for easy meals all year long.*

Nutritional yeast tastes nutty and salty, like many cheeses, but is dairy-free. It adds a rich umami flavor to foods, thanks to its glutamate content, along with a good dose of important brain health nutrients: selenium, folic acid, and B vitamins.

BREAKFAST SALAD WITH CRISPY POTATOES, SMOKED SALMON, AND JAMMY EGGS

SERVES 4

1 pound (455 g) fingerling potatoes, yellow, purple, or a mix (about 4 medium), or other small potatoes, scrubbed and cut lengthwise into ⅛-inch-thick (3 mm) slices (see Tip)

5 tablespoons (25 ml) extra-virgin olive oil

½ teaspoon sumac or paprika (see Tip)

½ teaspoon kosher salt, plus more for serving

¼ teaspoon freshly ground black pepper, plus more for serving

4 eggs

2 tablespoons fresh lemon juice

1 tablespoon chopped fresh dill, plus more for garnish

4 loosely packed cups (160 g) tender lettuces, such as butter, Bibb, or baby lettuces

5 ounces (140 g) thinly sliced smoked salmon

1 cup (200 g) Lemony Cashew Ricotta (page 373) or store-bought ricotta

¼ cup (30 g) raw hulled pumpkin seeds (pepitas), toasted (page 190)

¼ cup (35 g) hazelnuts, roasted and skinned, roughly chopped (page 190)

Salad for breakfast? Absolutely. You can—and should—make the first meal of the day a leafy green one, and a salad at that. In this recipe, the combination of crispy potatoes, smoked salmon, and boiled eggs gives tender lettuces a welcome breakfasty vibe. It does require a quick roast of the potatoes, though, so if you're pressed for time, save this recipe for a weekend.

Use this recipe as a template for future breakfast salads. In place of the potatoes, swap in leftover roasted vegetables like beets or cubes of squash. Try smoked trout for the salmon or cubes of feta instead of ricotta. As always, a generous wedge of avocado would be a good addition, too.

1. Preheat the oven to 400°F (200°C).

2. Toss the potatoes with 1 tablespoon of the oil on a rimmed baking sheet and spread them out so they are not touching. Sprinkle evenly with the sumac, ¼ teaspoon of the salt, and the pepper. Roast for 15 to 18 minutes, until brown and crispy.

3. Meanwhile, cook the eggs. Fill a medium bowl with ice and water. Bring a small saucepan of water to a boil. Gently lower the eggs into the boiling water using a slotted spoon. Reduce the heat to a low simmer and set the timer for 9 minutes. When the eggs are done, use the spoon to transfer them to the ice water. Once the eggs are cool enough to handle, roll them around on the counter to loosen the shell. Starting at the pointy end, peel the eggs and cut in half lengthwise.

4. Whisk the remaining ¼ cup (60 ml) olive oil with the lemon juice, dill, and remaining ¼ teaspoon salt in a small bowl.

5. Combine the lettuce and half the dressing in a large bowl. Toss to coat the leaves, then divide between serving plates or

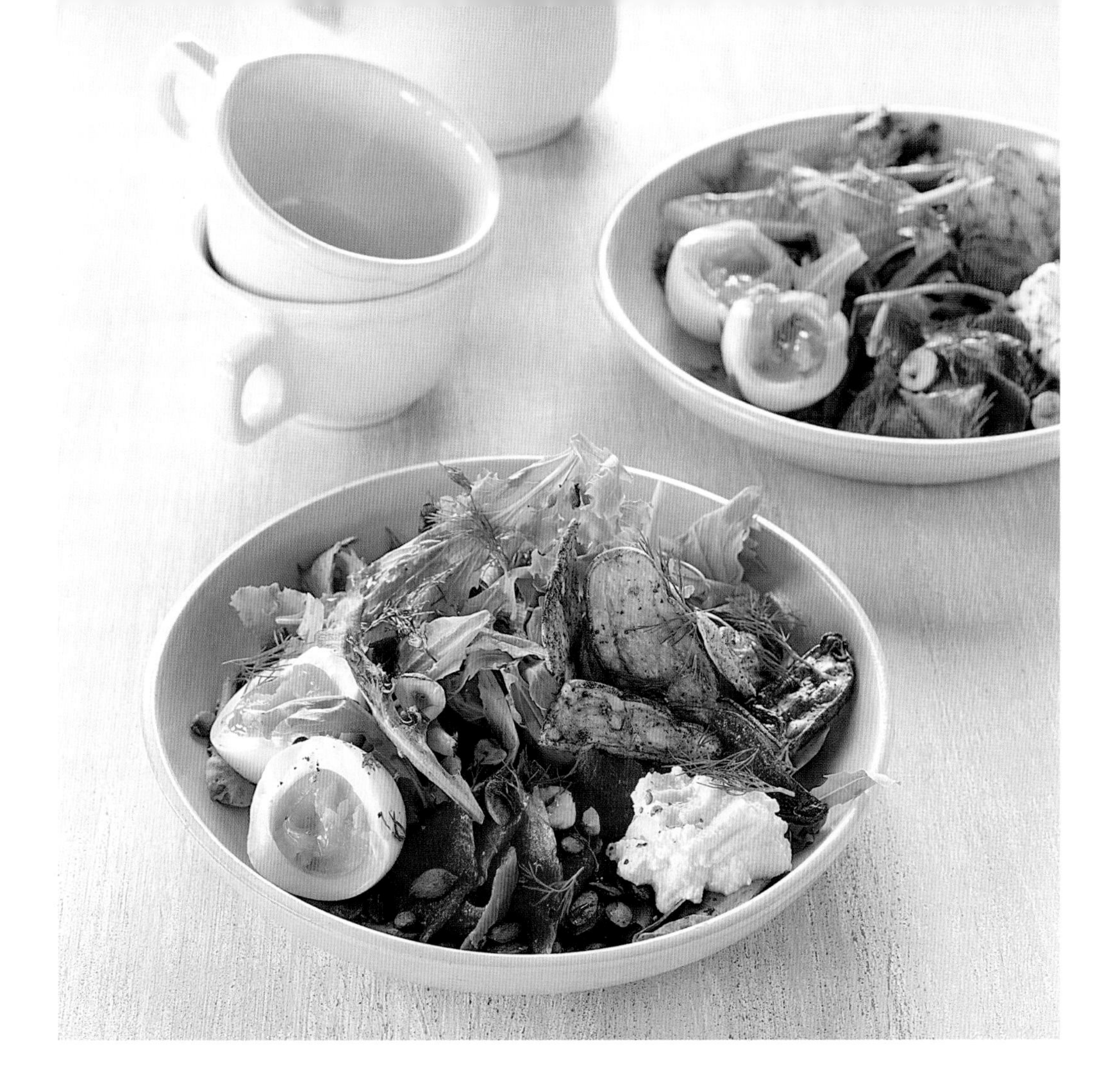

shallow bowls. Top each plate with roasted potatoes, smoked salmon, eggs, and a dollop of ricotta, dividing evenly. Drizzle with the remaining dressing, then sprinkle with the pumpkin seeds and hazelnuts, dividing evenly. Grind some pepper over top and sprinkle with more dill.

TIPS: *For the crispiest chips, soak the sliced potatoes in cold water for at least 30 minutes and up to overnight. Drain and pat completely dry before tossing with the oil. The baking time will depend on your oven and how thinly your potatoes are sliced.*

Sumac has a tart, lemony flavor that pairs well with potatoes and boiled eggs. If you can't find it, sweet or smoked paprika are good substitutes.

EASY GREENS SMOOTHIE

SERVES 2

1 medium banana (about 140 g), peeled, cut into pieces, and frozen

4 small ice cubes

2 cups (480 ml) unsweetened plant-based milk, homemade (page 363) or store-bought

1 small ripe avocado

One 1-inch (5 cm) piece fresh ginger, peeled and thinly sliced

One ½-inch-thick (1.25 cm) piece of lime (peel and all)

2 packed cups (100 g) baby spinach or tender spinach leaves

¼ cup (5 g) fresh mint leaves

1 teaspoon raw honey (optional)

2 teaspoons sesame seeds or hemp seeds (optional)

Getting your daily greens in shouldn't feel like a chore. Here you'll transform a generous serving of spinach with the bright flavors of ginger, lime, and mint. Avocado's mild flavor fades into the background but adds satisfying creaminess and body. For even more omega-3s, sprinkle seeds on top.

1. In the following order, layer the banana, ice cubes, milk, avocado, ginger, lime, spinach, mint, and honey (if using) in a blender and blend on high speed until smooth, about 1 minute.

2. To serve, divide between two glasses and sprinkle with sesame seeds, if using.

SCIENCE BITE:

EATING VS. DRINKING YOUR GREENS

Smoothies are a convenient addition to a brain-healthy dietary pattern. Blending greens breaks down the cell walls of plant fibers, which means your body will absorb them more quickly. It's best to get most of your greens by chewing them, a process that slows and stabilizes the entry of nutrients into the bloodstream and helps keep insulin levels from spiking. That being said, smoothies are a better choice than green juice, since juicing removes beneficial plant fibers from the drink.

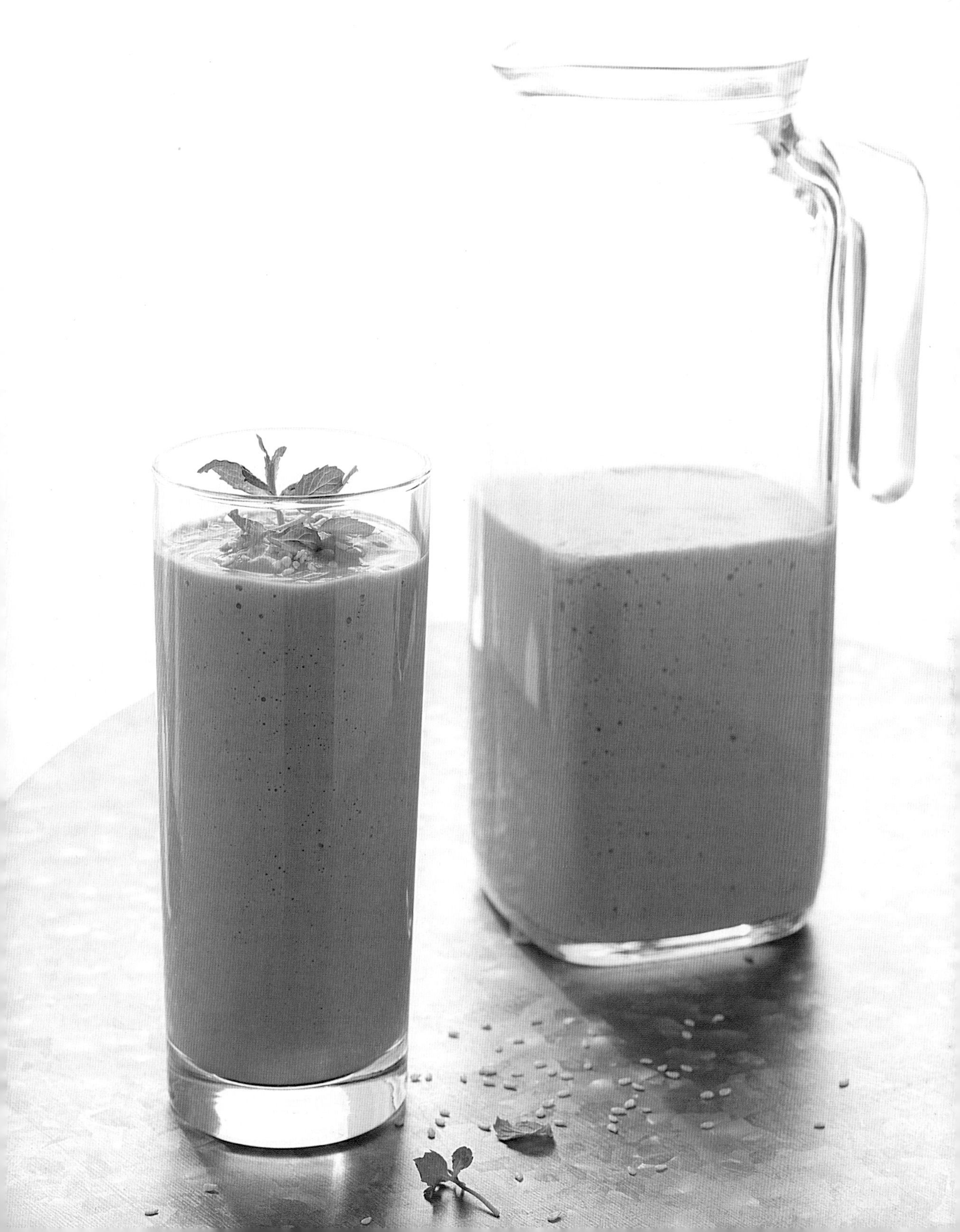

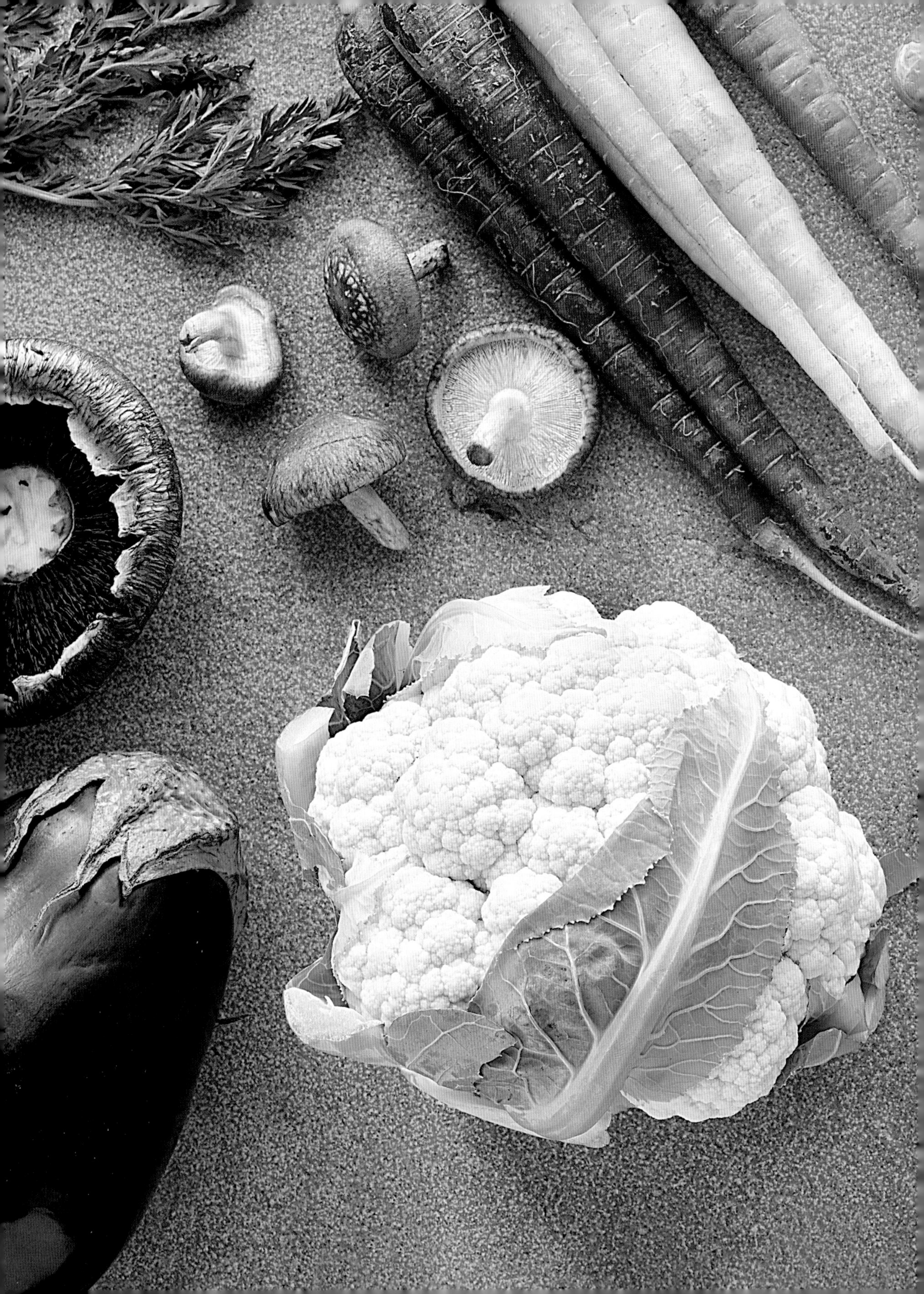

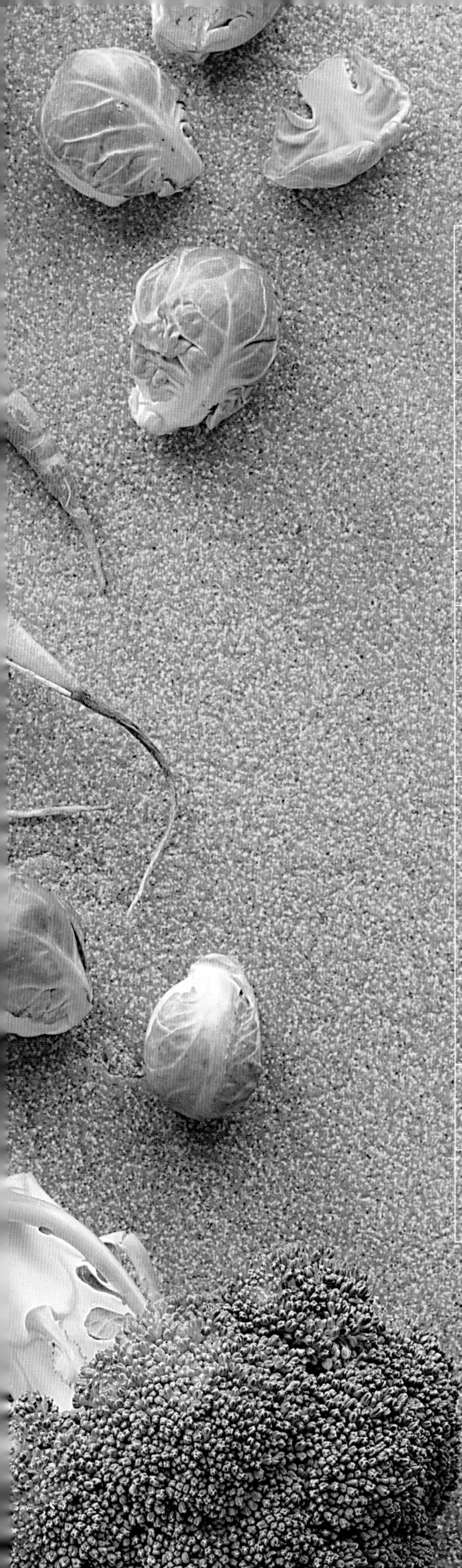

VEGETABLES

We now know that a brain-healthy diet should include at least three servings of vegetables (in addition to two servings of leafy greens) every day. In this chapter, vegetables become the crave-worthy dinner plate centerpiece they can—and should—be. Whether you already eat in a vegetable-focused way or are just testing it out with the occasional Meatless Monday, these recipes will inspire you to think of turning your veggies into the main course.

These dishes are hearty and satisfying, and in many cases, they have a familiar vibe. I like to think of them as brain-healthy makeovers of my favorite comfort foods—risotto, grilled cheese sandwiches with tomato soup, lasagna, fried rice, and fritters. One key to making vegetables the star of the show is reaching for bold-flavored pantry condiments that act like flavor bombs. I recommend you keep these on hand for quick, delicious veg-heavy meals: gochujang (Korean chili paste), Thai red curry paste, kimchi, dried mushrooms, chipotle chiles, and miso paste are all staples in the Brain Health Kitchen.

Except for a splash of fish sauce in the curry, the recipes in this chapter are entirely vegetarian. They get you in the groove of enjoying vegetables as a full meal. Of course, meat, fish and seafood, and poultry can be added to these dishes if you wish, though I recommend you view those proteins more like a condiment than a main dish—that means keeping meat to no more than 3 ounces (85 g) per serving. You are on the right track if three-quarters of your plate is vegetables and other plants.

SUPERSTAR VEGETABLES

Although it is impossible to narrow the rainbow of vegetables down to just a few, this chapter focuses on my favorites as seen through the lens of brain health. These have the most solid data to prove them as part of a diet that protects against age-related cognitive decline, and it just so happens they're some of the tastiest vegetables, too.

With each recipe, you'll learn how to retain the nutrient density of your vegetables by using cooking methods that keep their brain-friendly plant compounds from seeping out. The vegetables in this chapter are superstars because they possess one or more of these benefits:

- **Rich in flavonoids.** This broad family of compounds that reside in plant pigments has proven to be important for fending off Alzheimer's. Flavonoids are also the basis for viewing your diet as a "rainbow" of diverse plants since they're responsible for the colors; vibrant green, soothing purple, cheerful red, sunny orange, and/or golden yellow veggies are code for flavonoid density.

- **High in fiber.** When you ingest the recommended amount of fiber (between at least 30 and 40 grams per day), your food is not just more satisfying, it has the power to bind up harmful blood cholesterol, slow down the absorption of sugars, and provide fuel for the trillions of microbes that live in your gut. Plus, your body absorbs more of the flavonoids, which ride piggyback onto the fiber through your digestive tract.
- **Cruciferous.** Vegetables in this family (including cauliflower, broccoli, broccoli rabe, and Brussels sprouts) are rich in disease-fighting sulforaphanes. These compounds bump up production of the

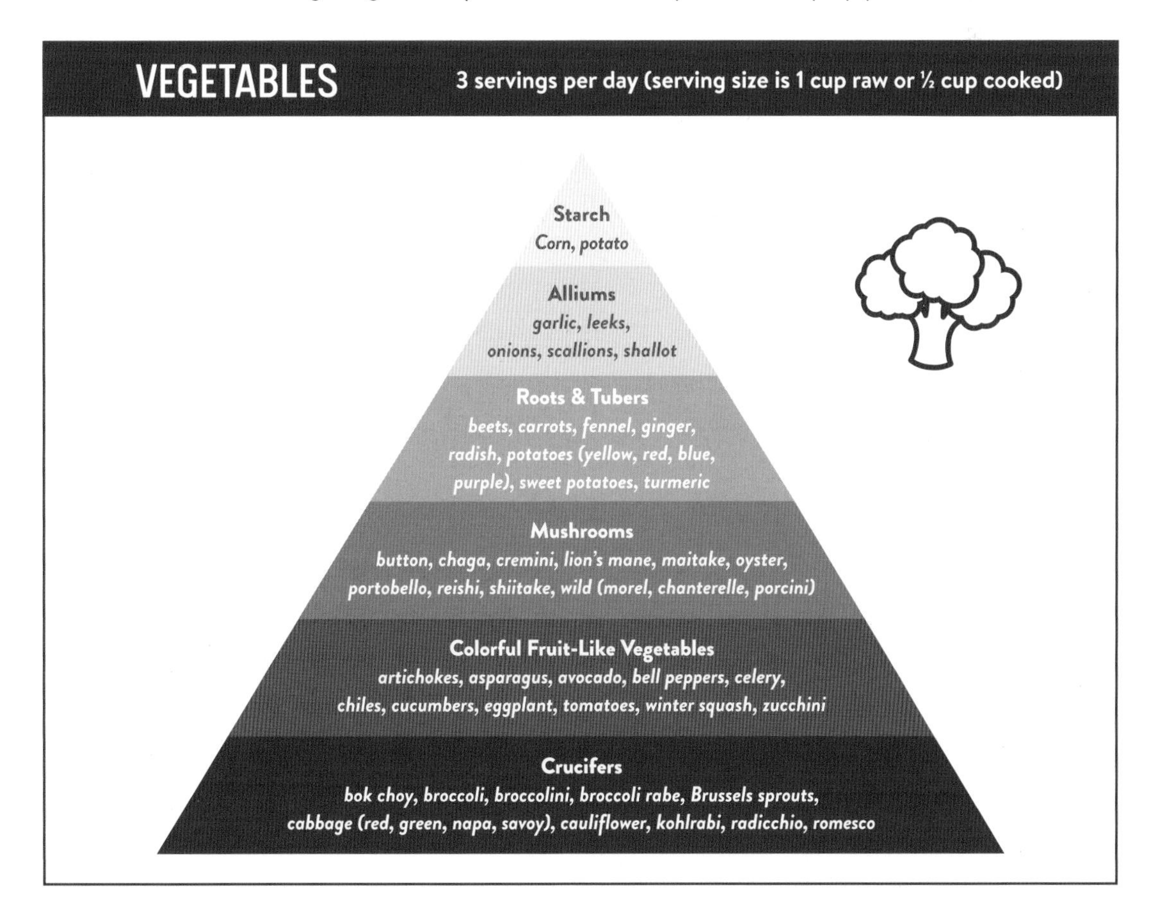

neurotransmitter acetylcholine (a key player in memory and learning), activate a pathway that makes antioxidants more available, quell harmful oxidative stress in the brain, and boost the production of brain-derived neurotrophic factor (BDNF) that enhances brain cell growth and repair.

- **Potent aromatics.** These flavor boosters from the allium family of vegetables (garlic, onions, shallots, scallions) are not only packed with beneficial phytonutrients, they also create hunger-inducing aromas and complex layers of flavor in your cooking, along with the type of prebiotic fiber your gut microbes need to thrive.

You'll also notice some honorary vegetables in the mix. These are not technically vegetables at all but, in fact, are savory fruits we treat like vegetables, such as avocados, tomatoes, and eggplant. Mushrooms, which are neither fruits nor vegetables—they are part of the fungi kingdom—are important for providing antioxidants (like ergothioneine and glutathione) shown to protect brain cells from the effects of aging.

ORGANIC OR NOT?

Certain vegetables concentrate pesticide residue more than others, which makes organic a must when you're choosing bell peppers, carrots, celery, cherry tomatoes, cucumbers, green beans, hot peppers, potatoes, snap peas, sweet potatoes, tomatoes, winter squashes, and zucchini.

Some conventionally grown vegetables harbor smaller amounts of pesticides, which tend to congregate on vegetable skin and near stems. These include asparagus, avocados, broccoli, cabbages, cauliflower, eggplant, mushrooms, onions, and sweet corn. Be sure to clean these vegetables well by rinsing thoroughly with fresh water, and consider peeling them. That said, many of the brain-healthy nutrients are concentrated in the skin, so if you can afford it, buy organic and keep the skin on.

The bottom line: The benefit of boosting your diet with a wide diversity of vegetables far outweighs the potential harm from small amounts of pesticide residue on conventional produce. So if organic vegetables are too expensive, go for the best veggies you can find, scrub them clean, peel if you must, and rinse well.

EGGPLANT STEAKS WITH MISO-MAPLE BRUSSELS SPROUTS SLAW

SERVES 4 TO 6

- **¼ cup (60 ml) fresh orange juice**
- **4 tablespoons extra-virgin olive oil**
- **2 tablespoons white miso paste**
- **1 tablespoon pure maple syrup**
- **1 large garlic clove, minced (about 1 teaspoon)**
- **¼ teaspoon freshly ground black pepper**
- **¾ pound (340 g) Brussels sprouts, shredded (about 2 cups) (see Tip)**
- **4 to 5 small radishes, thinly sliced**
- **¼ cup (40 g) pickled ginger, finely chopped (from a jar; see Tip on page 263)**
- **2 medium globe eggplants (each about 1½ pounds/680 g), sliced into 1-inch (2.5 cm) planks lengthwise, flesh scored crosswise on an angle**
- **3 tablespoons gochujang (fermented Korean chili paste)**
- **1 tablespoon water**
- **¼ cup (60 ml) plain, unsweetened Greek yogurt**
- **¼ teaspoon kosher salt**
- **4 to 6 eggs**
- **1 tablespoon unhulled sesame seeds, toasted**

Meet your new favorite way to eat eggplant: thick steak-like slabs that are roasted until mahogany brown. After slashing the surface of each "steak" in a crosshatch pattern, you'll smear the flesh with gochujang (Korean chili paste), which seeps into the nooks and crannies as the eggplant roasts to create deep flavor and a delightful, crispy texture.

The peel of purple eggplant is rich in anthocyanins—the same phytonutrient that famously makes blueberries good for the brain. So whenever possible, don't peel your eggplant. When cutting into steaks, be sure to include the convex end pieces. Keep an eye on them while baking as they may cook a little faster than the middle pieces.

1. Set an oven rack in the center position and preheat the oven to 425°F (220°C). Line a rimmed baking sheet with parchment paper.

2. Whisk together 2 tablespoons of the orange juice and 2 tablespoons of the oil with the miso, maple syrup, garlic, and pepper in a large bowl. Add the Brussels sprouts, radishes, and ginger and toss to coat; set aside, tossing occasionally, while you prepare the eggplant.

3. Place the eggplant slices on the prepared baking sheet. Stir together 2 tablespoons of the gochujang, 1 tablespoon of the oil, and the water in a small bowl to make a spreadable sauce. Using a spoon or a brush, coat the eggplants with the sauce, dividing evenly, being sure to get it between the hatch marks. Bake for 16 to 20 minutes, until the eggplant skin is collapsed and crispy, the flesh is soft, and the surface is a dark cocoa brown.

continued

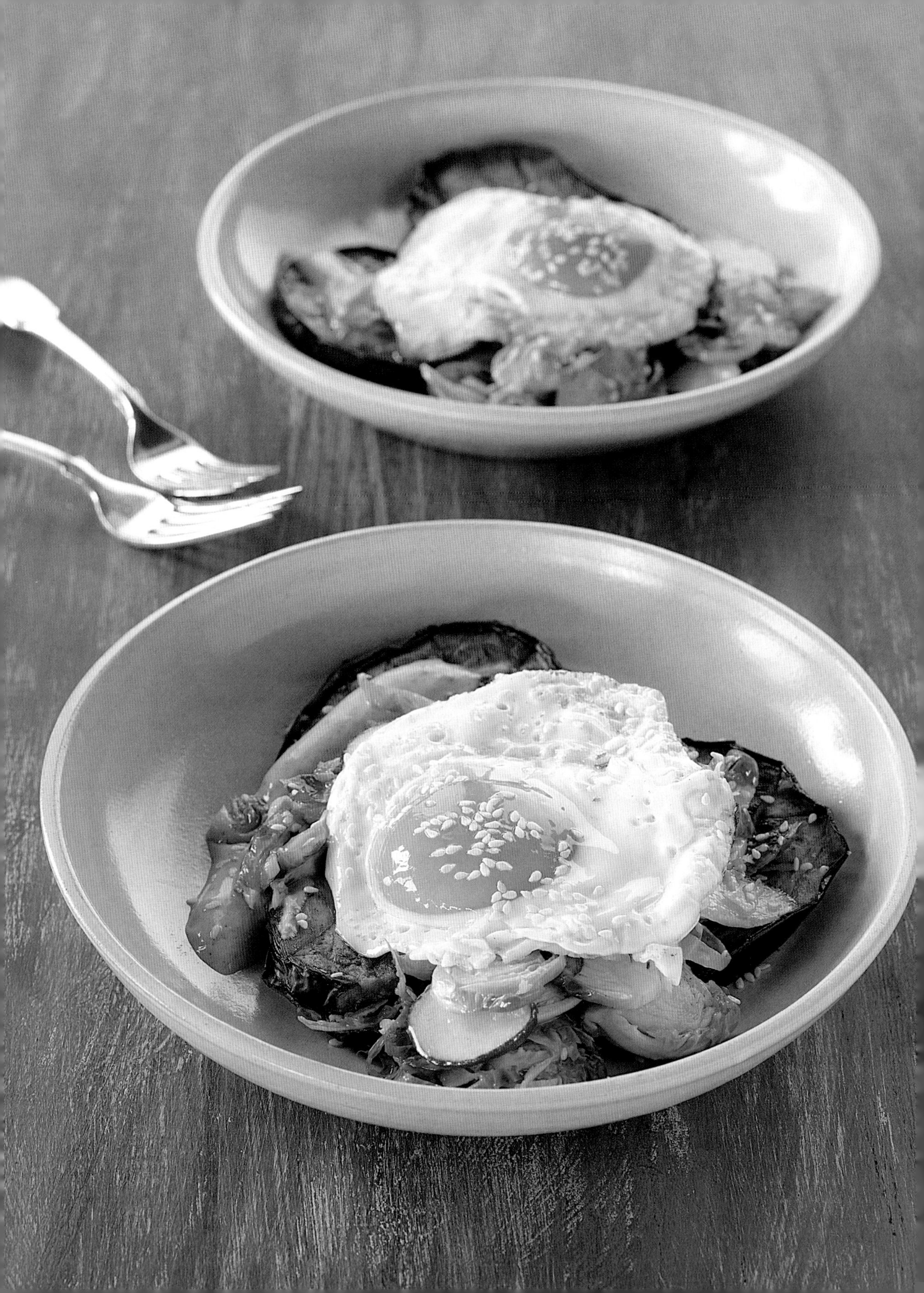

4. Meanwhile, stir together the remaining 2 tablespoons orange juice, remaining 1 tablespoon gochujang, the yogurt, and the salt in a small bowl.

5. Just before serving, warm the remaining 1 tablespoon oil in a large nonstick skillet over medium-low heat. Crack in the eggs and cook until the whites are cooked through and the yolk is set, 3 to 5 minutes.

6. Transfer the roasted eggplant steaks to plates and top with a generous dollop of the yogurt sauce. Give the Brussels sprouts salad a toss and divide between the plates. To finish, top each plate with a fried egg and sprinkle with the sesame seeds.

TIP: *A food processor fit with a slicing blade makes quick work of shredding Brussels sprouts. Just turn the machine on and drop the sprouts through the top feeding tube.*

SCIENCE BITE:

NIGHTSHADES ARE ANTI-INFLAMMATORY FOODS

Eggplants are part of the Solanaceae family of flowering plants, also known as nightshades. (Fun fact: Eggplants are actually berries!) Maybe you've read that nightshades cause inflammation in the body, that the lectin in their seeds is toxic to the gut lining, or that their oxalates will give you kidney stones. Not true! Eggplant, as well as other nightshades (which include white potatoes, bell peppers, tomatoes, tomatillos, cayenne pepper, and paprika) are actually anti-inflammatory for most people. In fact, animal studies show that over time, this anti-inflammatory action may counteract the detrimental effect of bombarding brain cells with chronically elevated blood sugar.

Nightshade allergies and sensitivities are very rare—less than 1 percent of the population. Allergies are caused by glycoalkaloids, a compound naturally produced by all nightshade plants. This is a natural, plant-produced pesticide that helps the plant fight against pathogens, which may also be the clue to its pro-inflammatory action: it can stimulate an immune response in people. Cooking nightshades reduces their glycoalkaloids content by half, eliminating most mild nightshade sensitivities.

BETTER-FOR-YOU GRILLED CHEESE SANDWICH

SERVES 4

1 small winter squash (butternut, kabocha, or delicata) (1 pound/455 g), sliced ½ inch (1.25 cm) thick (see Tip)

1 medium yellow onion (about 10 ounces/285 g), thinly sliced

2 tablespoons extra-virgin olive oil, plus more if needed

1 teaspoon kosher salt

1 cup (200 g) Lemony Cashew Ricotta (page 373) or store-bought ricotta

1 cup (4 ounces/115 g) grated Gruyère cheese

¼ teaspoon freshly ground black pepper

8 slices whole-grain bread

One 15-ounce (425 g) can artichoke hearts, packed in water, drained and quartered

This grilled cheese checks off many comfort-food boxes—toasted bread and melty cheese to name two—with a strategic shift to more vegetables than cheese. Rings of roasted squash give the sandwich substance. Stirring together Gruyère with either a dairy or plant-based ricotta binds the sandwich together, keeping the saturated fat profile tipped toward brain health. If you use cashew ricotta and skip the Gruyère, you'll have an entirely plant-based dinner.

A grilled cheese sandwich dipped into creamy tomato soup is a welcome, nourishing dinner for all ages. For the accompanying tomato soup, see page 120.

1. Set an oven rack in the center position and preheat the oven to 425°F (220°C). Line a baking sheet with parchment paper.

2. Toss the squash, onion, 1 tablespoon of the oil, and ¼ teaspoon of the salt on the prepared baking sheet, making sure both sides of the squash pieces are well coated. Bake for 20 to 24 minutes, until the squash is tender and the onions are golden brown. Slip off and discard the squash skin, if you like (see Tip).

3. Reduce the oven temperature to 300°F (150°C). Place the vegetables back in the oven to keep warm.

4. Combine the ricotta, Gruyère, and pepper in a small bowl. Spread the mixture on one side of each piece of bread, dividing evenly, then top four of the bread slices with the squash and onions, followed by the artichokes. Cover with the remaining four slices of bread and press gently so everything sticks together.

5. Warm the remaining 1 tablespoon oil in a large nonstick skillet over medium heat. Add two sandwiches to the pan and

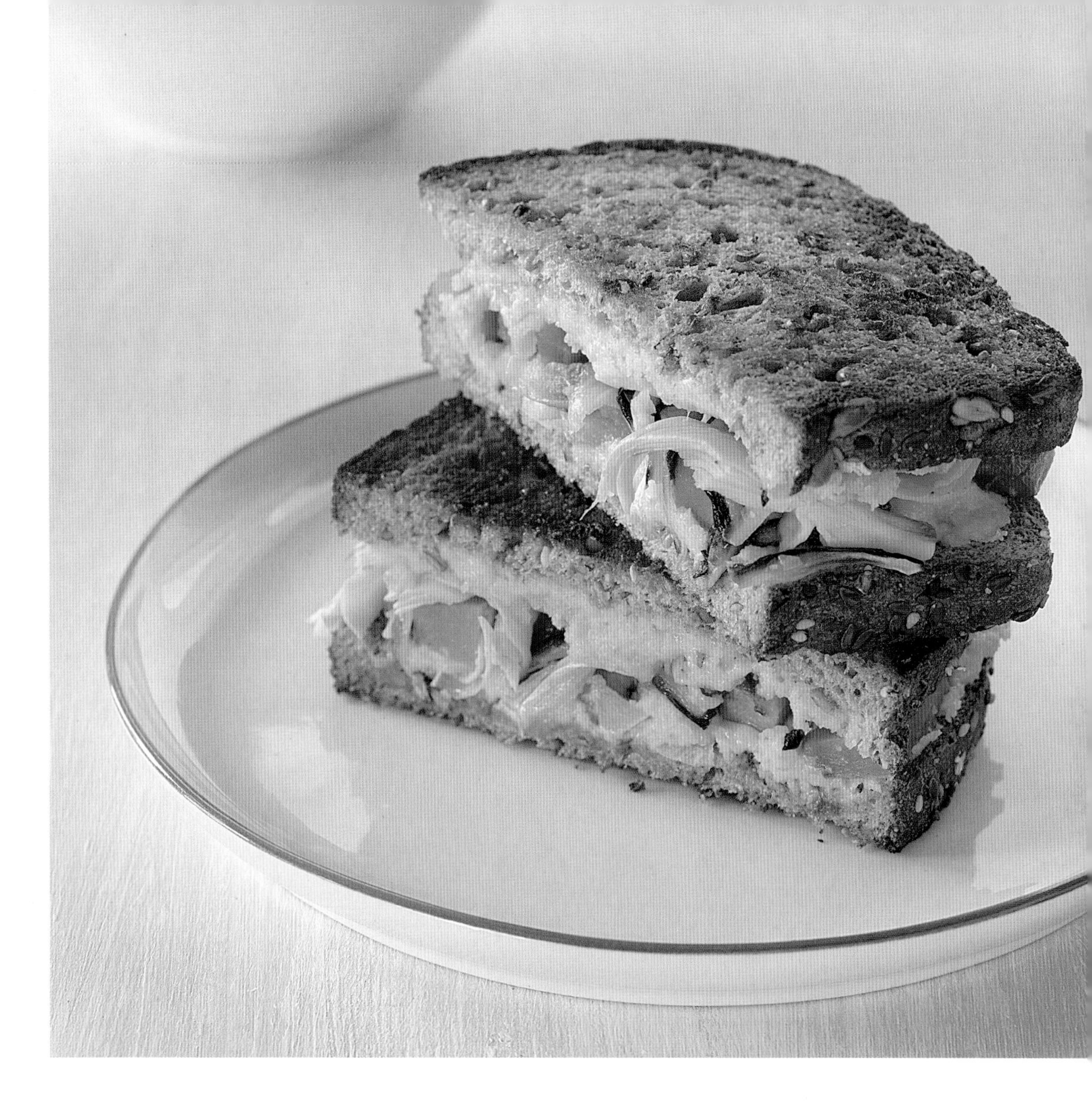

cook until the bread is toasty brown and the cheese is soft, 4 to 6 minutes on each side. Transfer to the pan in the oven to keep warm while you make the remaining sandwiches, adding a drizzle more oil, if needed. Serve warm.

TIP: *All squash skin is edible (and a good source of fiber and vitamins A, C, and E), but some are tastier than others. Delicata, red kuri, and kabocha squashes are good choices to enjoy with the peel on. Others, like acorn and butternut squash, have a tougher, more fibrous skin that you may want to discard. It's easier to slip off the skins after roasting.*

CREAMY TOMATO SOUP

SERVES 4 AS A SIDE

2 tablespoons extra-virgin olive oil, plus more to finish

2 large garlic cloves, chopped (about 2 teaspoons)

Two 28-ounce (988 g) cans crushed or whole peeled tomatoes (preferably San Marzano)

1 cup (150 g) raw cashews

½ teaspoon kosher salt

Flaky salt (optional)

½ cup (10 g) fresh basil leaves, plus a few small leaves for garnish

Simmering cashews along with the canned crushed tomatoes softens them into an easily blended, creamy soup that provides healthy fats from the nuts and boosts the nutrition of the tomatoes.

1. Heat the oil in a medium saucepan over medium heat. Add the garlic and cook until golden, 1 to 2 minutes. Pour in the tomatoes, cashews, and kosher salt. Bring to a boil then reduce to a gentle simmer, stirring often. Cook until the liquid has reduced slightly and the cashews are softened, about 30 minutes.

2. Carefully transfer the soup to a blender (cover the lid with a kitchen towel to prevent splatters) and blend on low speed for 10 seconds, then work up to high speed until the soup is more orange than red and completely smooth, 2 to 3 minutes. Add the basil and blend for about 30 seconds.

3. To serve, divide among four bowls, drizzle with olive oil, and sprinkle with flaky salt (if using). Garnish with basil.

SCIENCE BITE:

COOKING TOMATOES BOOSTS LYCOPENE

Unlike many plant foods, tomatoes actually become more nutritious after cooking. The process of heating the tomato breaks down cell membranes and frees up more lycopene for the body to absorb. In fact, cooked tomatoes provide 62 percent more lycopene than eating the same amount raw. Lycopene, one of the most potent antioxidants in the carotenoid family of phytonutrients, is what makes tomatoes red. You can also boost your lycopene absorption by enjoying raw tomatoes along with a brain-friendly fat, like a drizzle of extra-virgin olive oil or a slice of avocado.

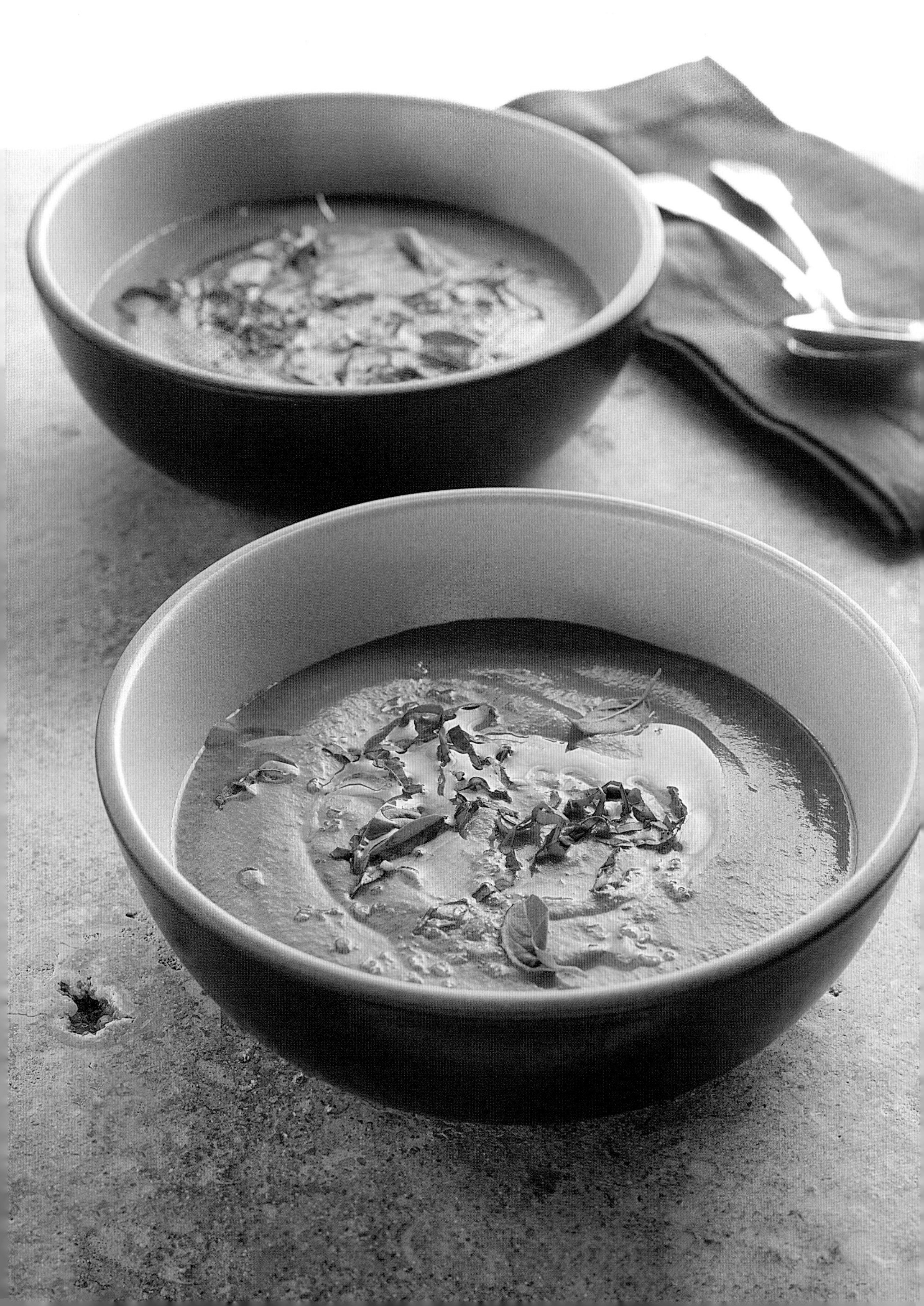

BUTTERNUT SQUASH AND COCONUT CURRY

SERVES 4 TO 6

1 cup (100 g) whole-grain red or brown rice, rinsed

One 13.5-ounce (398 ml) can unsweetened coconut milk

2 large red bell peppers (12 ounces/340 g total), diced (about 2 cups)

1 bunch scallions, white and light green parts thinly sliced

One 1-inch (2.5 cm) piece fresh ginger, grated (about 1 tablespoon)

2 large garlic cloves, minced (about 2 teaspoons)

2 to 4 tablespoons Thai red curry paste (more for a spicier curry)

4 cups (1 L) vegetable stock, chicken stock, or water

1 small butternut squash (about 1 pound/455 g), peeled, cut in half lengthwise, seeds removed, and cut into ½-inch (1.25 cm) half-moons

2 cups (230 g) thinly sliced kale leaves, fresh or frozen

2 tablespoons fish sauce

1 loosely packed cup (170 g) fresh cilantro leaves and tender stems, chopped, plus more leaves for garnish

¼ cup (60 ml) fresh lime juice

Lime wedges

Thanks to Thai red curry paste, a warming pot of deeply flavorful curry is a quick, brain-healthy dinner packed with tender winter squash and chewy rice. The secret to getting the sauce right is to use an abundance of aromatics—scallions, peppers, ginger, garlic—as the curry base. Coconut milk adds richness, and each bowl is packed with vegetables and lime juice for bright, fresh balance.

When delicata squash is in season, use it in place of the butternut; it's easier to prep, thanks to its edible, soft skin: no peeling required. The lazy cook in me also loves subbing in already peeled and cubed butternut squash from the grocery store (you'll need about 3 cups/225 g).

1. Bring a large pot of salted water to a rolling boil. Stir in the rice and let it boil, uncovered, until the grains are tender but still chewy, 25 to 35 minutes. Drain and return to the pot. Cover and set aside until the curry is done.

2. While the rice cooks, make the curry. Scoop 2 tablespoons of the coconut cream from the top of the can of coconut milk and melt it in a large pot over medium heat. Add the bell peppers, scallions, ginger, and garlic and cook, stirring often, until the vegetables are fragrant and soft, about 2 minutes. Add the curry paste and stir continuously until you have a smooth paste, about 1 minute. Slowly whisk in the remaining coconut milk and the stock. Increase the heat until the mixture is gently bubbling, then stir in the squash.

3. Reduce the heat to a gentle simmer, cover the pot, leaving the lid ajar, and cook, stirring often, until the squash is just tender, 22 to 30 minutes. Add the kale and cook until tender, about 5 minutes. Stir in the fish sauce and keep warm on the stove over low heat.

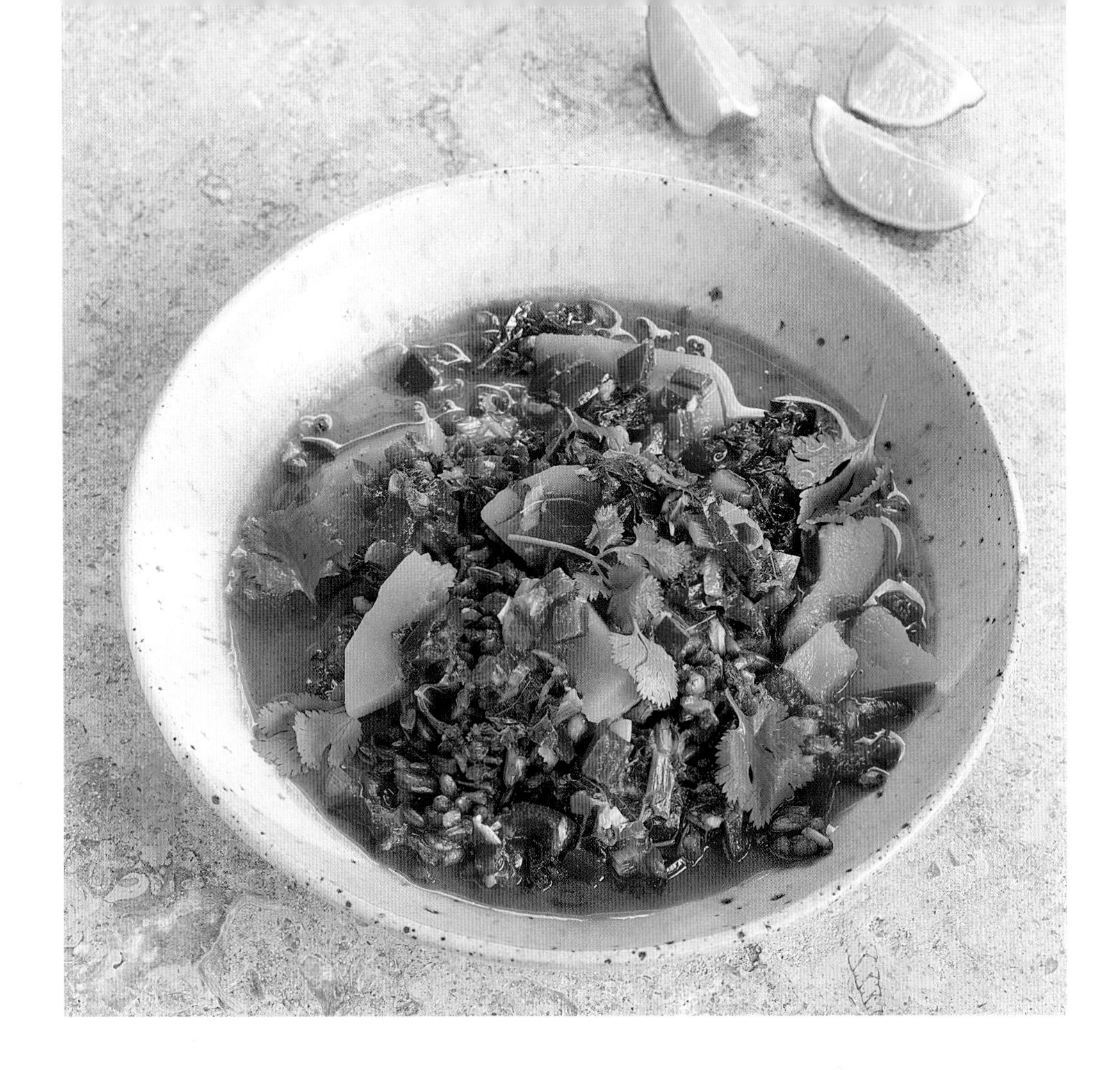

4. Just before serving, stir in the cilantro and lime juice. Scoop ½-cup (100 g) servings of rice into shallow bowls, spoon the curry over top, and sprinkle with cilantro leaves to garnish. Serve with lime wedges on the side.

TIP: *Cooking brown rice like pasta, as this recipe does, is quicker and more foolproof than the traditional absorption method. That's because you can sample the rice when it's almost done, as you would pasta, and avoid under- or overcooked grains. To cook brown rice the traditional way, bring 2½ cups (590 ml) water, 1 cup (100 g) brown rice, and ½ teaspoon salt to a boil. Reduce the heat to a low simmer, cover, and cook until tender but chewy, 50 to 60 minutes. Remove from the heat and let sit, covered, for 10 minutes, then fluff with a fork.*

MUSHROOM "BOLOGNESE" ON ZUCCHINI NESTS

SERVES 4 TO 6

1 cup (240 ml) boiling water

½ ounce (15 g) dried porcini mushrooms

3 medium zucchini (1 pound 5 ounces/ 595 g total), spiralized (about 6 cups) (see sidebar)

1 teaspoon kosher salt

¼ teaspoon freshly ground black pepper

2 tablespoons extra-virgin olive oil

1 large shallot (5 ounces/ 140 g), finely chopped (about ½ cup)

6 large garlic cloves, chopped (about 2 tablespoons)

12 ounces (340 g) mixed mushrooms, such as cremini, button, and shiitake, roughly chopped (about 6 cups)

2 tablespoons tomato paste

2 cups (480 ml) vegetable or chicken stock

1 cup (240 ml) dry white wine

2 teaspoons finely chopped fresh thyme, plus leaves for garnish

1 tablespoon white miso paste

Shaved Parmesan cheese (optional)

Mushrooms are an important part of a brain-healthy diet. Here you'll simmer different types of mushrooms in a Bolognese-inspired sauce, much like the traditional one, with lots of flavor boosters—aromatics, tomato paste, miso paste, and wine. The result is a lighter, quicker, and vegetable-focused sauce.

These "noodles" can be enjoyed raw or cooked. Swirl the zucchini into nests and bake them in the oven just enough to make the centers soft and the edges crispy. Or toss them raw with the hot sauce, to achieve the perfect consistency for a veggie noodle: tender with a toothsome bite.

1. Set an oven rack in the center position and preheat the oven to 350°F (175°C). Line a rimmed baking sheet with parchment paper.

2. Pour the boiling water over the dried mushrooms in a small bowl. Let steep for 15 minutes. Drain the mushrooms, reserving the soaking liquid, and coarsely chop when cool.

3. Meanwhile, assemble the zucchini nests. Scoop up about ½ cup (100 g) noodles at a time, then arrange into nine piles, or nests, on the prepared baking sheet. Sprinkle with ½ teaspoon of the salt and ⅛ teaspoon of the pepper, then drizzle with 1 tablespoon of the oil. Bake the nests for 10 to 12 minutes, until the zucchini noodles are soft and starting to brown around the edges.

4. Heat the remaining 1 tablespoon oil in a large skillet over medium heat. Add the shallot and the remaining ½ teaspoon salt and cook, stirring often, until the shallots are translucent, 4 to 6 minutes. Add the garlic, stirring until fragrant, about 30 seconds. Add the fresh mushrooms and cook, stirring often, until they are soft and starting to brown, 10 to 12 minutes.

continued

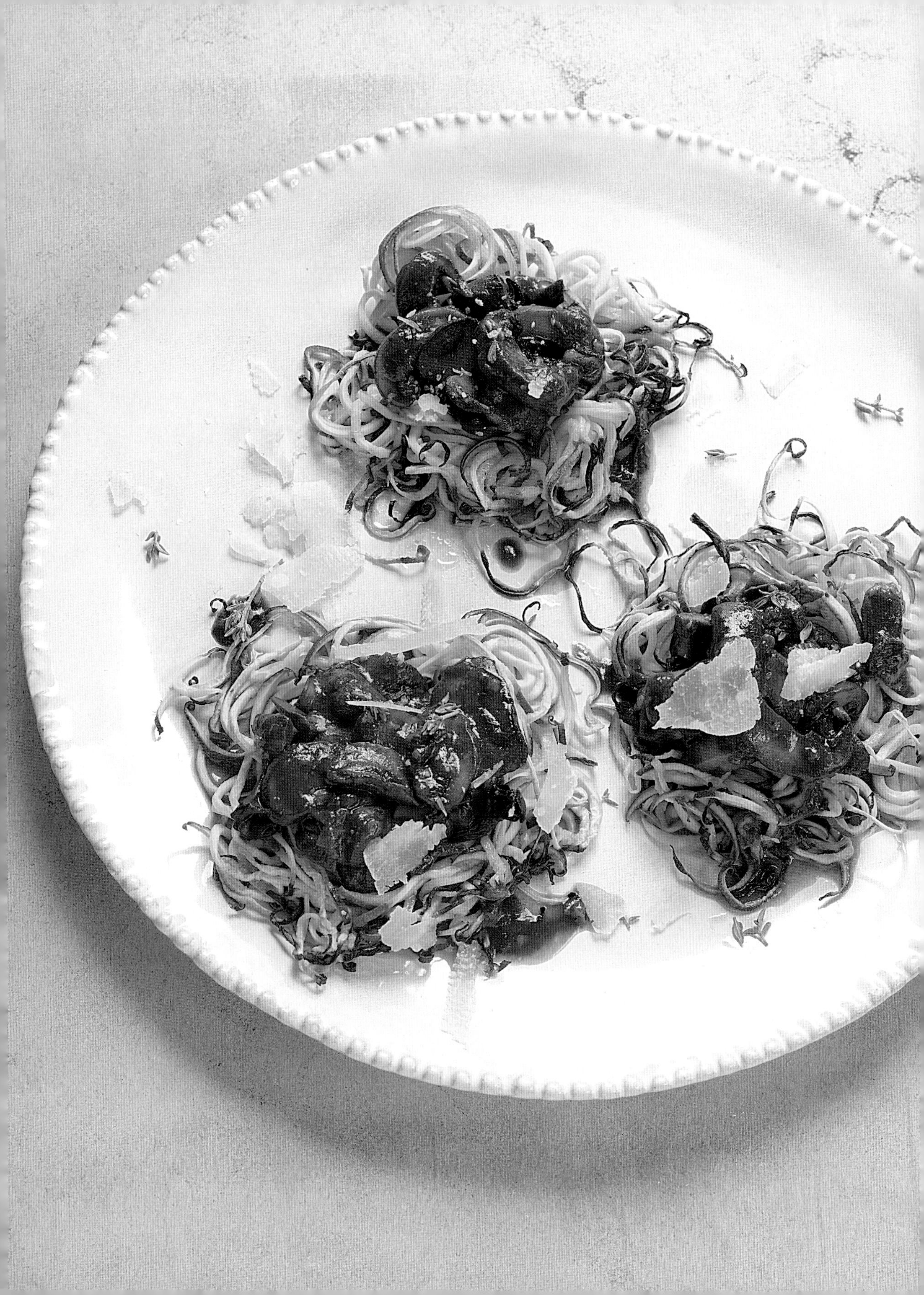

5. Push the mushrooms to one side of the pan and add the tomato paste to the other side. Pour in 2 tablespoons of the mushroom soaking water and whisk until smooth. Cook, stirring often, until the tomato mixture bubbles and thickens, about 2 minutes. Keeping the sautéed mushrooms to the side, stir in the rest of the mushroom soaking water plus the chopped soaked mushrooms, vegetable stock, wine, thyme, and remaining ¼ teaspoon pepper. Pull in the mushrooms from the side to mix with the sauce, then reduce the heat to a gentle simmer. Cook, stirring occasionally, until the sauce is reduced by half, about 30 minutes.

6. To finish the sauce, place the miso paste in a small bowl. Scoop out about ½ cup (120 ml) of the brothy part of the sauce and stir into the miso until no lumps remain. Pour the miso back into the sauce and stir to coat the vegetables. Cover the pot, turn off the heat, and let sit.

7. To serve, use a rigid spatula to transfer two or three nests to each plate. Make a well in the center of each one with a spoon and fill with ¼ to ⅓ cup (60 to 80 ml) mushroom sauce. Sprinkle with fresh thyme leaves and Parmesan, if using.

SPIRALIZING TIPS AND TRICKS

If you are new to spiralizing, zucchini are just the right shape and size to help you perfect the technique. Look for medium zucchini, about 6 to 8 inches (15 to 20 cm) long, that are straight, not curved. There's no need to peel. Trim off the stem and cut crosswise in half so you have two 3- to 4-inch (7.5 to 10 cm) pieces. Using a countertop spiralizer fitted with a "spaghetti"-shaped blade, place the cut end of the zucchini over the round blade and spiralize into noodle-shaped strands. Trim, if needed, with scissors into 6-inch (15 cm) strands.

Ready to branch out? Try spiralizing other vegetables:

- Potatoes and sweet potatoes: Make oven fries or savory waffles.
- Carrots: Toss into salads, stir-fries, and soups.
- Parsnips, turnips, rutabagas, celeriac: Toss with onions and roast in the oven as a bed for fish or chicken.
- Radishes and jicama: Tuck into tacos and salads.
- Kohlrabi: Use like noodles, raw or gently cooked. (Kohlrabi is like a cross between an apple and a parsnip.)

MUSHROOM AND WHITE BEAN SOCCA

MAKES 4

1 cup (115 g) chickpea flour

1½ cups (360 ml) water

⅓ cup (80 ml) extra-virgin olive oil

1 teaspoon kosher salt

¼ teaspoon freshly ground black pepper, plus more for serving

½ ounce (15 g) dried mushrooms, such as morels, shiitakes, or porcini (about ¼ cup)

1 tablespoon white miso paste

1 tablespoon grass-fed butter

½ pound (225 g) mushrooms, such as button, cremini, or a mix, sliced ½ inch (1.25 cm) thick

1 medium shallot (2½ ounces/70 g), thinly sliced (about ¼ cup)

½ cup (120 ml) unsweetened almond milk

1½ cups (275 g) white beans, such as cannellini or Great Northern, freshly cooked (page 215) or from one 15-ounce (425 g) can, rinsed

Microgreens

Socca is a thin, crêpe-like pancake served as a handheld snack in the south of France. Crispy on the outside and creamy on the inside, socca are made from protein-rich chickpea flour, so they are satisfying and naturally gluten-free, too. Here you'll load up thick socca with white beans, mushroom sauce, and miso butter before the batter finishes cooking.

Note that the batter has to sit at least 30 minutes before cooking, so if you're planning to make the recipe start to finish in one go, stir the batter together, then proceed with the rest of the ingredient prep. To get ahead on dinner, make and refrigerate the batter up to five days in advance.

1. Whisk together the flour, 1 cup (240 ml) of the water, 2 tablespoons of the oil, ½ teaspoon of the salt, and the pepper in a medium bowl. Set aside to let the flour hydrate and thicken, at least 30 minutes and up to overnight (tightly covered and refrigerated).

2. Preheat the oven to 250°F (120°C) and place a rimmed baking sheet on the center rack.

3. Place the dried mushrooms in a shallow bowl. Bring the remaining ½ cup (120 ml) water to a boil and pour over the mushrooms. Cover, allowing the mushrooms to steep, for about 5 minutes. Place a fine-mesh sieve over a measuring cup and pour the mushrooms and their liquid over top. Squeeze as much liquid as possible from the mushrooms and roughly chop the larger ones, leaving the small ones whole. Set the mushrooms and steeping liquid aside.

4. Stir together the miso paste and butter in a small bowl until no lumps remain; set aside.

continued

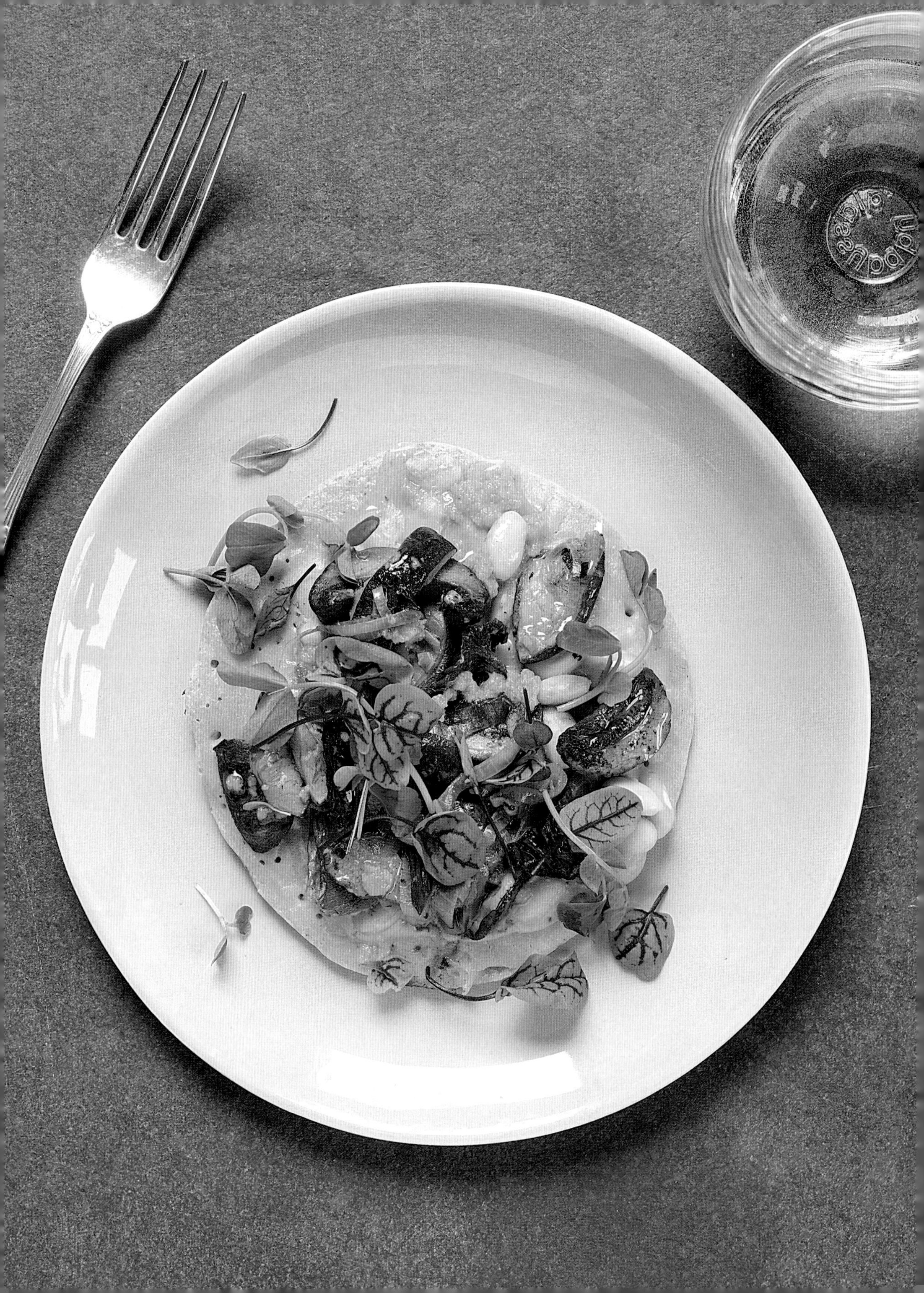

5. Warm 1 tablespoon of the oil in a medium skillet over medium heat. Add the shallots, sprinkle with ¼ teaspoon of the salt, and cook, stirring often, until soft and starting to brown, 5 to 7 minutes. Transfer to a plate and cover to keep warm.

6. Using the same skillet, warm 1 tablespoon of the oil over medium heat. Scatter the fresh mushrooms in the pan in an even layer, sprinkle with the remaining ¼ teaspoon salt, and cook, undisturbed, until starting to brown, 3 to 5 minutes. Add the shallots, reconstituted dried mushrooms, almond milk, and ½ cup (120 ml) of the mushroom steeping liquid. Cook over medium heat, stirring often, until the mushrooms are tender and the sauce starts to thicken, 5 to 7 minutes. Adjust the heat to its lowest setting and keep warm while you make the socca.

7. Warm a small nonstick skillet over medium-low heat with 1 teaspoon of the oil. Pour in ⅓ cup (80 ml) of the batter and swirl the pan until evenly distributed. Cook undisturbed until bubbles form on the surface of the batter, 1 to 1½ minutes. Scatter a heaping ⅓ cup (65 g) of the beans over the socca and cook until the center is set, another 1 minute. Top with ¼ cup (60 g) mushroom sauce and cook for another 30 seconds to warm through. Transfer to the baking sheet and keep in the oven while you cook the remaining socca. Repeat with the remaining batter; you should end up with four socca.

8. Transfer the socca to plates. Divide the miso butter evenly among the plates, and top with microgreens and more pepper, if you like.

BROCCOLI AND CAULIFLOWER FRITTERS WITH GARLICKY YOGURT AND TOMATOES

SERVES 4 TO 6

2 cups (1 pound/455 g) cherry tomatoes

2 tablespoons avocado oil

2 teaspoons fresh thyme leaves

1 teaspoon kosher salt

¾ teaspoon freshly ground black pepper

1 small head cauliflower (10 ounces/285 g), florets and stem chopped into 1-inch (2.5 cm) pieces

1 small head broccoli (10 ounces/285 g), florets and stem chopped into 1-inch (2.5 cm) pieces

1 egg, beaten

¼ cup (2 ounces/60 g) crumbled feta or goat cheese

¼ cup (30 g) oat flour, homemade (see sidebar on page 132) or store-bought

1 teaspoon ground cumin

2 medium garlic cloves, minced (about 1 teaspoon)

1 cup (240 ml) plain, unsweetened yogurt (coconut, whole milk, or nut-based)

2 tablespoons fresh lemon juice

Flaky salt (optional)

These easy, lacy-edged vegetable fritters are both tasty and brain healthy. The combination of two cruciferous vegetables—broccoli and cauliflower—will make these a welcome addition to your dinner rotation. While most vegetable fritters are heavy on binders like egg and cheese, these have just enough to achieve a comforting measure of richness while staying within the realm of brain-healthy quantities of dairy.

The patties will keep in the fridge for up to a day, so you can make them ahead of time and panfry just before eating. These fritters are versatile, too. Swap in goat cheese for the feta if you prefer. If you don't have oat flour, make these with another mild-flavored flour instead, such as chickpea or white whole wheat. Reheat leftover fritters in a microwave or conventional oven or on the stove and top with a fried egg for breakfast, or tuck them into whole-grain pitas (along with dollops of the addictingly good garlicky sauce) for a light lunch.

1. Set an oven rack in the center position and preheat the oven to 375°F (190°C). Line a plate with a paper towel.

2. Toss the tomatoes on a rimmed baking sheet with 1 tablespoon of the oil, the thyme, ¼ teaspoon of the kosher salt, and ¼ teaspoon of the pepper. Roast for 15 to 20 minutes, until the tomatoes are hot and starting to collapse. Set aside.

3. Meanwhile, place a steamer basket inside a large pot with a lid and fill with 2 inches (5 cm) of water. Add the cauliflower and broccoli and steam until soft, 10 to 12 minutes. Let sit in the steamer basket with the lid off to cool slightly.

continued

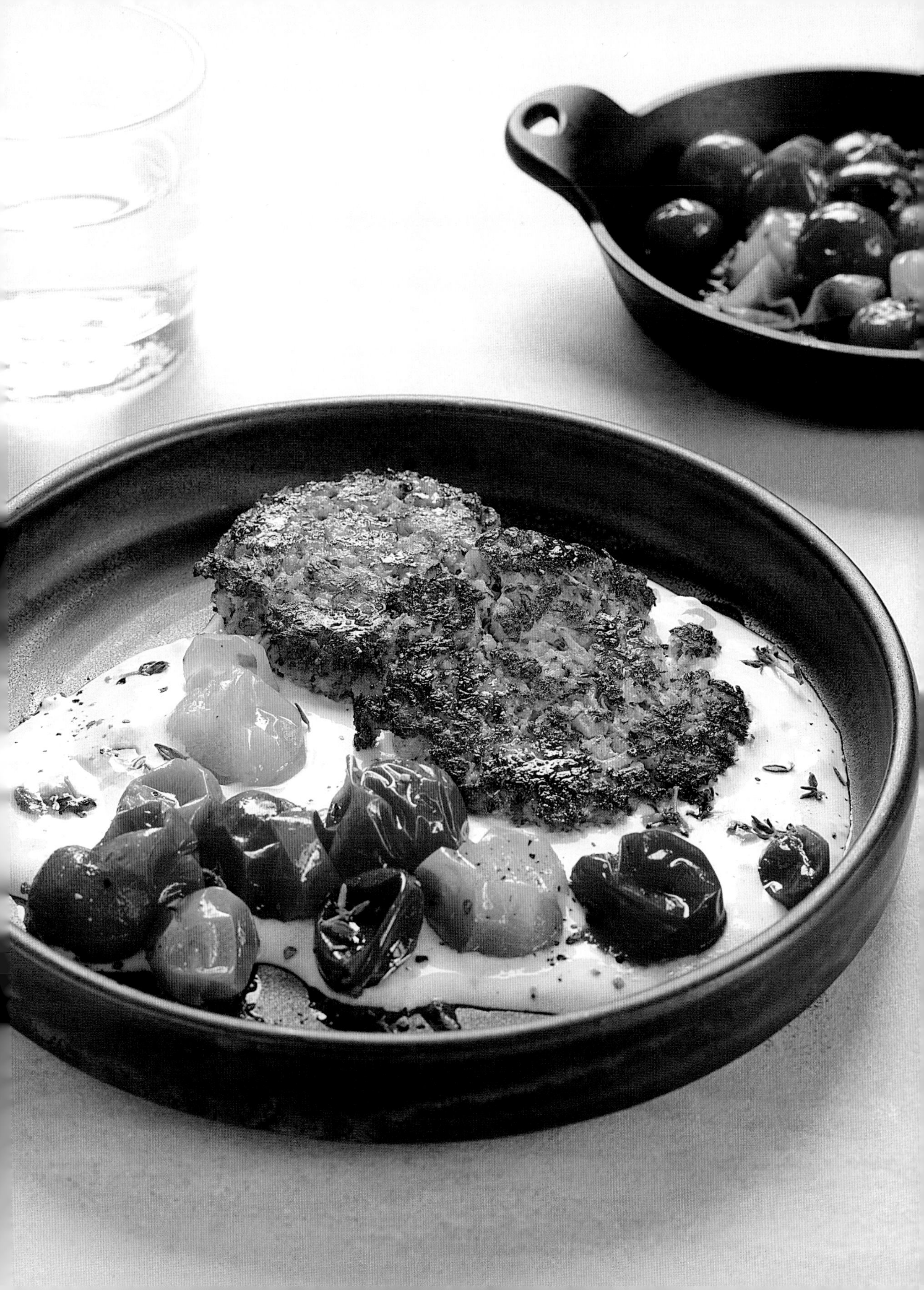

4. Combine the egg, feta, flour, cumin, half the garlic, ½ teaspoon of the kosher salt, and ¼ teaspoon of the pepper in a large bowl; stir to form a light batter. Add the broccoli and cauliflower. Use a potato masher or a large fork to mash the vegetables until they have a half-chunky, half-smooth consistency. Stir well until the vegetables are incorporated into the batter.

5. Heat the remaining 1 tablespoon oil in a large skillet over medium-high heat until shimmering. Working in batches, scoop ¼ cup (60 ml) of the batter, then compress it in your hands to make a patty. Carefully place in the oil, then repeat to cook four fritters at once, leaving about 2 inches (5 cm) of space between them and being careful not to overcrowd the pan.

6. Let the fritters cook undisturbed until browned on the bottom, 4 to 5 minutes. Flip the patties with a spatula and cook until browned on the second side, 2 to 3 minutes more. Transfer the fritters to the prepared paper towel–lined plate. Repeat with the remaining batter.

7. Stir together the yogurt, lemon juice, remaining garlic, remaining ¼ teaspoon kosher salt, and remaining ¼ teaspoon pepper in a small bowl.

8. To serve, divide the yogurt sauce between plates. Top with the fritters and roasted tomatoes, and flaky salt, if using.

MAKE YOUR OWN OAT FLOUR

It's easy to turn rolled oats (sometimes called old-fashioned oats) into a fiber-rich, gluten-free flour. Place oats in a blender and pulverize on medium-high speed into a powdery consistency, about 30 seconds. Fresh oat flour has a wonderful, nutty aroma and costs a fraction of what you'd pay at the grocery store—plus you can make as much or as little as you need. Blend 1½ cups (150 g) rolled oats to make 1 cup oat flour.

CAULIFLOWER AND KIMCHI FRIED RICE

SERVES 4

1 tablespoon avocado oil

2 medium carrots (8 ounces/230 g), scrubbed and diced into ¼-inch (6 mm) pieces (about 1 cup)

1 bunch scallions (2 ounces/ 60 g), thinly sliced, dark green parts reserved for garnish

2 large garlic cloves, minced (about 2 teaspoons)

One 12-ounce (340 g) bag frozen cauliflower rice (about 3¾ cups), or homemade (see sidebar)

1 cup (155 g) shelled edamame beans, frozen and thawed

2 tablespoons low-sodium soy sauce or tamari

4 eggs, lightly beaten

1 cup (150 g) cabbage kimchi, well stirred and roughly chopped, plus more for serving

½ cup (10 g) fresh cilantro leaves and tender stems, roughly chopped

1 avocado, sliced

Toasted sesame oil, for drizzling

If fried rice is a go-to one-pan supper in your house, I think you'll love this version using pebbly bits of cauliflower, or cauliflower "rice." Substituting cauliflower for actual white rice amps up the nutritional value, giving you twice as much fiber as well as a good dose of calcium, potassium, and sulforaphanes.

To make this dish brain healthier than traditional fried rice, you'll go easy on the oil and pack the dish with vegetables—carrots, scallions, edamame, and cabbage kimchi. An avocado on top adds a nice creamy contrast to the crisped cauliflower and spicy kimchi.

Lacto-fermented vegetables like kimchi are a wonderful addition to your brain-healthy eating because they may help cultivate a diverse collection of gut microbes, which are important for brain health. Typically made from napa cabbage, kimchi is a traditional food in Korean cooking, where it's used both as a condiment and as a key ingredient in recipes. Heady with garlic and spice, it can be mild or fiery: your choice. Look for kimchi in the refrigerated aisle of the grocery store, next to the tofu and jars of sauerkraut.

1. Warm 2 teaspoons of the avocado oil in a large skillet or wok over medium-high heat. Add the carrots and scallions and cook, stirring often, until the carrots are soft, 3 to 5 minutes. Add the garlic and cook until fragrant, about 30 seconds. Before opening the bag of frozen cauliflower rice, break up any large pieces with your hands. Then add the cauliflower rice and cook, stirring often, until soft and starting to brown, 4 to 6 minutes.

continued

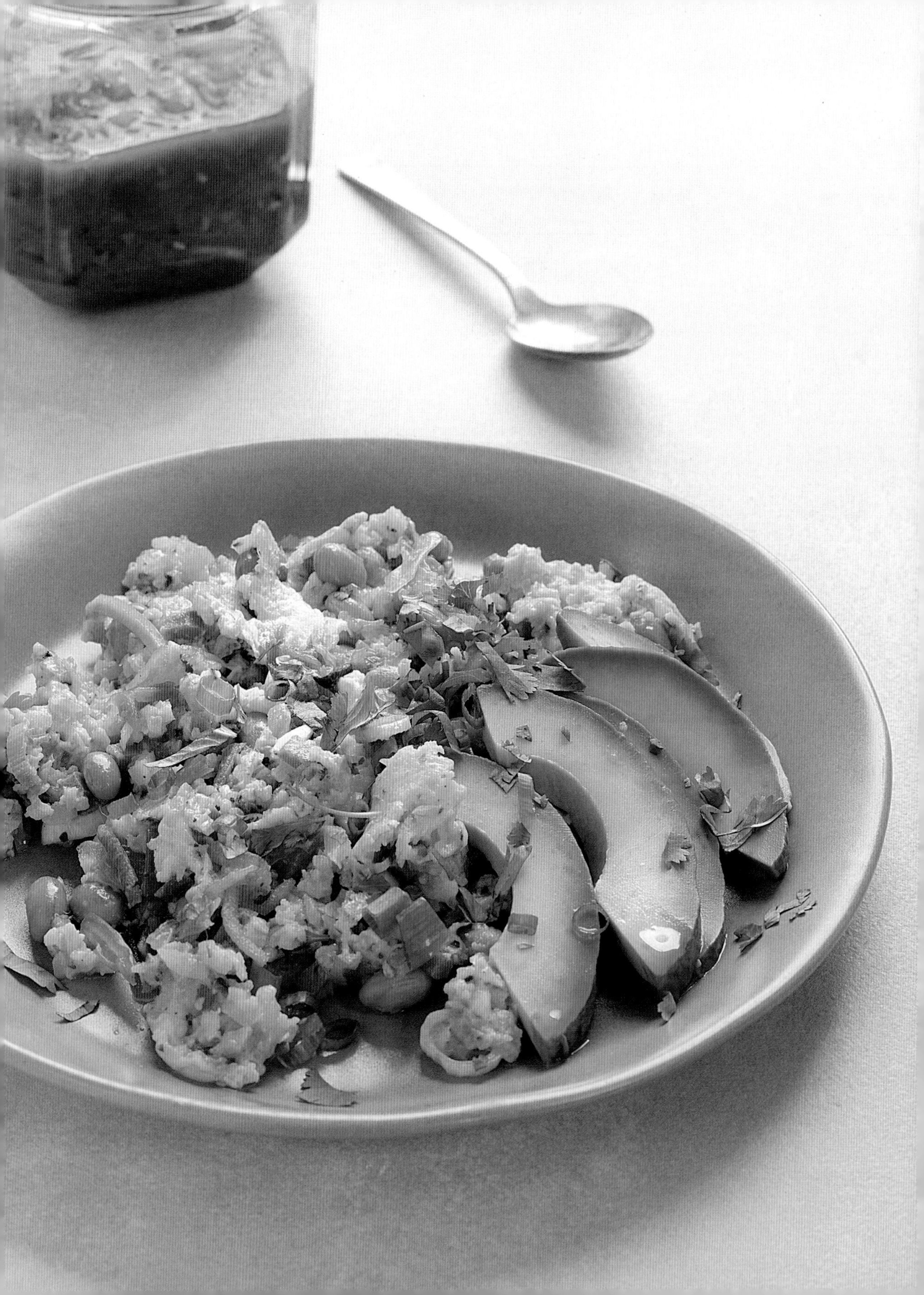

2. Stir in the edamame and soy sauce. Push the vegetables to one side of the pan; drizzle the other side with the remaining 1 teaspoon avocado oil, then pour in the eggs. Stir continuously, pulling the eggs from the edges toward the center until starting to set up, about 2 minutes.

3. Fold the eggs into the vegetables until evenly distributed throughout. Turn off the heat and stir in the kimchi and cilantro.

4. To serve, divide the cauliflower rice between shallow bowls, top with the avocado, add more kimchi (if you'd like), and drizzle with sesame oil.

MAKE YOUR OWN CAULIFLOWER RICE

You can make your own cauliflower rice quickly using a box grater or a food processor. You'll need one whole head of cauliflower. Using a sharp knife, separate the florets from the stalk. Trim and peel the stalk and cut into 2-inch (5 cm) pieces. Separate the florets into 2-inch (5 cm) pieces with your hands. Grate over the large holes of a box grater. Or, working in batches, place the cauliflower florets and stem in the bowl of a food processor, pulsing until the pieces are pebbly, roughly the size of Israeli couscous (a bit larger than rice). Leftover uncooked cauliflower rice keeps in an airtight container in the refrigerator for up to 3 days. To cook, sauté in a small amount of oil (like in this recipe), or steam in a pot fitted with a basket and filled with 1 inch (2.5 cm) of water over the stove for 3 to 5 minutes for tender "grains." To microwave, place in a bowl with 1 inch (2.5 cm) water, cover, and cook on high for about 3 minutes.

CRISPY CAULIFLOWER TACOS WITH CREAMY RED PEPPER SAUCE

SERVES 4

1 medium head cauliflower (1½ pounds/680 g), halved through the stem

2 teaspoons chili powder

½ teaspoon kosher salt

1 tablespoon avocado or extra-virgin olive oil

¼ cup (60 ml) water

1 cup (8 g) sugar snap peas, sliced diagonally

4 corn tortillas, warmed

Fresh cilantro leaves

Avocado, diced

Pickled jalapeños

1 lime, cut into 4 wedges

Tacos should be on regular rotation in your brain-healthy dinners—they're quick to make, fun to eat, and wonderful when packed with veggies. These cauliflower tacos get the crispy-creamy element just right with panfried slabs of cauliflower and a smooth roasted red pepper sauce. Heat lovers will relish the layers of spiciness, from the chili powder–dusted cauliflower and chipotle peppers in the sauce to the pickled jalapeños on top.

When purchasing tortillas, look for those made from non-GMO yellow corn, or corn in combination with other whole grains (like quinoa, wheat, or almond flour). Avoid any tortillas with added sugar (such as sucralose), unhealthy fats (hydrogenated palm or soybean oils), or other unfamiliar ingredients that sound like chemicals.

1. Cut the cauliflower into 3-inch (7.5 cm) cubes, each about ½ inch (1.25 cm) thick. Toss in a bowl with the chili powder and salt.

2. Heat a large nonstick skillet with a tight-fitting lid over medium heat. Add the oil, and when it starts to shimmer, add the cauliflower pieces, separating them so they do not touch. Once they become brown and crispy on one side, after about 3 minutes, flip them over. Cook until brown and crispy, then carefully pour the water into the skillet and cover. Remove from the heat and let the cauliflower steam in the pan for 1 to 2 minutes, or until easily pierced with a knife.

3. To build your tacos, divide the red pepper sauce, cauliflower, and peas between the tortillas. Top with cilantro, avocado, and a couple pickled jalapeños. Serve each plate with a lime wedge.

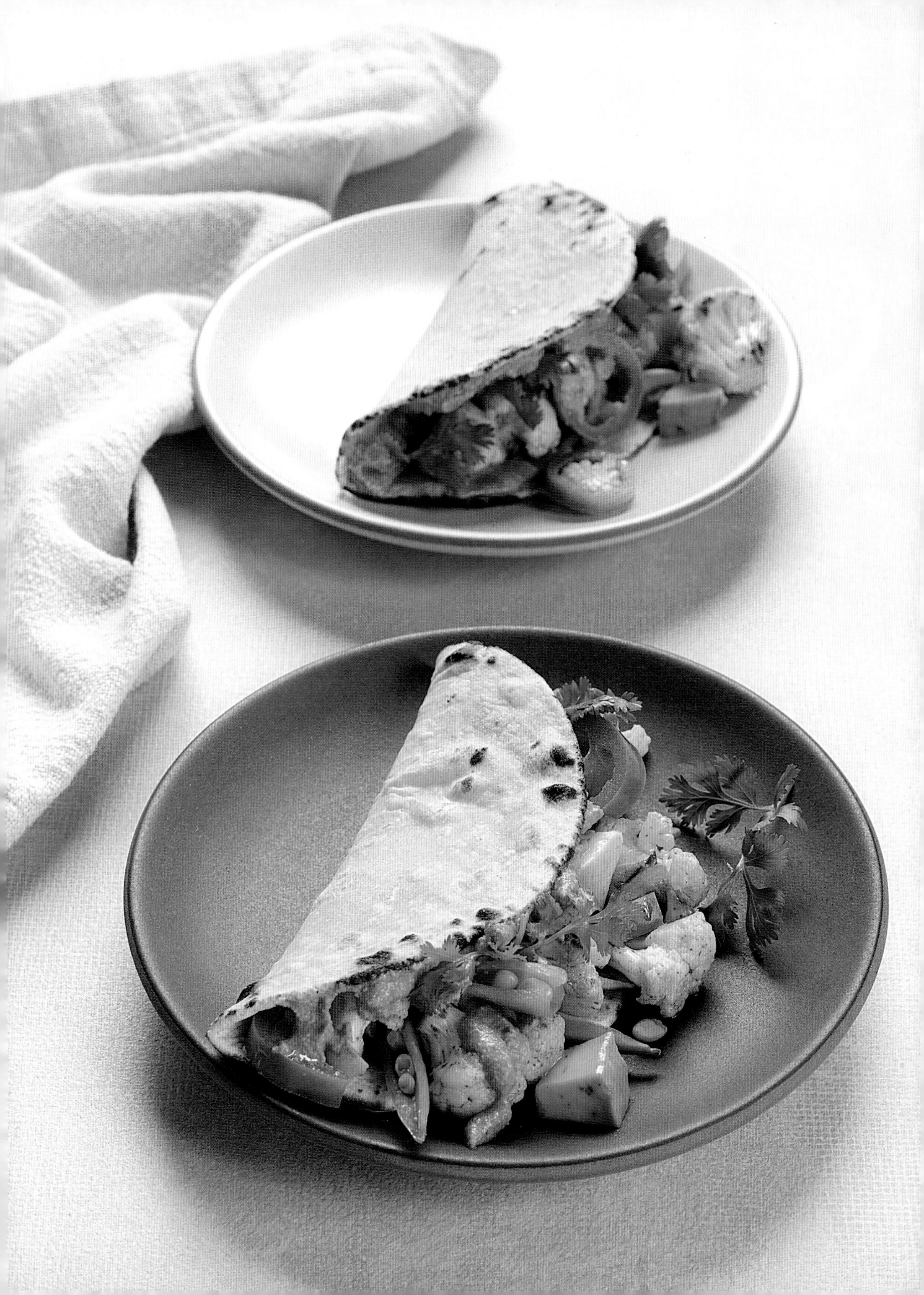

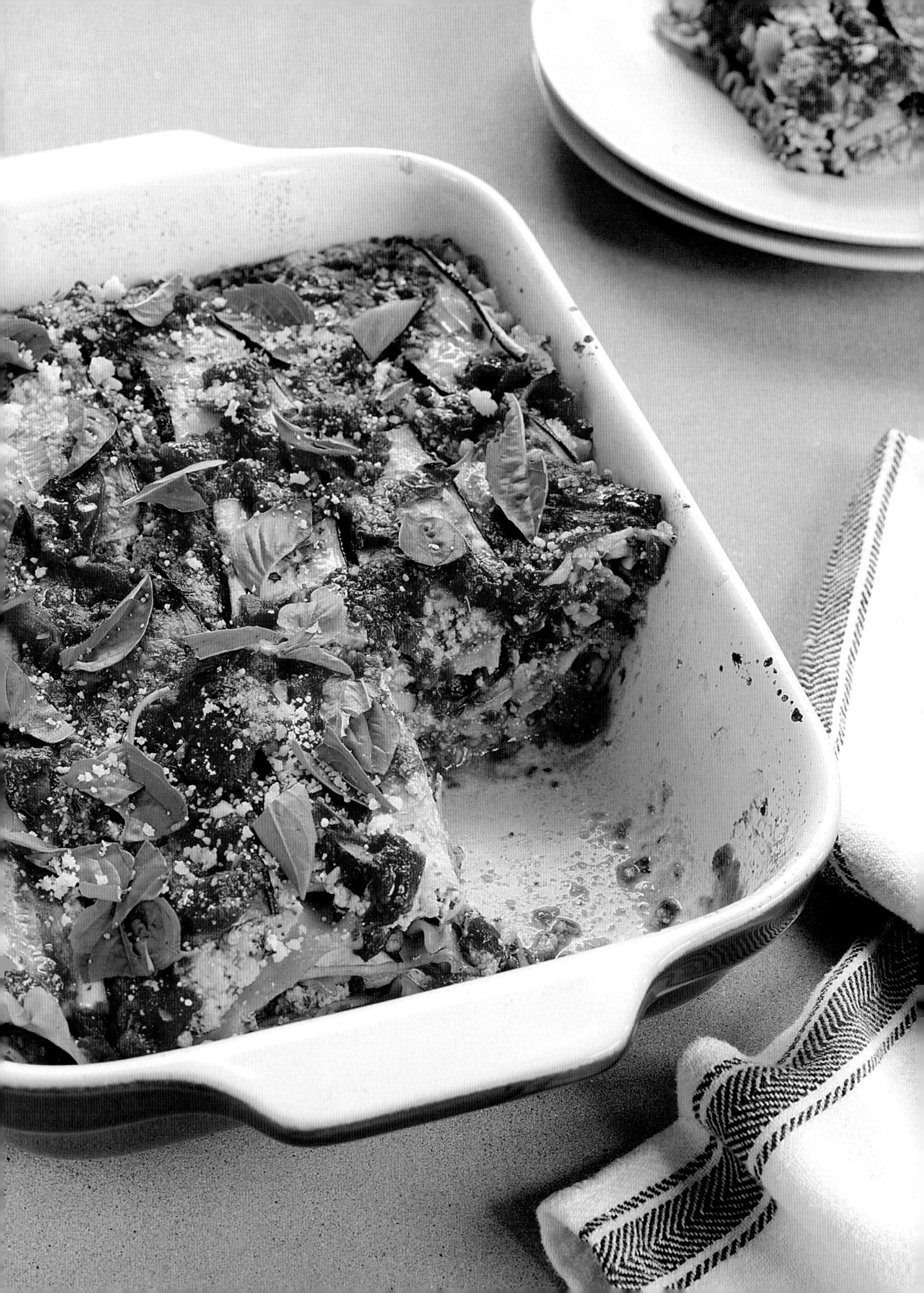

ZUCCHINI LASAGNA WITH SPINACH TOFU "RICOTTA"

SERVES 6

1 teaspoon dried oregano

1 teaspoon kosher salt

½ teaspoon crushed red pepper flakes

2 medium zucchini (14 ounces/400 g), cut in half through the middle then lengthwise into thin strips with a mandoline or sharp knife

2 tablespoons extra-virgin olive oil, plus more for the noodles

10 ounces (285 g) whole-grain, brown rice, or regular lasagna noodles (see Tips)

3 cups (750 g) Spinach Tofu "Ricotta" (recipe follows)

5 cups (1.2 L) marinara sauce, homemade (page 379) or from two 24-ounce (710 ml) jars (see Tips)

Fresh basil, torn

Grated Parmesan cheese (optional)

This vegetable-focused lasagna is both satisfying and fresh, thanks to some brain-healthy swaps to the old-school version. Crumbled tofu stands in for mozzarella, which, when amped up with plenty of lemon and garlicky sautéed spinach, creates a filling that tastes so much like ricotta you'd be hard-pressed to tell the difference. The result: an incredibly light lasagna with plenty of flavor.

You'll have a little extra marinara; spoon it over leftover lasagna.

1. Set oven racks in the upper- and lower-third positions and preheat the oven to 400°F (200°C). Line two baking sheets with parchment paper.

2. Stir together the oregano, salt, and red pepper flakes in a small bowl.

3. Place the zucchini in a single layer on the prepared baking sheets. Drizzle with the oil and flip each piece over to coat. Sprinkle 2 teaspoons of the oregano spice mix evenly over all the zucchini and bake for about 20 minutes, until soft in the middle and brown on the edges. Set aside eight or nine of the prettiest slices to top the lasagna.

4. Meanwhile, bring a large pot of salted water to a boil over high heat. Add the noodles, stirring occasionally, until the edges are soft but the center is still firm and white (about half the time the package recommends). Drain the pasta in a colander, drizzle with some oil, and toss to separate. See Tip (page 140).

5. Fill the bottom of a 9-by-13-inch (23 by 33 cm) baking dish with 1½ cups (360 ml) of the marinara. Lay a third of

the noodles in a single layer on top of the sauce. Dollop 1 cup (250 g) of "ricotta" over the noodles, spreading with a spoon to cover evenly. Working in the same direction as the noodles, layer a third of the zucchini on top of the ricotta. Repeat two more times each with 1 cup (250 ml) marinara, a third of the noodles, 1 cup (250 g) ricotta, and a third of the zucchini. Pour the remaining 1½ cups (360 ml) sauce over the top followed by the reserved zucchini. Sprinkle with the remaining ½ teaspoon oregano spice mix.

6. Cover the pan tightly with foil and bake for 45 to 55 minutes, until the lasagna is bubbling and the noodles are soft. Let the lasagna sit for about 10 minutes. Just before serving, sprinkle the top with basil and Parmesan, if using. Slice into 4-inch (10 cm) squares to serve.

TIPS: *Skip the dusting of Parmesan on top to make this recipe entirely dairy-free.*

My favorite gluten-free pasta (Jovial brown rice pasta) keeps its shape when baked. After boiling, be sure to lay the pasta out on a flat surface to keep it from curling up, then cover to keep from drying out.

You can streamline this dish by using marinara sauce from a jar and frozen spinach in the ricotta. When purchasing marinara, be sure to choose one that is low in sodium, added sugars, and saturated fats.

MORE USES FOR SPINACH TOFU "RICOTTA"

You'll find many uses for this lighter take on ricotta in savory dishes.

- Make zucchini rollatini—roasted zucchini slices smeared with the ricotta and rolled up, then baked in marinara.
- Use it in the Better-for-You Grilled Cheese Sandwich (page 118).
- Stuff into manicotti shells.
- Dollop on stuffed peppers.
- Tuck into an omelet with mushrooms.
- Smear on toasted whole-grain bread and top with roasted broccoli or olive-oil packed sardines.

SPINACH TOFU "RICOTTA"

MAKES 3 CUPS (750 G)

- **One 14-ounce (400 g) container extra-firm tofu, drained**
- **1 tablespoon extra-virgin olive oil**
- **2 large garlic cloves, minced (about 2 teaspoons)**
- **4 loosely packed cups (160 g) baby spinach or 10 ounces (285 g) frozen spinach**
- **½ teaspoon kosher salt**
- **¼ cup (15 g) nutritional yeast**
- **¼ cup (60 ml) fresh lemon juice**
- **1 heaping tablespoon lemon zest**

1. Spread a clean kitchen towel on a rimmed baking sheet and place the tofu on half the towel. Fold the towel over to cover the tofu and press out as much water as possible. Top with a second baking sheet and weight it with something heavy, such as a cast-iron pan or two large cans of tomatoes. Let the tofu sit at room temperature until drained of water, at least 20 minutes.

2. Meanwhile, if using fresh spinach, heat the oil in a large skillet over medium heat. Add the garlic and cook until starting to soften (but not changing color), about 30 seconds. Add the spinach, sprinkle with the salt, and cook, stirring often, until the spinach is wilted, 3 to 5 minutes. (Alternatively, if using frozen spinach, place in a bowl with ¼ cup/60 ml water and the garlic, cover, and microwave on high for 4 minutes. Drain, chop, and squeeze dry.) Transfer the spinach to the bowl of a food processor.

3. Unwrap the tofu and squeeze out as much water as you can; break into pieces with your hands and add to the processor with the nutritional yeast, lemon juice, and lemon zest. Pulse until the "ricotta" is smooth but with large flecks of green, 20 to 30 seconds.

4. Use immediately, or keep in the fridge in an airtight container for up to 3 days. Drain off any water that accumulates, if needed, before using.

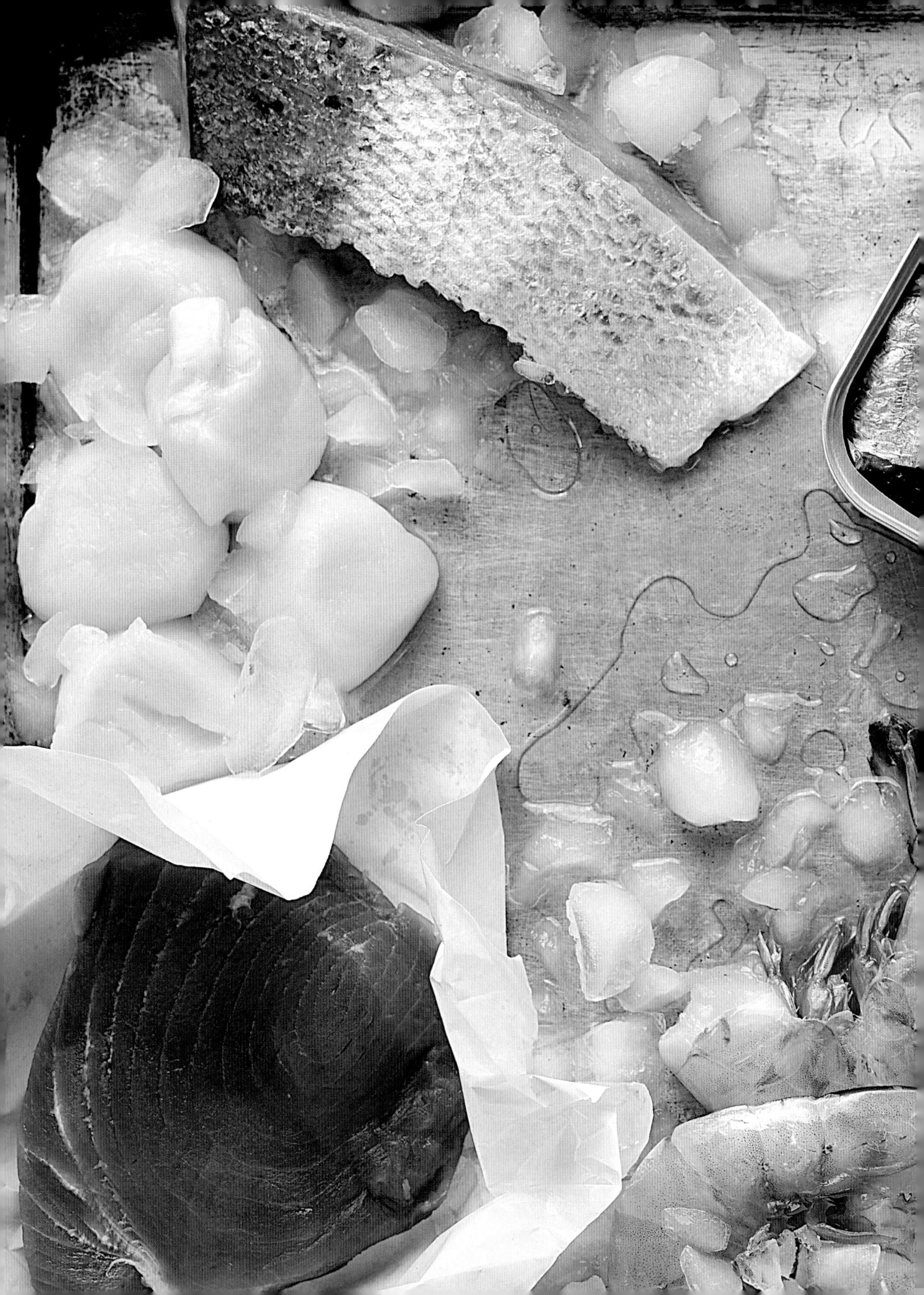

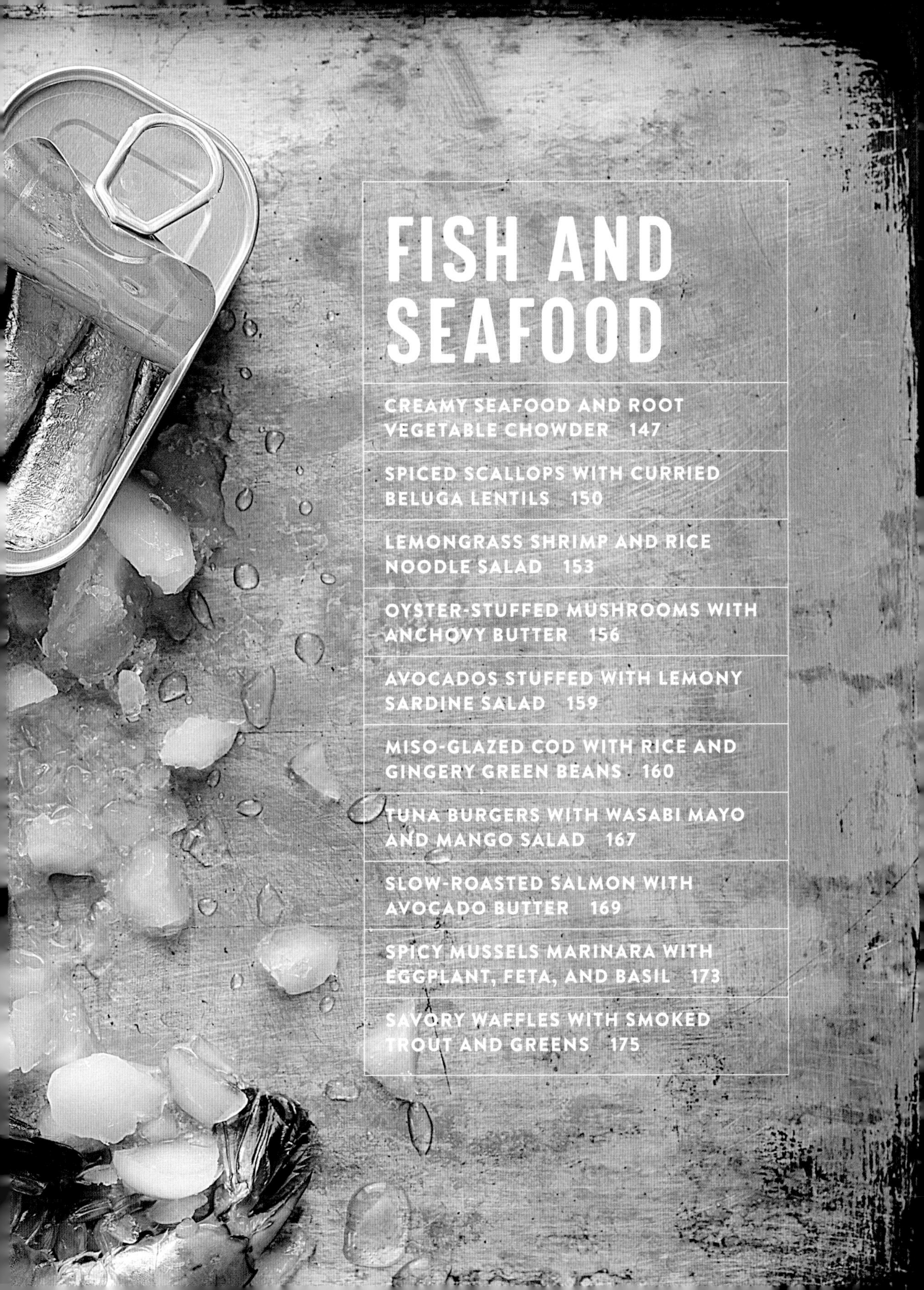

FISH AND SEAFOOD

Fish and seafood are considered good-for-the-brain foods because of the connection between vital compounds found in fish—like omega-3 fatty acids—and brain health. Over the past twenty-five years, dozens of studies have shown seafood's brain-specific benefits. Fish eaters perform better on memory tests and experience less cognitive decline when compared to those who eat less fish. And people who enjoy fish on a regular basis are less likely to develop Alzheimer's disease.

One reason is this: fish and seafood provide the two types of omega-3 fatty acids)—DHA (docosahexaenoic acid) and EPA (eicosapentaenoic acid)—that are crucial for brain health. They're considered particularly critical because the body doesn't produce this type of fatty acid; you must get it from food, primarily fish and seafood. The brain requires these particular omega-3s to repair and build brain cells throughout life.

Besides DHA and EPA, other key brain health nutrients are found in fish and seafood, like selenium, vitamin D, and vitamin B12. Arguably the single most important vitamin for brain health, B12 is essential for building the myelin sheath that protects nerve cells.

If you already enjoy fish and seafood as part of your brain-healthy way of eating, this chapter is packed with recipes that will help you increase the variety of seafood you consume. Just like with eating plants, it's important for brain health to mix it up. Eating a variety of seafood—bivalves, crustaceans, little fish, oily cold-water fish, and freshwater fish—ensures you will get enough of the key brain health nutrients they offer. Adding bivalves like oysters, scallops, clams, and mussels into your seafood rotation, for instance, ensures you get enough vitamin B12. A deficiency in B12 can lead to depression, cognitive impairment, and peripheral nerve disease. Cold-water fish, like salmon and arctic char, excel at providing DHA. And by choosing fish low on the food chain, like sardines and anchovies, you get a whole package of nutrients and brain-healthy fats while alleviating the intense demand for larger fish like tuna that are hard to source sustainably.

So if you already love making tuna fish salad, for example, try a brain-healthier upgrade using canned sardines in the Avocados Stuffed with Lemony Sardine Salad (page 159). If shrimp is your go-to, you'll love the Lemongrass Shrimp and Rice Noodle Salad (page 153). If cooking fish intimidates you, the ease of making mussels (page 173) at home might surprise you.

BRAIN-FRIENDLY COOKING TECHNIQUES

The beneficial DHA, EPA, and vitamin D in fish are stored in their fat—that's why cold water oily fishes, like wild-caught salmon and arctic char, are especially good for your brain. But if your fish is grilled over high heat or seared in a very hot pan, those delicate nutrients seep out. Frying fish and seafood not only destroys beneficial fats, it also racks up advanced glycation end products (AGEs), damaging by-products of high-heat cooking (see page 280). It's far better to cook fish and seafood with gentle, lower-heat methods.

Don't worry; you can still enjoy crispy, delicious fish with brain-friendly cooking techniques. When grilling, use a low, indirect heat. Even better, protect the fish and seafood with a barrier from the heat—a cedar plank, sheet pan, or grill basket work well. Avoid searing your fish over high heat in a pan. If you gently braise instead, your fish will not only cook up perfectly flaky and

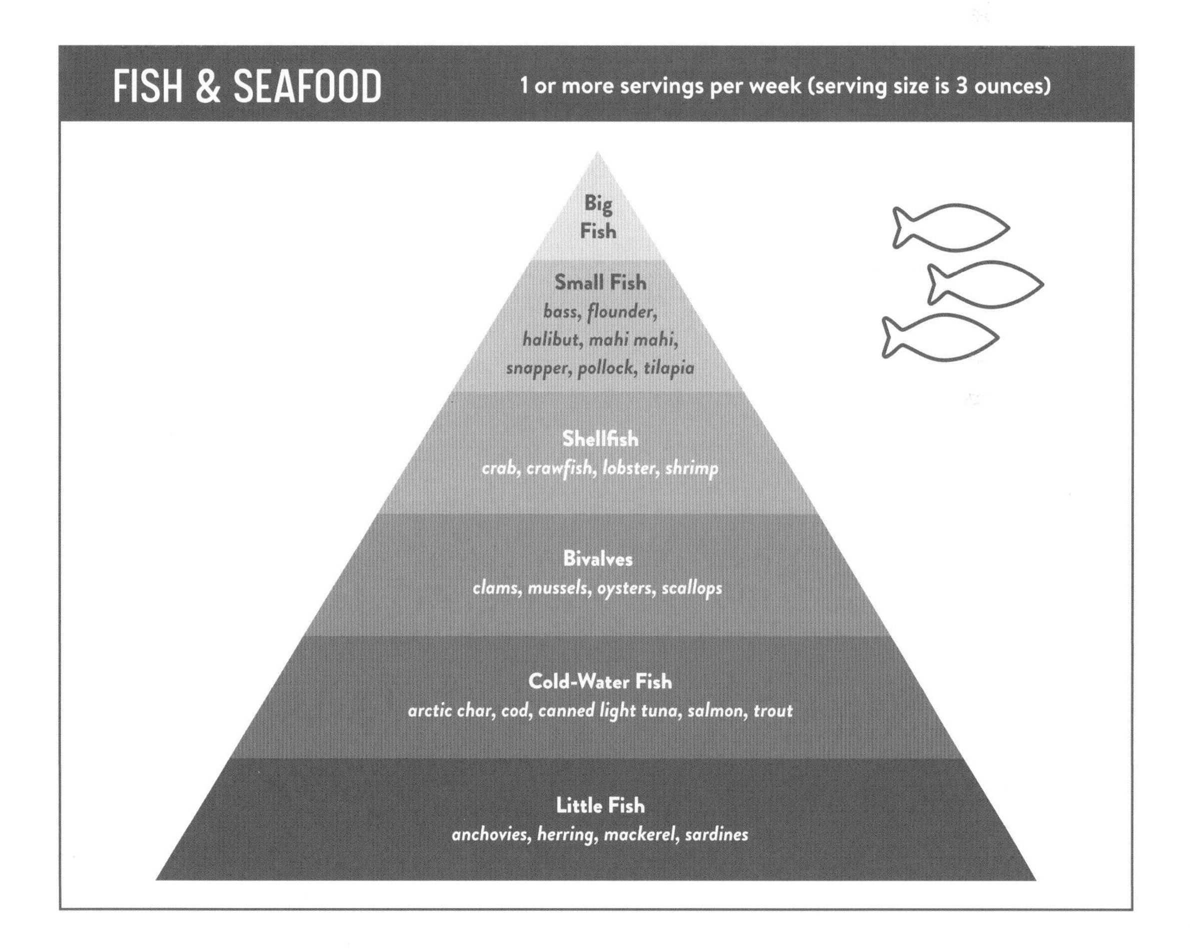

tender, it will retain its brain-boosting nutrients. Or try a low temperature "slow roast"—an incredibly easy, hands-off preparation.

While you should limit fried food—especially fried fish and seafood—in a brain-healthy diet, you can get a similar crispy result by pan-frying or roasting. Use a coating of nuts (as in the Pumpkin Seed Crusted-Salmon on page 192) or breadcrumbs (see the Panfried Cod with Collard Greens and Crispy Lemons on page 99), to serve as a layer of protection from the heat.

A SIMPLE STRATEGY FOR CHOOSING FISH AND SEAFOOD

Many home cooks find buying and preparing seafood confusing, and the stakes can feel high since quality fish is expensive. Questions abound. Should you choose wild-caught or farmed fish? (See page 152.) Fresh or frozen? (Frozen is often best. Most of the fish at the fish counter, unless you live near the sea, has been frozen and defrosted.) Alaska or Atlantic? (Alaska has particularly high standards for harvesting fish sustainably so is almost always a good choice; fish and seafood from the Atlantic vary tremendously.) Does organic designation mean anything with seafood? (Don't bother looking for a certified organic label; the US Department of Agriculture has not yet set these standards for aquatic species. If you find a fish labeled "organic," it is probably farmed fish from Europe.) And if you think quality seafood is out of reach financially, consider tinned fish, especially sardines, anchovies, and mackerel (learn more on page 148).

Purchasing seafood means balancing the immense health benefits with other concerns like exposure to environmental toxins. On one hand, you want to provide your brain with the type of fish and seafood rich in DHA and EPA. On the other, you want to protect your brain from exposure to mercury, a known neurotoxin that accumulates in certain species. In addition, the health of our oceans is in a precarious state, so you want to make sure your fish and seafood choice won't contribute to the depletion of that delicate ecosystem.

Some fish (like anchovies, American shrimp, and mussels) are a better choice than others—for brain health, planetary health, and your grocery bill. See pages 164 and 165 to understand which fish you can eat often and which fish should be enjoyed less frequently.

CREAMY SEAFOOD AND ROOT VEGETABLE CHOWDER

SERVES 4 TO 6

2 pieces bacon

1 tablespoon extra-virgin olive oil

1 small onion (8 ounces/ 230 g), finely chopped (about 1 cup)

4 cups (1½ pounds/680 g) mixed root vegetables, peeled, cut into ½-inch (1.25 cm) pieces

1½ teaspoons smoked paprika

1 teaspoon kosher salt

½ teaspoon freshly ground black pepper, plus more for serving

4 cups (1 L) unsweetened almond, cashew, or oat milk

10 ounces (285 g) cooked clams, canned and rinsed or frozen

One 3- to 4-ounce (90 to 120 g) can mussels

1 tablespoon fresh marjoram leaves, plus more for garnish

One 10-ounce (280 g) fillet white flaky fish (such as halibut, cod, or monkfish)

If you get in the habit of stocking your pantry with different kinds of tinned seafood, this hearty chowder comes together quickly. Mussels packed in extra-virgin olive oil have a fresh, briny quality and retain all the nutrient density of fresh mussels. Here they form the backbone of flavor for this chowder along with clams and a smoky paprika. This recipe allows you flexibility to include a variety of root vegetables; I like a mix of celery root, carrot, and sweet potato.

You may notice that this is the only recipe in the book that includes bacon. Yes, bacon! Cooked up crisp and crumbled atop the finished dish as a condiment, a small amount goes a long way. Because bacon is a processed meat that has been associated with health problems, it's meant to be enjoyed infrequently, if at all, in a brain-healthy diet. Feel free to omit the bacon. Your seafood chowder will still be delicious, but you may need to adjust the salt in the finished dish.

1. Place the bacon in a large pot over high heat and cook, stirring often, until crispy and brown, 4 to 6 minutes. Drain off the fat, crumble into small pieces, and set aside as a topping for the chowder.

2. Reduce the heat to medium, add the oil and onion to the pot, and cook, stirring often, until the onion is translucent, 5 to 7 minutes. Add the root vegetables, paprika, salt, and pepper. Stir to coat the vegetables with the spices and cook until the vegetables are soft, 5 to 7 minutes.

continued

3. Add the milk and bring to a low simmer (do not let it boil, or the milk may separate). Cook, stirring occasionally to make sure nothing sticks to the bottom of the pan, until you can easily pierce the vegetables with a knife, 12 to 18 minutes.

4. Stir in the clams, mussels (along with any oil, if olive oil–packed), and marjoram. Bring the chowder back up to a gentle simmer and place the fish on top. Cover the pot with the lid ajar and cook until the fish easily flakes with a fork, about 6 minutes. Flake and stir the pieces into the pot.

5. To serve, divide the chowder between bowls, then sprinkle the reserved bacon over top along with marjoram and pepper, if you like.

BUYING TINNED SEAFOOD

Peruse the canned fish aisle at the supermarket and you'll find some of the most affordable, tasty, and healthful fish in the sea. And because they are low on the food chain, these tiny fish are more sustainable, too. Skip the canned shrimp and crab (better purchased at the seafood counter), but stock up on light tuna, little fishes, and bivalves. The little fishes—anchovies, sardines, herring, mackerel—provide good doses of DHA and EPA. Bivalves like mussels, oysters, and clams are some of the richest sources of vitamin B12. Be sure to check the sodium content, especially in smoked seafood, which you should avoid if on a low-sodium diet. Rinsing your canned seafood before eating or cooking helps somewhat, since much of the salt is in the oil or water used to pack the can.

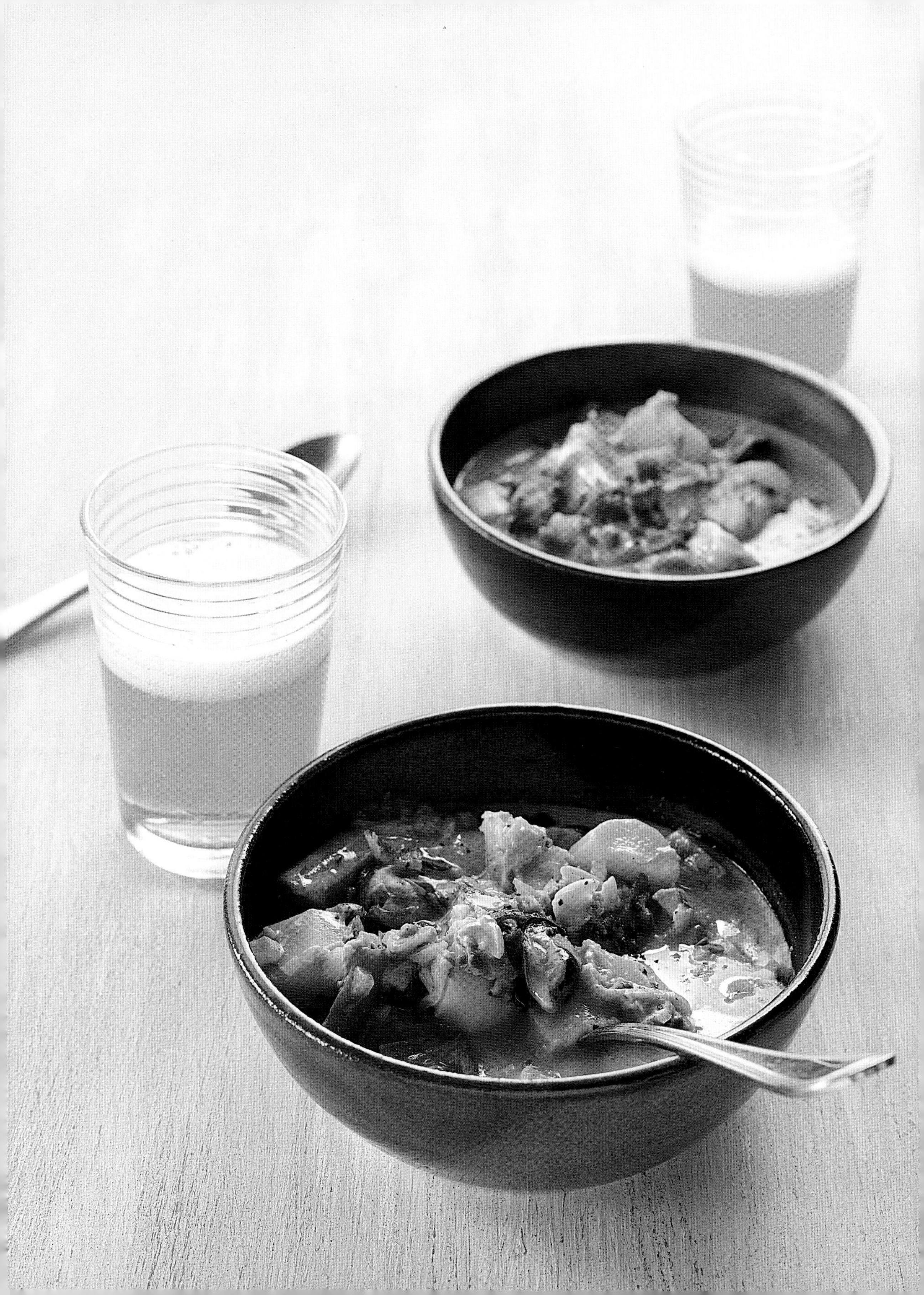

SPICED SCALLOPS WITH CURRIED BELUGA LENTILS

SERVES 4

2 tablespoons avocado oil

1 tablespoon curry powder

¾ teaspoon kosher salt

½ teaspoon freshly ground black pepper

1 large garlic clove, minced (about 1 teaspoon)

One 13.5-ounce (398 ml) can unsweetened coconut milk

¾ cup (180 ml) water

1 cup (200 g) black beluga or French green lentils, rinsed

2 teaspoons ground ginger

2 teaspoons ground turmeric

1 bunch scallions (4 ounces/115 g), white and light green parts thinly sliced

2 pounds (910 g) sea scallops (about 18 total), patted dry (see Tip)

5 loosely packed cups (200 g) baby spinach

Flaky salt (optional)

Scallops are a home run for brain health. They're low in mercury and rich in omega-3 fatty acids, vitamin B12, selenium, zinc, and a full set of amino acids. And it doesn't take much time or effort to turn fresh scallops into a satisfying meal. In fact, the less you do to them, the better. Here they get a dusting of ground ginger and turmeric before being briefly seared and served on a bed of coconut milk–braised lentils with wilted spinach. Black beluga lentils hold their shape nicely after cooking, but easier-to-find green lentils (sometimes called French or du Puy) work just as well.

1. Warm 2 teaspoons of the oil in a large pot over medium heat. Stir in the curry powder, ½ teaspoon of the kosher salt, and ¼ teaspoon of the pepper and cook, stirring constantly to avoid burning, until the oil is golden and fragrant, about 30 seconds. Add the garlic and continue to cook for another 30 seconds. Whisk in the coconut milk and water and bring to a boil. Stir in the lentils, then reduce the heat to a gentle simmer. Cook with the lid ajar, stirring often to make sure nothing sticks to the pot, until the lentils are tender, 20 to 25 minutes. Cover and set aside.

2. Stir together the ginger, turmeric, and the remaining ¼ teaspoon each kosher salt and pepper in a small bowl. Add the scallops and toss to coat.

3. Heat 1 teaspoon of the oil in a large nonstick skillet over medium-high heat. Add the scallions and cook, stirring often, until soft and brown on the edges, about 2 minutes. Scrape into a small bowl. Add the remaining 1 tablespoon oil to the pan, heat until just shimmering, then carefully place the

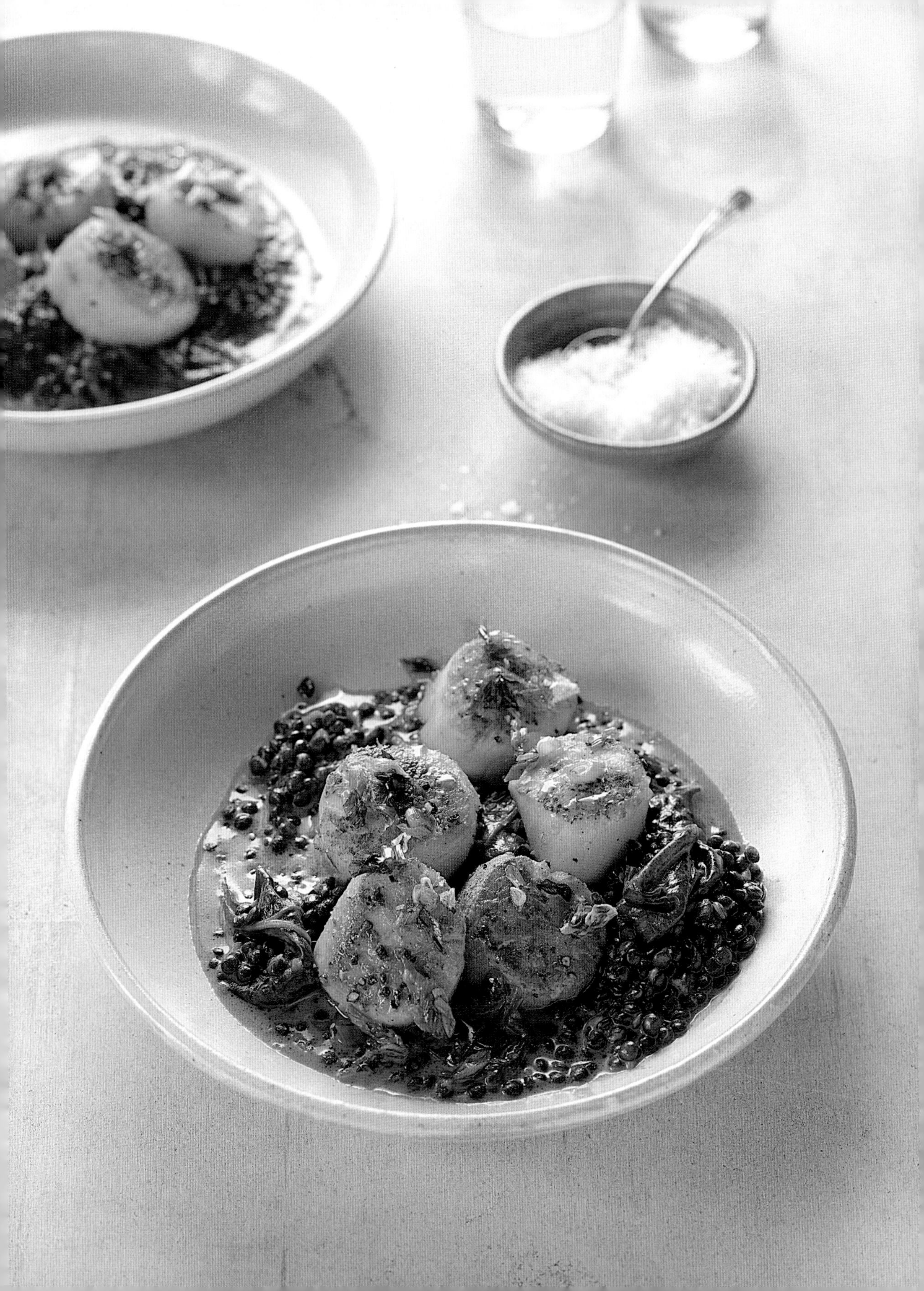

scallops in a single layer. Cook, undisturbed, until the scallops are golden brown on the bottom, about 3 minutes. Turn them over and cook on the other side for 2 minutes until golden brown.

4. Fold the spinach into the lentils, allowing the warm lentils to wilt the leaves slightly. To serve, divide the lentils and spinach between shallow bowls. Top with the scallops, sprinkle with the scallions, and finish with flaky salt, if using.

TIP: *Purchase scallops fresh from the seafood counter of your grocery store or fishmonger and cook them the same day. Fresh scallops are pearly white to beige and have a clean, briny aroma. Avoid any that are bright white, which means they may have been packed in water and absorbed excess weight. For this dish, look for sea scallops—the large variety sometimes referred to as U-10 (meaning up to 10 per pound). You could also use bay scallops (the tiny ones) or diver scallops, which are medium-size, but keep an eye on them when searing as they will be done faster.*

WILD-CAUGHT VS. FARMED

Wild-caught seafood is usually—but not always—a better choice than farmed. That's because wild fish tend to have more of the brain-friendly omega-3s (like DHA) and less saturated fat. Farmed salmon, for example, has three times the saturated fat of wild-caught salmon, as well as about 50 percent more calories. Although wild fish may harbor environmental pollutants, farmed fish can have alarming levels of pollutants, depending on the method of farming. Farmed mussels, oysters, and clams are an exception; advances in cultivating these bivalves have progressed to the point that these farms actually improve the oceans where they live. When shopping for fish—wild or farmed—always question the source, either by reading the small print on the package or asking the person behind the fish counter. If it's unclear, consult the Monterey Bay Aquarium Seafood Watch website (or phone app; see Resources, page 390), which constantly evaluates which fish are plentiful enough to consume and whether their fishing or farming methods cause harm to habitats or other wildlife.

LEMONGRASS SHRIMP AND RICE NOODLE SALAD

SERVES 4

- **¼ cup (60 ml) fresh lime juice**
- **¼ cup (60 ml) rice vinegar**
- **1½ to 2 teaspoons sambal oelek (Indonesian fresh chili paste)**
- **½ pound (225 g) Forbidden Rice noodles (or thin, pad Thai–style rice noodles)**
- **1 tablespoon avocado oil**
- **1 large shallot (5 ounces/140 g), finely chopped (about ½ cup)**
- **3 tablespoons finely chopped lemongrass, pale, tender centers only**
- **One 1-inch (2.5 cm) piece fresh ginger, grated (about 1 tablespoon)**
- **3 large garlic cloves, chopped (about 1 tablespoon)**
- **1 pound (455 g) medium shrimp (about 30), peeled and deveined (see Tip)**
- **3 medium carrots (12 ounces/340 g), shaved into ribbons with a vegetable peeler**
- **2 loosely packed cups (80 g) tender lettuces (butter, Bibb, or baby romaine), torn into bite-size pieces**
- **2 cups (60 g) chopped fresh mixed herbs (mint, basil, and cilantro leaves), plus more for garnish**
- **½ cup (70 g) raw peanuts, roughly chopped**
- **Lime wedges**

Think of this fresh and crunchy salad as a cross between shrimp pad Thai and a spicy noodle salad. Although I love traditional pad Thai, with its stir-fried noodles and tangy tamarind sauce, at home I am more likely to go light on the noodles and heavy on the vegetables. This dish is especially good with Forbidden Rice noodles, a purple-black variety made from anthocyanin-rich Forbidden Rice (aka black). If you can't find it, use regular rice or brown rice noodles instead.

There's really no substitute for the intense, citronella-like aroma and flavor that fresh lemongrass adds to the shrimp. In a pinch, you can get by using lemongrass paste in a tube (use 2 tablespoons paste for 3 tablespoons freshly chopped). The good news is, most grocery stores now carry fresh lemongrass stalks. Look for them in the produce section next to the ginger.

1. Stir together the lime juice, vinegar, and 1½ teaspoons of the sambal oelek (more if you prefer a spicier dish) in a large bowl. Set aside, reserving 2 tablespoons of the dressing to drizzle on the finished dish.

2. Bring a large pot of water to a boil. Add the noodles and cook, stirring occasionally until tender, 5 to 6 minutes. (Or follow the package directions, as some rice noodles will cook by soaking in hot water.) Drain well, add to the bowl with the dressing, toss, and set aside.

3. Heat the oil in a large nonstick skillet over medium heat. Add the shallot, lemongrass, and ginger and cook until the shallot is translucent, 5 to 7 minutes. Add the garlic and the shrimp, stir to coat with the lemongrass mixture, and cook until the shrimp are just pink on both sides, about 4 minutes total. Turn off the heat and set aside.

continued

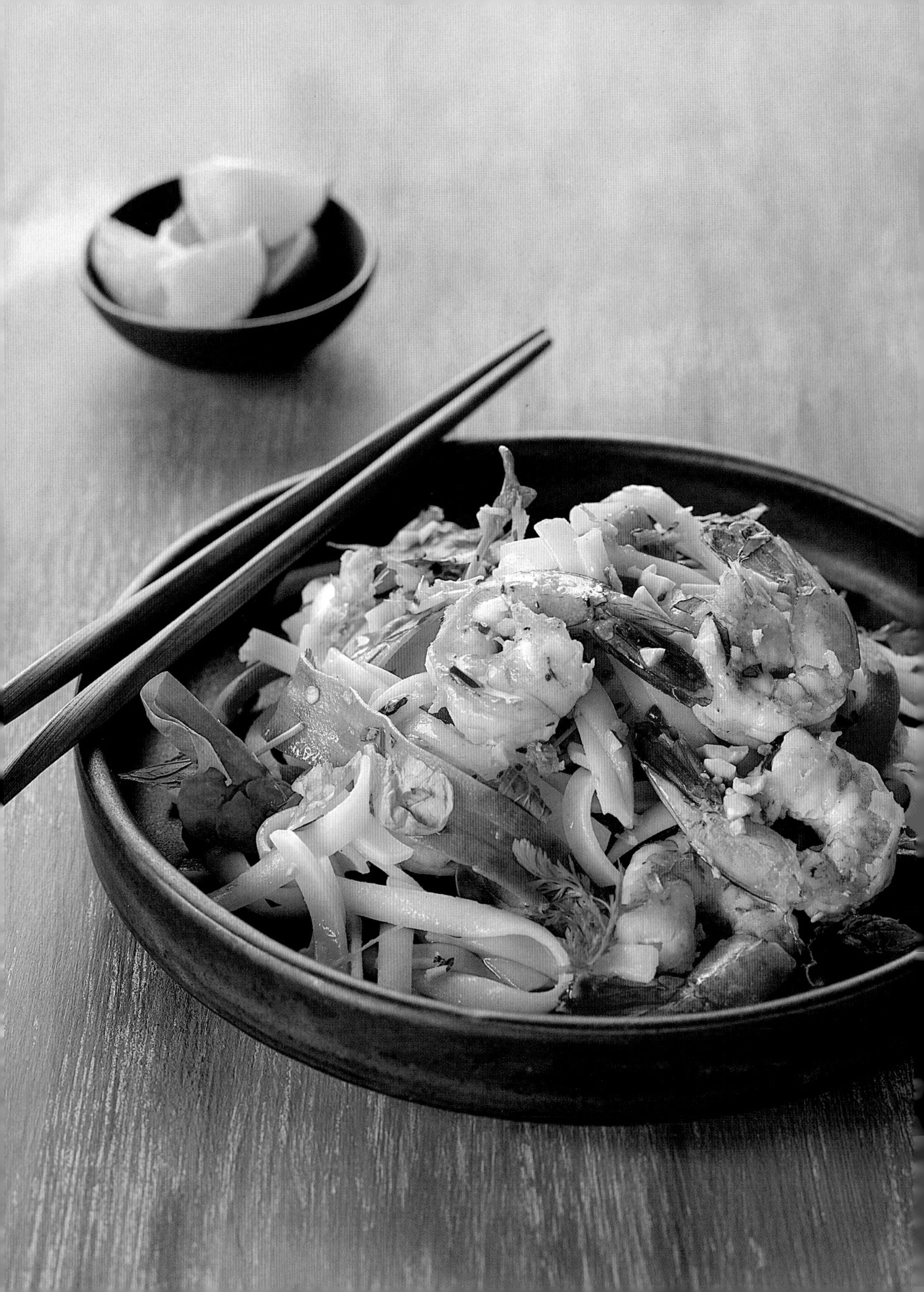

4. Add the carrots, lettuce, and herbs to the bowl of noodles. Toss well and divide among shallow bowls. Top with the shrimp, then sprinkle with the peanuts and more herbs. Just before serving, drizzle with the reserved dressing. Serve warm, at room temperature, or chilled, with lime wedges alongside.

TIP: *When purchasing shrimp, look for American wild-caught shrimp. Shrimp imported from other countries is more likely to be contaminated with environmental toxins, fraudulently labeled, and the result of unethical labor practices. If purchasing frozen shrimp at the grocery store, look for peeled, tail-on shrimp for the best product. Cleaning the shrimp of its innards takes only a minute and ensures your shrimp will be safe to eat. Just take a sharp knife along the back and under the belly and remove any dark-colored debris. Or ask the fishmonger at the grocery store to clean them for you. As for canned shrimp: don't buy it. Most is imported from countries with questionable farming practices and heavy use of antibiotics.*

SCIENCE BITE:

ASTAXANTHIN IN SHRIMP

Shrimp is rich in the antioxidant astaxanthin, a member of the carotenoid family of nutrients. Animal studies have documented that astaxanthin exerts impressive neuroprotective effects on cognition and memory. Its antioxidant power is active right where the brain is most vulnerable to amyloid deposition—in the hippocampus. Scientists hope to prove that getting enough astaxanthin in the diet has the same neuroprotective properties in human brains, and it is being evaluated as a possible therapeutic agent for Alzheimer's and Parkinson's diseases. Besides shrimp, crab and scallops are also rich in astaxanthin.

OYSTER-STUFFED MUSHROOMS WITH ANCHOVY BUTTER

SERVES 8 TO 12 AS AN APPETIZER

- **1 pound (455 g) medium-size button or cremini mushrooms (about 24)**
- **1 tablespoon extra-virgin olive oil**
- **¼ teaspoon kosher salt**
- **¼ teaspoon freshly ground black pepper, plus more to finish**
- **4 to 5 anchovy fillets, preferably packed in olive oil, finely chopped, or 2 teaspoons anchovy paste**
- **4 tablespoons unsalted butter, at room temperature**
- **1 large garlic clove, minced (about 1 teaspoon)**
- **1 tablespoon fresh lemon juice**
- **One 3- to 4-ounce (90 to 120 g) can small smoked oysters, drained and coarsely chopped**
- **2 tablespoons finely chopped fresh flat-leaf parsley leaves**
- **2 tablespoons finely chopped roasted red bell pepper (from a jar)**
- **¼ cup (30 g) panko breadcrumbs**

These petite mushroom caps are packed with big flavor thanks to a combination of smoky oysters, roasted red peppers, and umami-rich anchovy butter. This recipe offers an alternative to the cheese-and-cracker party staple. Making a double batch is a good idea because they always get devoured, even by people who aren't fond of oysters and anchovies. And while stuffed mushrooms are irresistible little party bites, you could also serve them with a side salad for a light dinner.

1. Set an oven rack in the center position and preheat the oven to 400°F (200°C). Line a baking sheet with parchment paper.

2. Separate the mushroom caps from the stems, reserving the stems for another use (like stock, page 374). Arrange the mushroom caps on the baking sheet with the stem side facing up. Drizzle with the oil and sprinkle with the salt and black pepper. Set aside.

3. Mash together the anchovies, butter, garlic, and lemon juice in a medium bowl. Fold in the oysters, parsley, roasted pepper, and 2 tablespoons of the breadcrumbs. Divide the stuffing evenly between the mushroom caps (about 1 heaping teaspoon each, depending on their size) and press it gently with your fingers. Top with the remaining 2 tablespoons breadcrumbs. Bake for 15 or 20 minutes, until the tops are golden brown. (For a crunchier topping, broil for 5 minutes just before serving.)

4. Just before serving, top each mushroom with more black pepper, if you like.

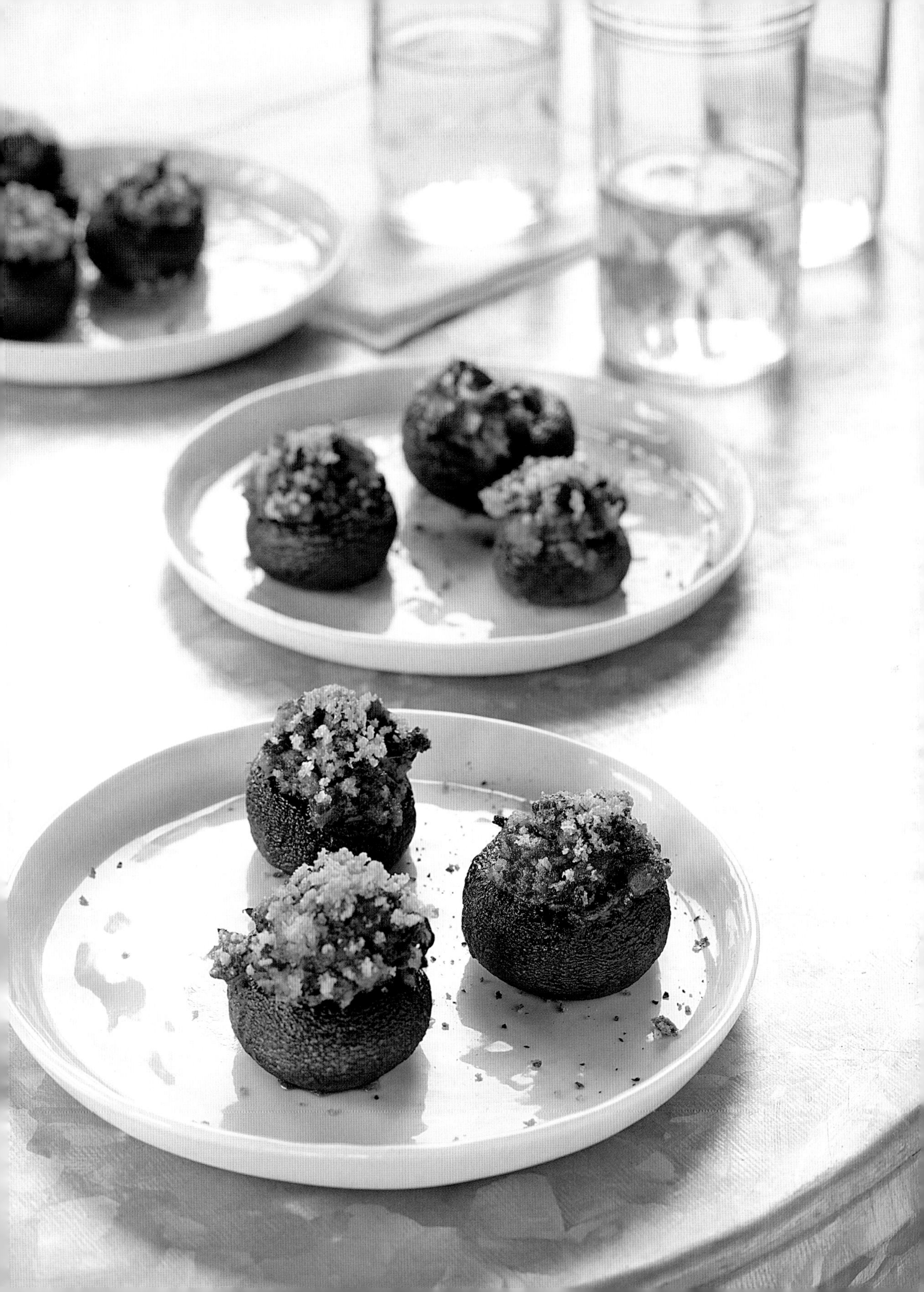

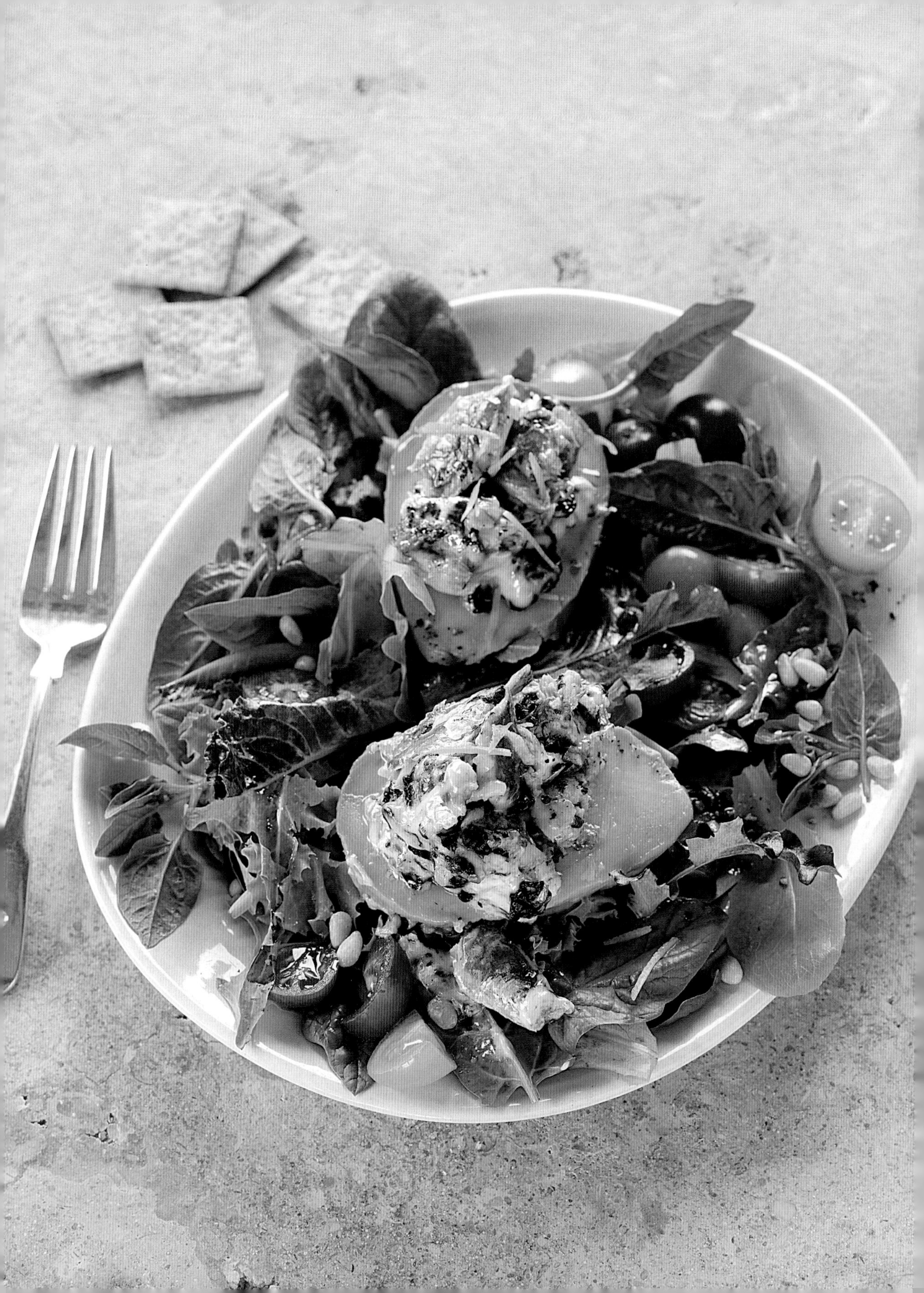

AVOCADOS STUFFED WITH LEMONY SARDINE SALAD

SERVES 4

- Two 4-ounce (120 g) cans boneless, skinless oil- or water-packed sardines, preferably wild-caught, drained
- ¼ cup (40 g) dried currants or golden raisins
- ¼ cup (60 ml) fresh lemon juice
- 2 tablespoons vegan mayo or Almost Instant Cashew Cream (page 370)
- 1 tablespoon lemon zest
- 1 medium garlic clove, minced (about ½ teaspoon)
- ½ teaspoon kosher salt
- ¼ teaspoon freshly ground black pepper
- 3 tablespoons extra-virgin olive oil
- 5 loosely packed cups (200 g) mixed baby greens
- 1 medium tomato (6 ounces/170 g), diced, or 1 cup (170 g) cherry tomatoes, halved
- 4 avocados, halved
- ½ cup (60 g) pine nuts, lightly toasted
- Flaky salt (optional)
- Whole-grain crackers, for serving

Here's an easy dish to bring you into the tinned seafood fold (or convince you to swap sardines for tuna if you're already a fan). Canned sardines beat tuna when it comes to brain health: they have more omega-3s per serving, more calcium, potentially less mercury exposure, and (in my opinion) better flavor. Scooping the salad into halved avocados adds not only a touch of nostalgia but turns the salad into a satisfying and attractive meal.

1. Place the sardines in a small bowl and break them up into pieces with a fork. Toss with the currants, 2 tablespoons of the lemon juice, the mayo, lemon zest, garlic, ¼ teaspoon of the kosher salt, and the pepper. Set aside.

2. For the dressing, stir together the oil, remaining 2 tablespoons lemon juice, and remaining ¼ teaspoon kosher salt in a small bowl.

3. Toss the greens, tomato, and half the dressing in a large bowl. Divide between four plates and place two avocado halves alongside. Fill each avocado with 2 tablespoons of sardine salad and drizzle with the remaining dressing. Sprinkle with the pine nuts, flaky salt (if using), and more pepper, if you like, and serve with whole-grain crackers.

MISO-GLAZED COD WITH RICE AND GINGERY GREEN BEANS

SERVES 4

1 cup (210 g) brown rice

1 tablespoon avocado oil

1 medium shallot (2½ ounces/70 g), finely chopped (about ¼ cup)

12 ounces (340 g) green beans, trimmed (about 4 cups)

One 1-inch (2.5 cm) piece fresh ginger, grated (about 1 tablespoon)

1 cup (240 ml) rice vinegar

1 cup (240 ml) dry sake

2 teaspoons pure maple syrup

¼ cup (75 g) white miso paste

½ cup (120 ml) warm water

Four 4- to 6-ounce (115 to 170 g) Atlantic or black cod fillets

Pickled ginger, thinly sliced

2 tablespoons unhulled sesame seeds, black, white, or a mix, toasted

This recipe is inspired by the famous miso-marinated black cod by chef Nobu Matsuhisa. I've streamlined the dish so that it takes no more than thirty minutes, start to finish, and upped the brain health virtue of the sauce by significantly reducing the sugar and salt. The cooking method here—a gentle poaching in the caramel-like sauce—is also more brain friendly because the low heat helps preserve the cod's omega-3 fatty acids, vitamin D, and vitamin B12, all of which seep out or go up in smoke with high-heat cooking.

White miso paste is a key ingredient here, adding both earthy flavor and body to the sauce. Sometimes called sweet miso or kyoto shiro miso, it is made from fermented soybeans and rice. Find it in the refrigerated section near the tofu at the grocery store.

1. Bring a large pot of salted water to a boil. Add the rice and stir. Boil, uncovered, until the rice is chewy and tender, 28 to 32 minutes. Drain in a colander, then return to the pot. Cover the pot and set it away from the heat.

2. Meanwhile, heat the oil in a large skillet over medium-high heat. Add the shallot and cook, stirring often, until translucent and starting to brown, 5 to 7 minutes. Add the green beans and ginger and cook until the beans are just starting to soften, about 5 minutes. Set aside in the pan.

3. Combine the vinegar, sake, and maple syrup in another large skillet and bring to a boil over high heat. Reduce the heat to a gentle simmer and cook until the sauce coats the back of a spoon, 15 to 20 minutes. Whisk the miso paste into the warm water until smooth, then whisk the mixture into the sauce. Keeping the sauce at a gentle simmer, nestle the cod

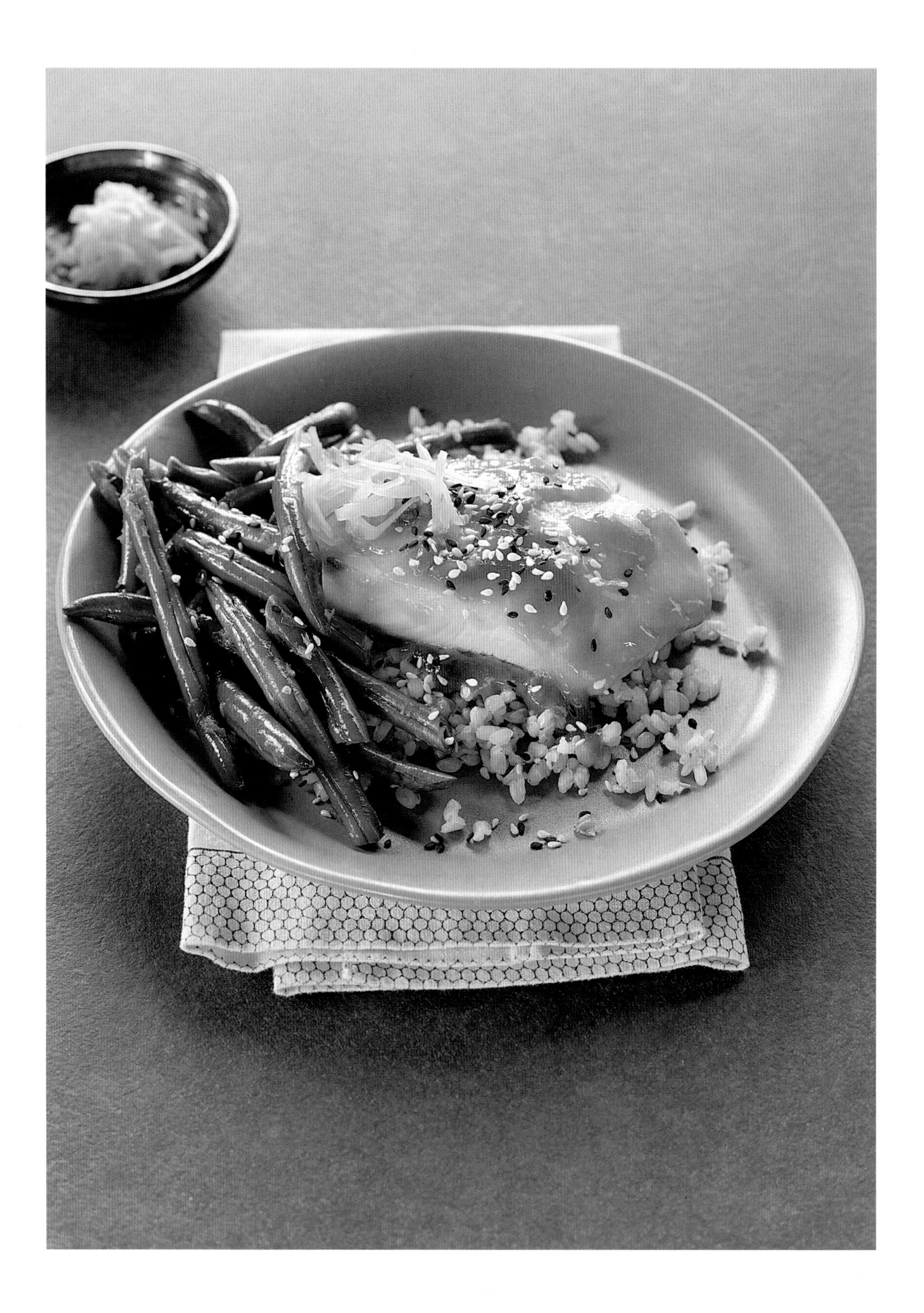

in the pan atop the sauce. Cook, with the lid ajar, until the fish is opaque and easily flakes with a fork, 8 to 12 minutes.

4. Just before serving, finish the green beans by quickly stirring over medium-high heat. Add ¼ cup water and cover until the beans are crisp-tender, about 3 minutes.

5. To serve, divide the rice between shallow bowls, then top each with a piece of fish, any sauce left in the pan, some green beans, pickled ginger, and sesame seeds.

FISH OR OMEGA-3 SUPPLEMENTS?

Getting enough of the brain-friendly omega-3s—DHA and EPA—is important for fending off Alzheimer's and other dementias. But what if you don't eat fish and seafood? Or what if you don't have access to quality seafood, or just don't get enough? Taking a supplement to meet your DHA and EPA requirements may be a good idea.

The science of omega-3 supplementation is still evolving. So far, studies have failed to prove supplements protect the brain to the same degree that eating fish and seafood does. This may be a function of the dose—many studies employed a smaller dose (under 2 grams) than the 4 to 6 grams per day (from food) associated with less shrinkage of the brain based on MRI studies. And it may be that only certain subsets of people will benefit from supplementing, such as those who carry the ApoE4 Alzheimer's risk gene.

A recent study is more promising. When participants were given more than 2 grams of DHA and EPA per day, the supplement group had 28 percent more DHA and 43 percent more EPA crossing the blood brain barrier compared to a placebo group. Still, those who carry an ApoE4 risk gene may struggle to get enough; uptake was three times higher for those without this gene. Researchers are hot on the trail to test not only higher doses for ApoE4 carriers, but also more efficient forms, like phospholipid-based omega-3s.

It may make sense to augment your brain-protective dietary pattern with a supplement of DHA and EPA. While the ideal dose has not yet been clearly determined, evidence indicates that more than 2 grams per day of fish oil-derived DHA and EPA can meaningfully increase these beneficial nutrients in our brains. Because too much omega-3s in the bloodstream can accentuate blood-thinning medications, like aspirin and warfarin, it's important to discuss this with your physician.

What if you follow a vegan or vegetarian dietary pattern? You may be wondering if you can get adequate levels of DHA and EPA into the brain by eating only plant foods. Plants provide a different type of omega-3s—ALA, or alpha-linolenic acid, found in nuts, seeds, and vegetable oils. But there's a catch: ALA must be converted to DHA to get to the brain. Only 1 to 5 percent of the ALA you consume reaches the brain as DHA. That's not nearly enough to supply the brain's omega-3 requirements.

You could get your DHA and EPA from the same source fish do—sea vegetables like edible seaweeds, such as nori and kombu. Or look for a DHA and EPA supplement made from a plant-based algal oil. We still don't know if plant-based DHA and EPA supplements are as effective as the ones made from fish oil, but researchers are looking into this.

The bottom line: Be sure to supply your brain with the omega-3s it requires to thrive—especially if you carry the ApoE4 gene. You can do this by eating at least one high-quality fish or seafood meal each week, taking a supplement, or both.

CHOOSING THE BEST SEAFOOD FOR YOUR BRAIN AND THE PLANET

All the fish in the sea (that you are most likely to find at the supermarket) has been broken down into three categories, as seen through the lens of brain health: Brain-Friendliest Fish, Enjoy on Occasion, and Enjoy Rarely, if at All.

BRAIN-FRIENDLIEST FISH: These fish have it all. They score high marks for environmental sustainability (Monterey Bay Aquarium Seafood Watch–approved; see Resources, page 390) and are less likely to harbor mercury and other pollutants, such as PCBs (polychlorinated biphenyls) and pesticides. And they are rich in DHA, the most important omega-3 for brain health.

The small fish on the bottom of the food chain like anchovies and herring are an especially savvy choice in this category: big on flavor, nutrient-dense (especially for their size), and some of the best seafood bargains. Enjoy these one or more times each week.

- American shrimp (wild-caught; see the Tip on page 155)
- Anchovies (wild-caught, Adriatic Sea, see the sidebar Anchovies: Whole, Fillets, and Paste on page 92)
- Arctic char (wild-caught or farmed)
- Catfish (USA farmed or wild-caught from Chesapeake Bay)
- Clams (wild-caught or farmed)
- Cod (wild-caught, Alaskan)
- Halibut (wild-caught, Alaskan)
- Herring (wild-caught)
- Lake trout (wild-caught, USA)
- Light tuna (aka skipjack tuna, canned)
- Lobster (wild-caught, see Monterey Bay Aquarium Seafood Watch for best choice)
- Mussels (farmed)
- Oysters (farmed and some wild-caught)
- Rainbow trout (wild-caught and some farmed, USA)
- Salmon (wild-caught, Alaskan)
- Sardines (wild-caught, Pacific, look for the Marine Stewardship Council stamp of approval)
- Scallops (wild-caught or farmed)
- Sole (wild-caught and farmed)

CHOOSING THE BEST SEAFOOD FOR YOUR BRAIN AND THE PLANET	
ENJOY ON OCCASION: These fish are good sources of lean protein, DHA, EPA, and other key brain health nutrients like selenium, zinc, iodide, and vitamin D. Because some are large fish that eat smaller fish, they may bioaccumulate mercury. As long as you are not pregnant, you can enjoy these fish about once a month.	• Ahi tuna (fresh) • Albacore tuna (canned) • Crab (wild-caught, Alaskan, see Monterey Bay Aquarium Seafood Watch for other good sources) • Monkfish (wild-caught, USA) • Octopus (wild-caught, Alaskan) • Rockfish (aka Pacific snapper, wild-caught, USA)
ENJOY RARELY, IF AT ALL: These are mostly large predator fish that can potentially rack up high levels of mercury in their flesh. These are the fish to avoid entirely if you are pregnant because mercury is particularly harmful to developing fetuses, as well as babies and young children. Enjoy these as an occasional treat, if at all. These are all wild-caught fish that may have suffered from overfishing. While swordfish is making a comeback, it's best to check Monterey Bay Aquarium Seafood Watch for up-to-date sourcing.	• Barracuda • King mackerel (aka kingfish, wild-caught, USA and Mexico) • Marlin • Shark • Swordfish • Tilefish

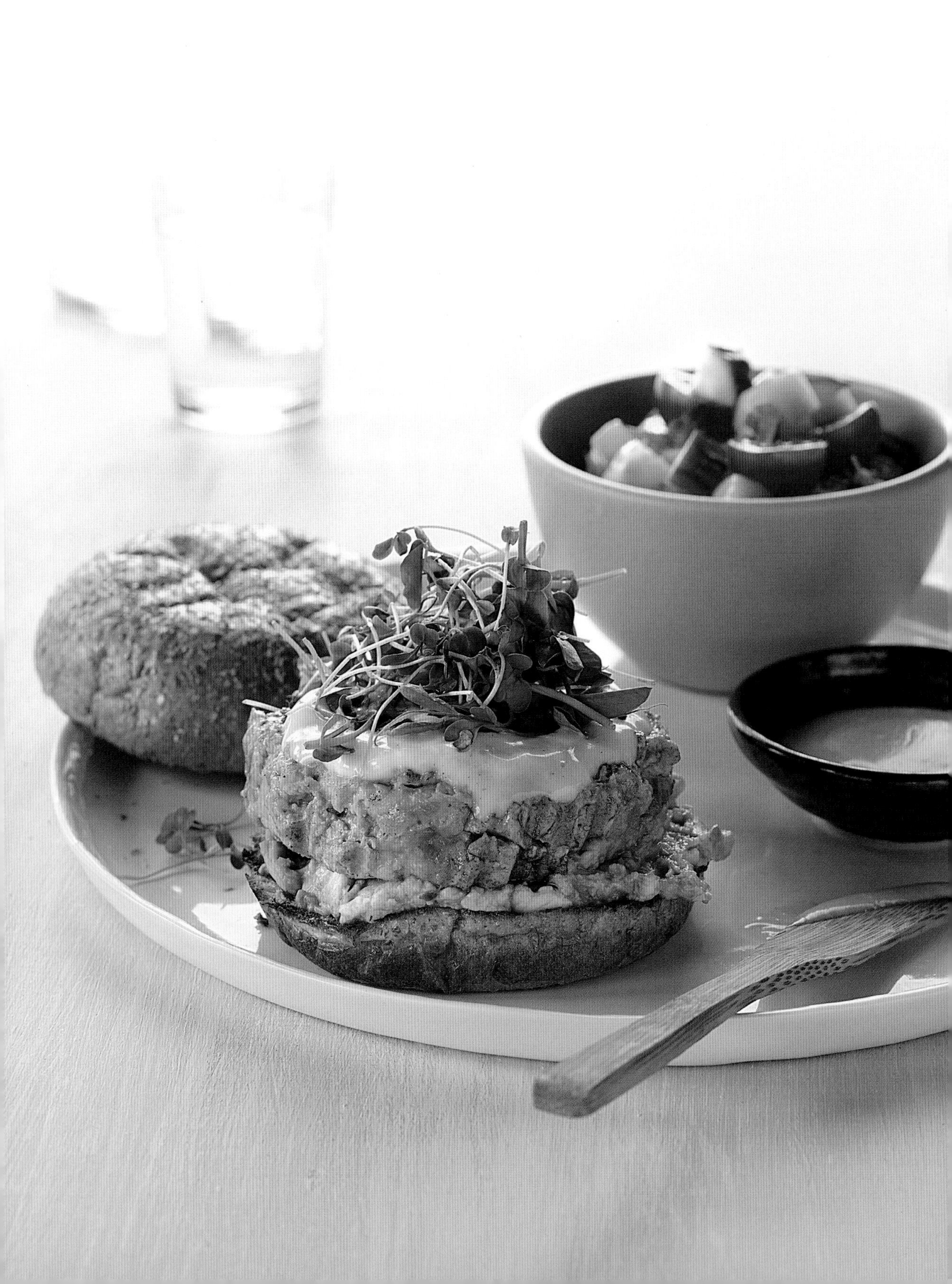

TUNA BURGERS WITH WASABI MAYO AND MANGO SALAD

SERVES 4

- **1 pound (455 g) fresh ahi tuna, cut into 1-inch (2.5 cm) pieces**
- **2 teaspoons wasabi powder**
- **2 teaspoons water**
- **1 tablespoon finely grated fresh ginger (from a 1-inch/2.5 cm piece)**
- **1 large garlic clove, minced (about 1 teaspoon)**
- **1½ teaspoons kosher salt**
- **½ cup (120 ml) vegan mayo or Almost Instant Cashew Cream (page 370)**
- **1 teaspoon low-sodium soy sauce**
- **½ teaspoon sriracha or other hot sauce**
- **2 tablespoons fresh lime juice**
- **2 tablespoons extra-virgin olive oil**
- **1 ripe mango, peeled and cut into ½-inch (1.25 cm) cubes**
- **1 Persian cucumber, cut into ½-inch (1.25 cm) cubes**
- **2 cups (340 g) cherry tomatoes, halved**
- **2 tablespoons fresh mint leaves**
- **1 avocado, mashed**
- **4 sprouted-grain or whole-grain hamburger buns or English muffins, toasted**
- **½ cup (15 g) microgreens (optional)**

If you love sushi, poke bowls, and a medium-rare ahi tuna steak, these burgers are for you. Although fresh tuna is a great source of lean protein and brain-friendly fats, I recommend limiting your intake of larger species of tuna like ahi to once a month. (See Science Bite, page 168.) By turning ahi tuna into a burger, a small amount of fish goes a long way.

Like most burgers, the toppings are key. Here smashed avocado below and a creamy wasabi mayo on top is a crave-worthy pairing.

To create the ideal texture for the burgers, you will need to partially freeze the tuna before pulsing in a food processor. Use that time to prep the wasabi mayo and mango salad.

1. Place the tuna pieces in a single layer on a plate or pie tin and freeze for 30 minutes.

2. Stir together 1 teaspoon each of the wasabi powder and water in a small bowl to make a smooth paste. Scrape the paste into the bowl of a food processor with the partially frozen tuna, ginger, garlic, and 1 teaspoon of the salt. Pulse about 15 times, until the tuna starts to come together in a ball (being careful not to overprocess), until you have a mostly chunky, partly smooth mixture. Divide the mixture into four equal portions and use wet hands to shape into 1-inch-thick (2.5 cm) patties. Place on a plate, cover, and refrigerate until you are ready to grill.

3. Meanwhile, stir together the remaining 1 teaspoon each wasabi powder and water in a small bowl to make a smooth paste. Stir in the mayo, soy sauce, and sriracha. Set aside.

continued

4. Whisk together the lime juice, 1 tablespoon of the oil, and the remaining ½ teaspoon salt in a medium bowl. Add the mango, cucumber, tomatoes, and mint; toss well and set aside.

5. Set a grill pan over medium-high heat (or heat a grill to medium over direct heat). Brush both sides of each tuna patty with the remaining 1 tablespoon oil and place on the grill pan or grill. Cook until the bottoms are firm, about 3 minutes. Flip and cook until both sides are firm to the touch and lightly browned, an additional 3 minutes, or until the internal temperature reaches 105°F (40.5°C) for rare or 110°F (43°C) for medium-rare.

6. Divide the avocado between the bottom halves of the buns. Top each with a tuna burger, a dollop of wasabi mayo, some microgreens, and the top halves of the buns. Serve with the mango salad alongside.

SCIENCE BITE:

MERCURY LEVELS IN FISH AND BRAIN HEALTH

Because large predator fish like tuna can accumulate mercury, it is best to limit consumption to no more than once a month. For adults, however, in particular those over age sixty-five, the brain health benefit of eating seafood outweighs potential harm from mercury exposure. Limiting mercury is most important in early stages of life. A 2015 study from Rush University's Memory and Aging Project sheds light on the impact of mercury on the brain in older adults. Nearly one thousand participants in northeastern Illinois were examined for how much fish and seafood they consumed, whether or not they developed Alzheimer's, and, after they passed, the impact of eating seafood on their brains at autopsy. Those who consumed more fish and seafood were less likely to develop Alzheimer's or another dementia despite the fact that they accumulated more mercury in their brains. In other words, eating fish translated to fewer cases of Alzheimer's.

SLOW-ROASTED SALMON WITH AVOCADO BUTTER

SERVES 4 TO 6

2 small fennel bulbs (8 ounces/230 g), thinly sliced, fronds reserved for garnish

Two 15-ounce (425 g) cans chickpeas, drained (about 3 cups)

1 large lemon, thinly sliced, seeds removed

½ cup (120 ml) water

¼ cup (60 ml) extra-virgin olive oil, plus more for drizzling

1 teaspoon kosher salt

One 1½-pound (680 g) whole salmon fillet, skin-on (preferably wild-caught), about 1 inch (2.5 cm) thick (see Tip)

¼ teaspoon freshly ground black pepper

1½ cups (230 g) peas (fresh or frozen)

2 large, ripe avocados, mashed (about 1 cup)

3 tablespoons fresh lemon or lime juice

2 tablespoons unsalted butter, preferably grass-fed, at room temperature

2 tablespoons fresh flat-leaf parsley leaves

1 medium garlic clove, minced (about ½ teaspoon)

Slow-roasting salmon is not only a brain-friendlier method than cooking over higher heat, it's practically foolproof, turning out perfectly cooked salmon every time. Think tender, rosy-hued fish infused with flavor from the lemons and the fennel. It's a streamlined dish that comes together quickly, too, thanks to pantry staples like canned chickpeas and frozen peas. And because the salmon roasts in the same sheet pan as the vegetables, cleanup is fast.

Once you put the salmon in the oven, mix up the avocado butter (a recipe handed down to me from my mother). It's wonderful slathered on grilled corn or peak-season sliced tomatoes. It's also fantastic served on other fish and seafood. Dollop it on grilled shrimp or cod fillets, or fold it into tuna or sardine salad. Because avocado butter freezes well, it's a good way to use up a bunch of ripe avocados that need to be eaten. Of course, if you don't feel like getting out a food processor, you can use a fork to mash the avocado with the butter and the other ingredients, adding the chopped parsley last.

1. Set an oven rack in the center position and preheat the oven to 300°F (150°C).

2. Toss the fennel, chickpeas, lemon, water, 2 tablespoons of the oil, and ½ teaspoon of the salt on a rimmed baking sheet until evenly coated, then spread into an even layer. Top with the salmon, skin side down, and pour the remaining 2 tablespoons oil over top. Sprinkle the salmon with pepper and ¼ teaspoon of the salt.

3. Bake for 20 to 28 minutes, stirring in the peas after 10 minutes, until the salmon is just turning opaque. (If using an instant-read thermometer, take the temperature in the

thickest part of the fish: 125°F/50°C for medium-rare; up to 140°F/60°C for well done.)

4. Meanwhile, combine the avocados, lemon juice, butter, parsley, garlic, and the remaining ¼ teaspoon salt in the bowl of a food processor. Process until completely smooth. Keep in the refrigerator until ready to eat.

5. To serve, divide the salmon and vegetables between plates and spoon a tablespoon of any pan sauce over top. Top each piece of fish with 2 tablespoons avocado butter, some of the reserved fennel fronds, and a drizzle of oil. Top with more pepper, if you like.

6. To store extra avocado butter, transfer to an airtight container with a piece of waxed paper or parchment paper pressed onto the surface of the butter to prevent browning. It will keep like this for up to 3 days in the refrigerator or 3 months in the freezer.

TIP: *You can use fillets of salmon, too. Four- to 6-ounce (115 to 170 g) portions work well. Start checking for doneness after 15 minutes, especially if you prefer your salmon rare.*

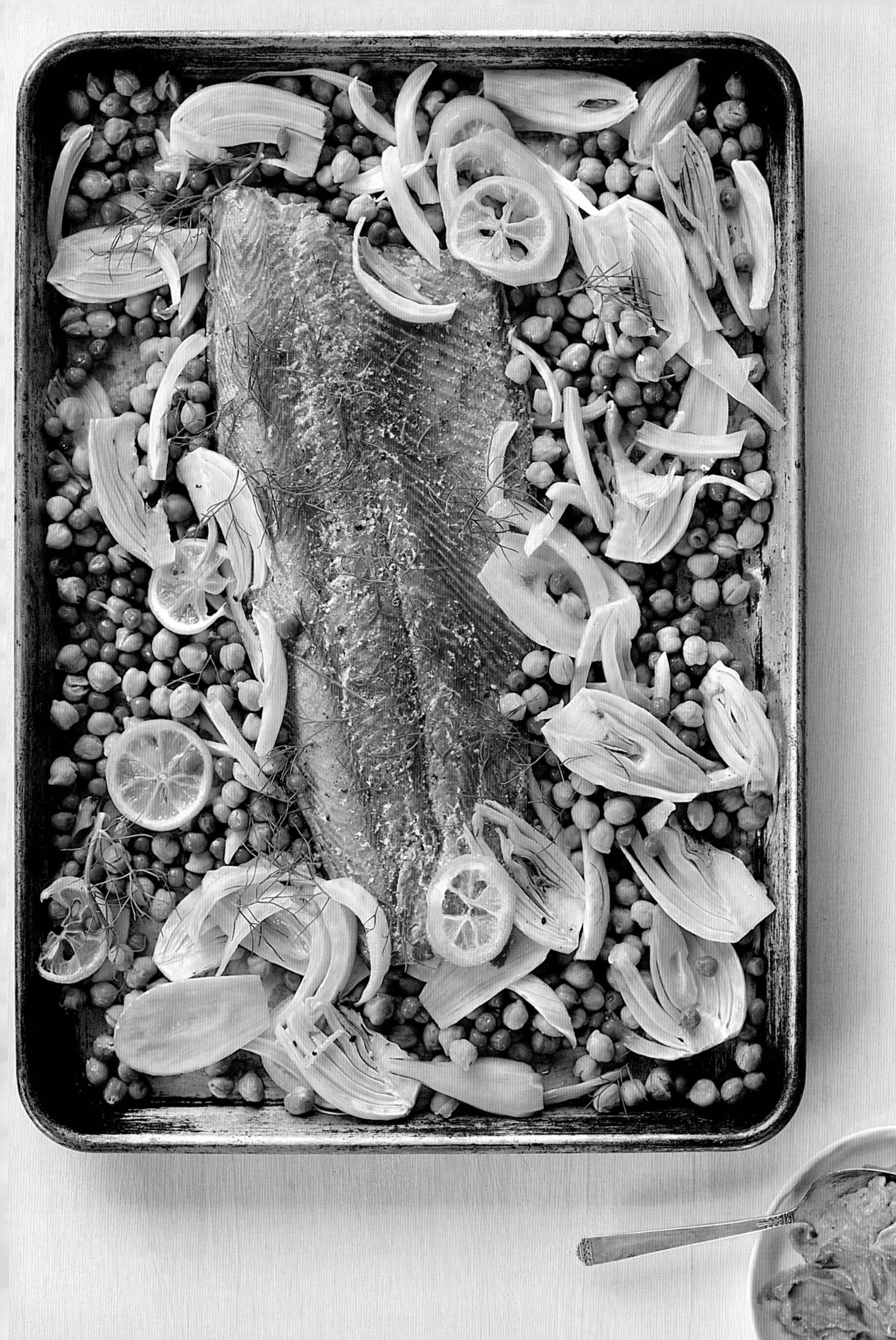

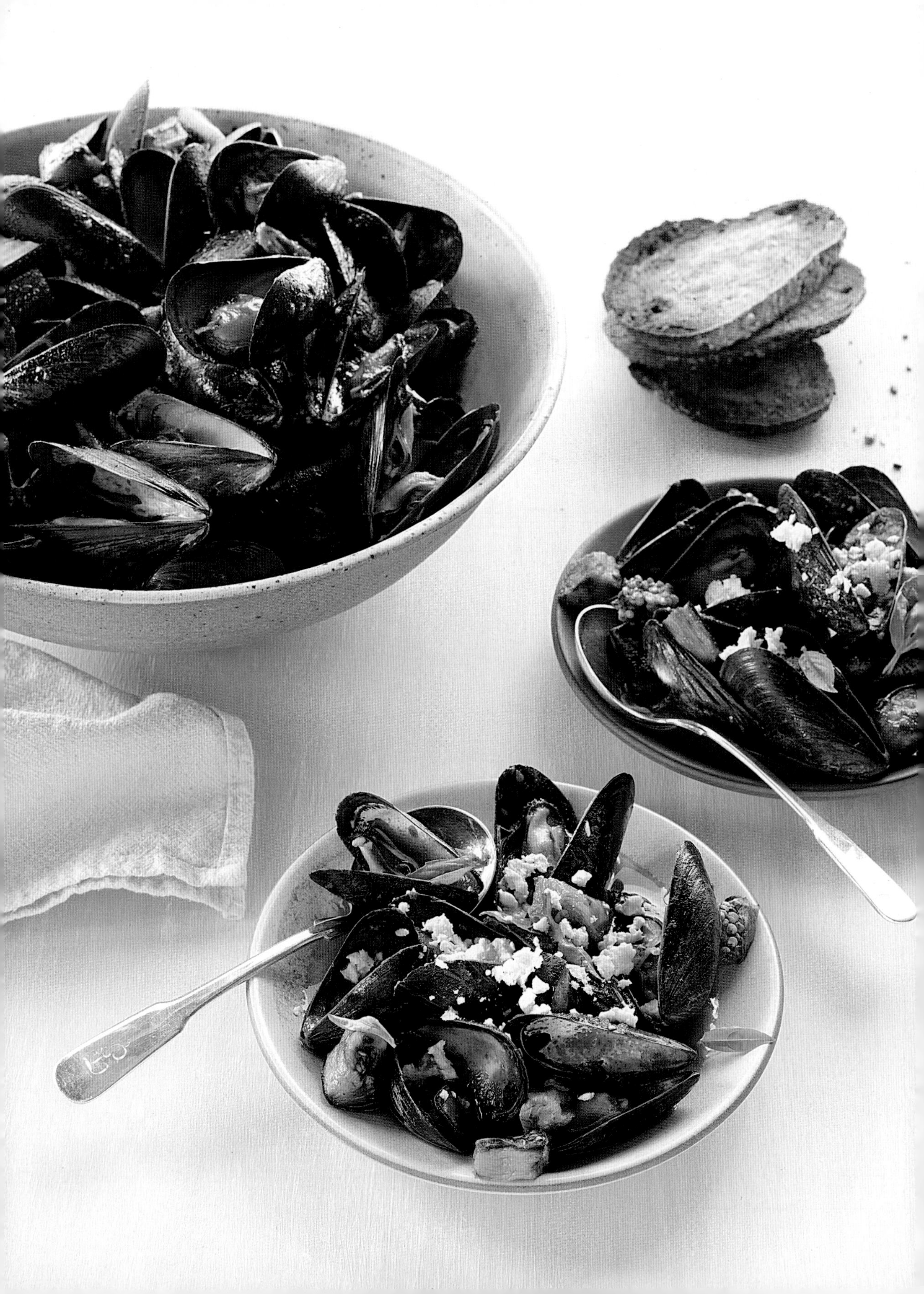

SPICY MUSSELS MARINARA WITH EGGPLANT, FETA, AND BASIL

SERVES 4

1 large globe eggplant (1 pound/455 g), cut into 1-inch (2.5 cm) cubes

3 tablespoons extra-virgin olive oil

1¼ teaspoons kosher salt

1 large garlic clove, chopped (about 1 teaspoon)

One 15-ounce (425 g) can crushed tomatoes

1½ cups (360 ml) dry white wine

¼ teaspoon crushed red pepper flakes

2 pounds (910 g) mussels, scrubbed (see Tip)

½ cup (115 g) feta, crumbled

1 cup (20 g) fresh basil leaves, torn

Toasted whole-grain bread, for serving

If you've never steamed a pot of mussels at home, you'll be pleasantly surprised to learn how easy it is. This dish starts with a simple wine-spiked marinara that simmers while cubes of eggplant roast in the oven. The eggplant nestles alongside the mussels in the sauce so that everything is infused with delicious garlic and tomato flavor. While it can be tricky to tell when other seafood dishes are done, with mussels it couldn't be easier—when most of the shells have opened up, they are ready to eat.

Serve as an appetizer or add a green salad for a light supper.

1. Set an oven rack in the center position and preheat the oven to 400°F (200°C). Line a rimmed baking sheet with parchment.

2. Place the eggplant on the prepared baking sheet and toss with 2 tablespoons of the oil and 1 teaspoon of the salt. Roast for 25 to 30 minutes, until the cubes are crispy on the edges and starting to brown.

3. Meanwhile, heat the remaining 1 tablespoon oil in a large heavy saucepan with a tight-fitting lid over medium-high heat. Add the garlic and cook until golden brown and fragrant, about 1 minute. Add the tomatoes, wine, red pepper flakes, and the remaining ¼ teaspoon salt. Bring to a boil then reduce the heat to a gentle simmer, stirring occasionally, until the sauce thickens enough to coat the back of a spoon, 20 to 25 minutes.

4. Stir in the mussels and the roasted eggplant. Adjust the heat to maintain a gentle simmer and cover. Cook with the lid

on until nearly all the mussels have opened, 6 to 8 minutes. (Discard any mussels with tightly closed shells.)

5. Divide the mussels and their sauce between shallow bowls and scatter the feta and basil over top. Serve with toasted bread.

TIP: *Purchase mussels at the seafood counter of the grocery store or from a fishmonger you trust. Always purchase live mussels; avoid the frozen ones on the half shell. Their shells should be tightly closed (open ones have already died) and smell like the sea—fresh, clean, and briny—and be packed up in a bag of ice. Keep them in the refrigerator for up to 48 hours, changing the ice as needed. Just before steaming, rinse and scrub off their "beards"—aka the scraggly bits that cling to the shell's opening.*

SCIENCE BITE:

BIVALVES AND VITAMIN B12

Vitamin B12 (aka cobalamin) is a major player in your brain health. It's crucial for building the myelin sheath that wraps around nerve cells, protecting them from oxidative stress. It helps dial back the amount of homocysteine in the body, a key driver of inflammation in the brain. B12 deficiency states are associated with depression, cognitive impairment, and peripheral neuropathies. The good news is that when B12 deficiency is the sole reason for dementia, it can be treated, and reversed, with supplements and food.

You need only a small amount of vitamin B12 to be healthy. In fact, the recommended dietary allowance according to the National Institutes of Health is just 2.4 micrograms per day, or the amount in 3 ounces (85 g) of oysters, clams, or mussels. And because vitamin B12 is stored in the liver, whenever you consume more than you need (like when you enjoy a dozen oysters on the half shell), your body will save the rest for later. But if you follow a vegan or vegetarian diet, a nutrient-poor omnivorous diet, or have certain medical conditions that impair its absorption, a B12 deficiency can result. Besides bivalves, foods that offer vitamin B12 include eggs, dairy products, wild salmon, and some fortified foods, like soy milk and cereal.

SAVORY WAFFLES WITH SMOKED TROUT AND GREENS

SERVES 4 TO 6

½ cup (140 g) plain, unsweetened Greek yogurt

¼ cup (60 ml) fresh lemon juice

½ teaspoon kosher salt

2 cups (255 g) chickpea flour

2 teaspoons baking powder

½ teaspoon ground turmeric

¼ teaspoon freshly ground black pepper, plus more for serving

1 cup (240 ml) unsweetened almond, cashew, or oat milk

2 eggs, at room temperature

1 tablespoon lemon zest

6 tablespoons (90 ml) extra-virgin olive oil, plus more for the waffle iron

1 medium zucchini (7 ounces/200 g), grated and squeezed dry (about 1¼ cups; see Tip)

¼ cup (15 g) grated yellow onion

4 loosely packed cups (160 g) fresh mixed greens, such as baby romaine and arugula

12 ounces (340 g) wild-caught smoked trout, flaked

Lemon wedges

Waffles probably don't come to mind when you think of eating for brain health, but these savory golden ones pack in superstar ingredients like chickpea flour, vegetables, turmeric, and almond milk. The zucchini strands help create lacy, crisp edges, and the turmeric and black pepper combo adds antioxidant power and spice. On top, flaked smoked trout gives the dish a brunchy appeal, along with a day's full dose of DHA and EPA.

Depending on your waffle maker and how many people are eating, you might have extra waffles. Stored in an airtight container, the waffles keep well in the freezer. Just pop the frozen waffles in a toaster for a quick, protein-packed snack—or a fancy breakfast for one. I like them topped with sliced avocado and a poached egg, subbing in smoked salmon for the trout.

Note that you'll need to zest the lemon before juicing. To make the waffles dairy-free, omit the lemon and yogurt topping and use Almost Instant Cashew Cream (page 370) instead.

1. Preheat the oven to 300°F (150°C) and place a rimmed baking sheet in the oven.

2. Stir together the yogurt, 2 tablespoons of the lemon juice, and ¼ teaspoon of the salt in a small bowl; set aside.

3. Whisk together the chickpea flour, baking powder, turmeric, pepper, and remaining ¼ teaspoon salt in a medium bowl.

4. In a separate small bowl, whisk the milk, eggs, lemon zest, remaining 2 tablespoons lemon juice, and 4 tablespoons of

the oil until combined. Whisk into the flour mixture until no lumps remain, then fold in the zucchini and onion.

5. Heat a waffle iron at the medium-high setting and brush with oil. Cook the batter according to the waffle maker's instructions. The waffles should be crispy and brown on the edges and easily pull away from the waffle iron. Timing will vary according to individual waffle makers.

6. Transfer cooked waffles to the baking sheet in the oven to keep warm. Repeat until all the batter has been used.

7. To serve, toss the greens with the remaining 2 tablespoons oil and a pinch of salt. Divide between plates. Top each plate with one or two waffles, then top with the smoked trout, dividing evenly, and a dollop of the lemon yogurt. Serve with lemon wedges and more pepper, if desired.

8. To store leftover waffles, keep them tightly wrapped in the freezer for up to 3 months. Pop in the toaster to warm, or heat in a 350°F (180°C) oven.

TIP: *Pass zucchini lengthwise over the large holes of a box grater to make long strands. If you have raw zucchini noodles left over from another dish (like the nests on page 124), you can sub them in for the same amount of grated zucchini.*

SCIENCE BITE:

SMOKED FISH, SODIUM, AND OMEGA-3S

Smoking at low temperatures can be one of the more brain-friendly ways to prepare fish. That's because smoked fish—salmon, trout, mussels, and mackerel—retain concentrations of omega-3 fats comparable to fresh fish. However, the process of smoking fish also adds salt. Be sure to keep portion sizes to less than 3 ounces (85 g) total each week, especially if you are on a low-sodium diet.

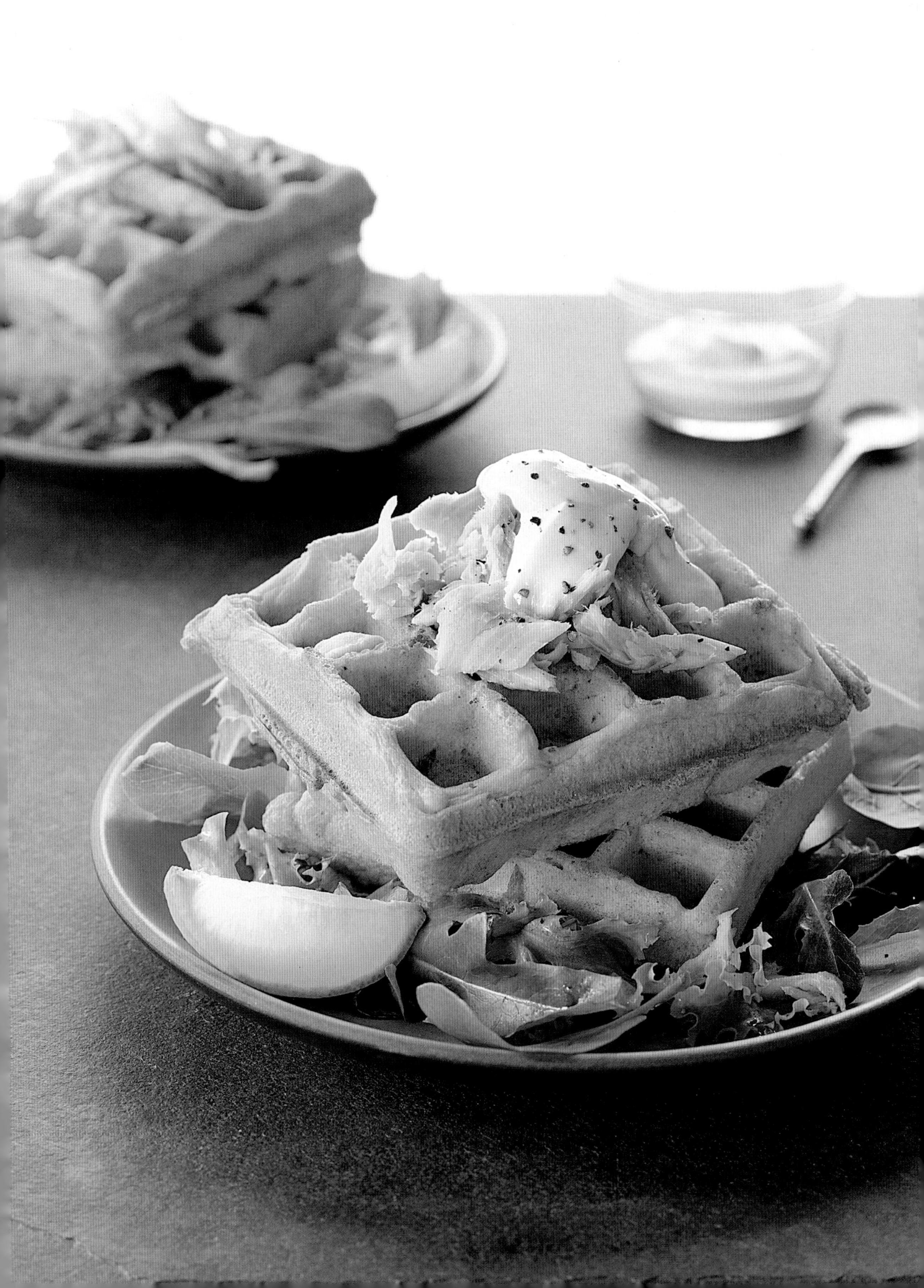

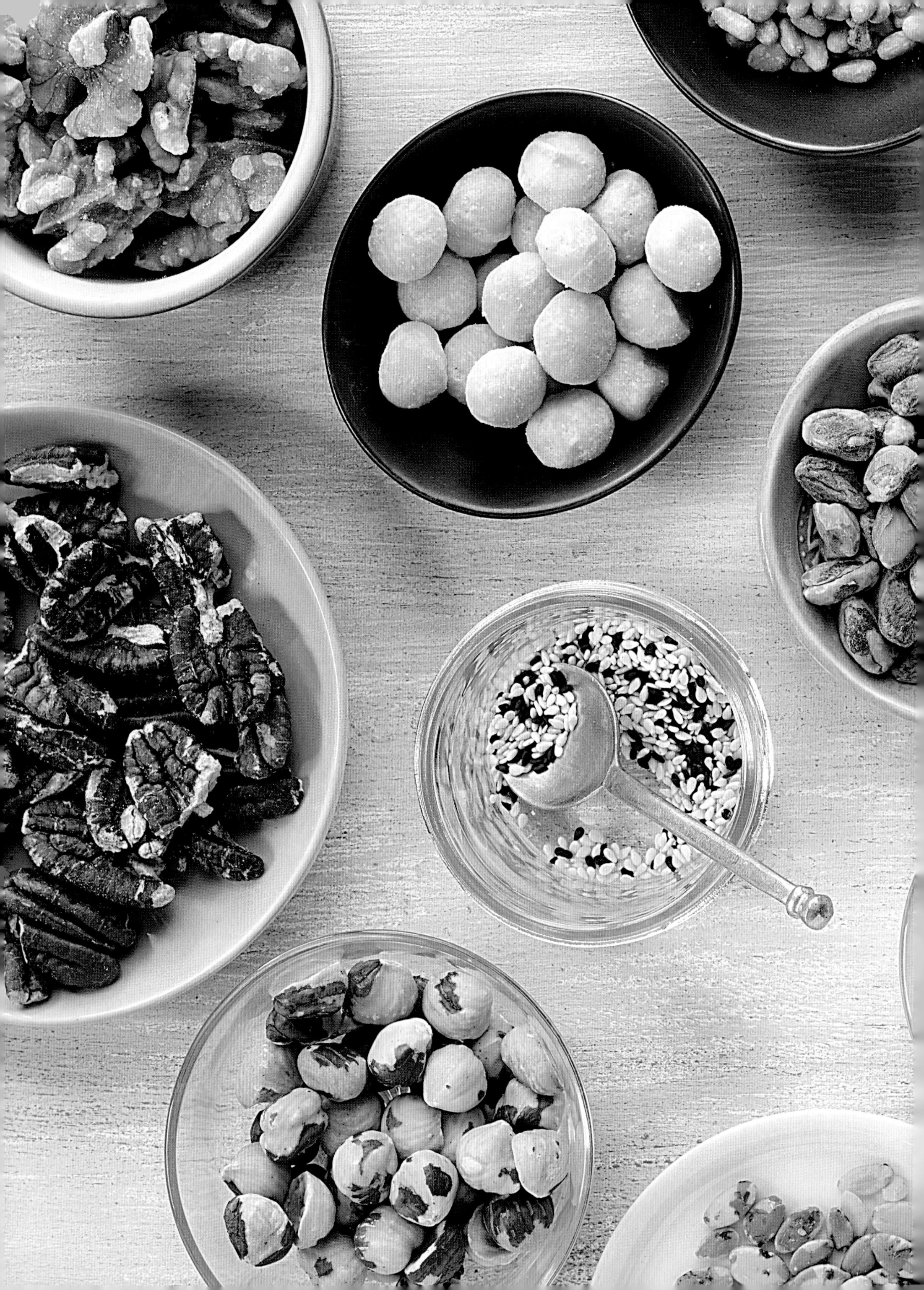

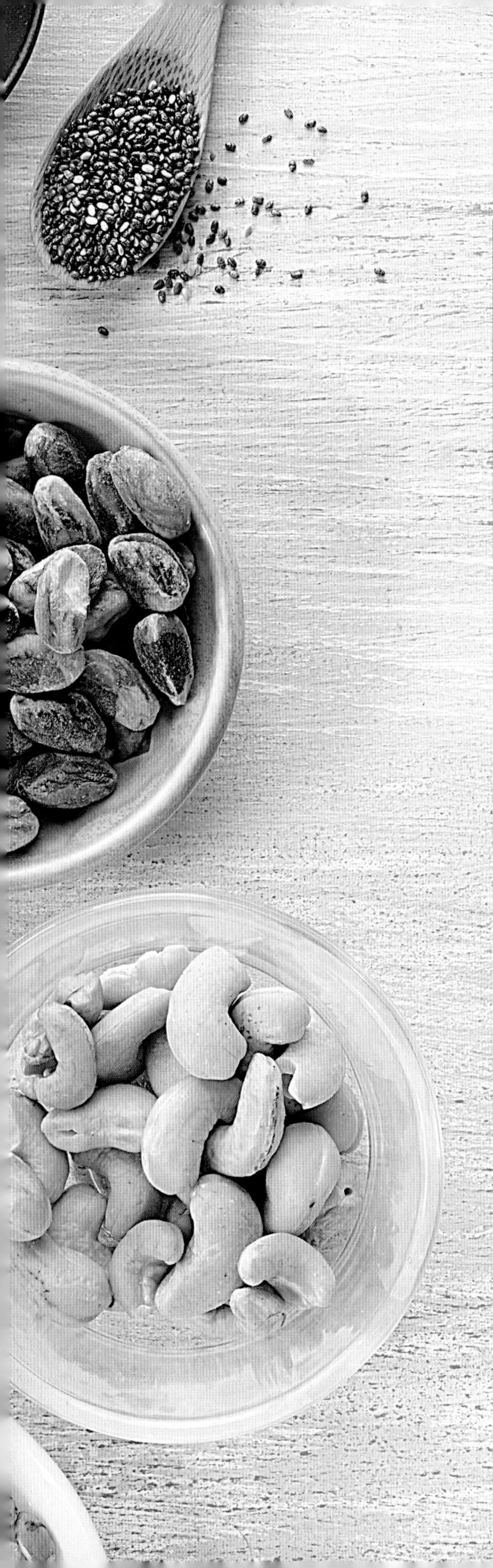

NUTS AND SEEDS

I was the kid who wouldn't touch a chocolate chip cookie if it was studded with walnuts. If sesame seeds graced any food, I scraped them off. Same with almonds, pecans, and pistachios (my dad's favorite snack). I wasn't allergic to nuts and seeds, just a picky eater. Now I'm the person who soaks cashews to make DIY nut milk and cashew cream, turns walnuts into a crumbly Parmesan-like topping, and liberally sprinkles food with a rainbow of seeds. In fact, nuts and seeds are the secret of my brain-healthy cooking because they add creamy texture and body to foods, thanks to their satiating fats.

Snacking on nuts at least four times a week has been proven in many prospective studies to reduce the risk of heart disease (like heart attack and stroke), help maintain a healthy weight at midlife, and contribute to dementia-free longevity. In numerous large-scale, prospective studies of healthy older adults, eating nuts was consistently associated with better performance on cognitive tests, with folks who consumed nuts four times weekly outperforming those who ate nuts just a few times a month.

Nuts are one of the ten brain-healthy food groups from the MIND diet study (page 17), which demonstrated that healthy adults who consume four or more ¼-cup (40 g) handfuls of nuts each week are up to 53 percent less likely to be diagnosed with Alzheimer's. In the Green MED diet study (see page 18), adding an extra serving of walnuts to the Mediterranean diet was a polyphenol-boosting strategy that resulted in brain volume gains over time.

Seeds have a similar brain-healthy fat and nutrient composition as nuts but haven't been studied as rigorously regarding long-term health benefits. For that reason, I advise supplementing your diet with seeds *in addition to* enjoying at least four handfuls of nuts each week. Think of seeds as a bonus brain-healthy food group, ready for you as a satisfying snack, a creamy condiment, or a flourish to give your home-cooked meals an extra pop of color and crunch. Because both nuts and seeds are calorie-dense, be aware of how easy it is to overdo it if you are watching your weight.

SHOPPING FOR NUTS AND SEEDS

Look for high-quality nuts and seeds in the bulk or baking sections of your grocery store. Because nuts and seeds are packed with brain-healthy fats (like the omega-3 fatty acid alpha-linolenic acid) and antioxidants (especially vitamin E), they are highly perishable. Buy only the amount of nuts and seeds you think you'll need in the next six months. Sometimes the freshest nuts and seeds at the best price are from large retailers and online grocery stores because they have a high turnover and are less likely to be languishing on the shelves getting stale. See Resources (page 390).

Steer clear of the snack aisle when shopping for nuts and seeds. That's where you'll find the industrially produced ones that are laden with a long list of inflammatory oils, stabilizers, artificial flavors, added sugars, and excess salt. And because they are often processed with high-heat methods, these snacks rack up AGEs (advanced glycation end products, page 280), glycotoxins associated with accelerated brain aging.

Whenever possible, purchase your nuts and seeds raw (untoasted and unsalted) rather than roasted, since raw nuts retain more of their healthy fats

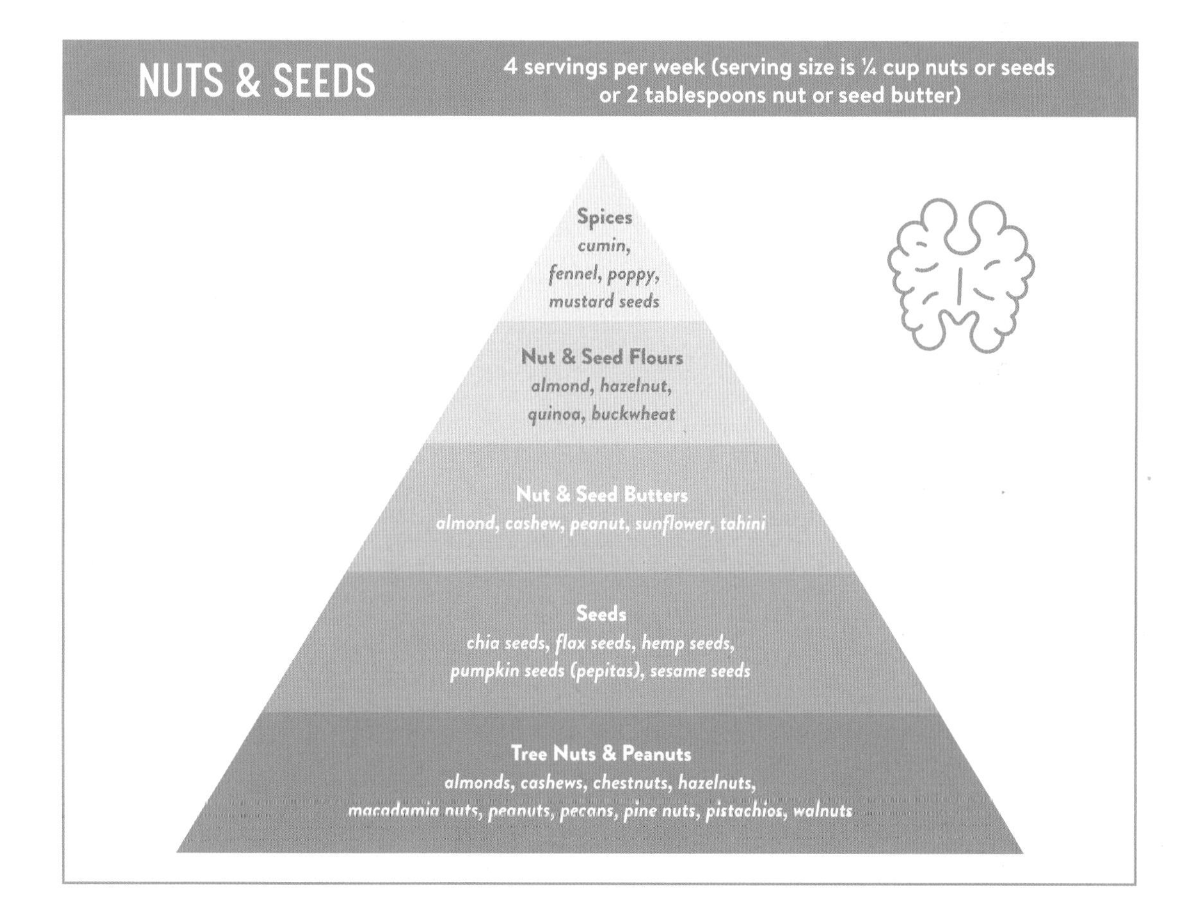

and antioxidants. Raw nuts are usually fresher, too, so they will taste better and last longer in your pantry. Toasting them yourself (to boost flavor and texture) allows you to control how much heat you apply and minimize any loss of nutrients. (See page 190 for toasting instructions.)

Most nuts grown in the United States, however, are not truly "raw" even if it says so on the label. That's because nuts are pasteurized to reduce bacterial contamination (like salmonella). Rest assured that pasteurization does not damage the nuts' delicate fats or affect the taste in any way. Though nuts imported from Italy and Spain are often unpasteurized, take care—they may be stale or fraudulently labeled. So if you are looking for truly raw nuts (because you want to sprout them, for example), seek out small-scale farmers at farmers' markets where regulations allow them to sell unpasteurized nuts.

ORGANIC OR NOT?

Seek out fresh, high-quality nuts and seeds, organic if possible and you can afford it. The good news is, the benefit of consuming these brain-healthy nuts and seeds, even if not organic, outweighs any possible harm from trace amounts of pesticides. Because most nuts and seeds are encased in a hard shell when grown (like almonds and pine nuts), they offer a measure of protection against environmental toxins.

STORING NUTS AND SEEDS

When exposed to heat, sunlight, or oxygen, or when sitting in your cabinet for too long after purchasing, the healthy fats and antioxidants in nuts and seeds can become rancid. That's one reason it's better to buy only as many as you need for the next few months, preferably whole, not already chopped. And because nuts are porous, they can soak up flavors and smells from other foods stored near them.

Use airtight containers like mason jars or sturdy plastic bags to store nuts and seeds. They'll last up to two months in a cold, dark place in your pantry; in the refrigerator for up to six months; or in the freezer for up to one year. Store nuts with the highest amount of fat—such as walnuts, pecans, and macadamias—in the freezer regardless of age.

ROASTED RED AND YELLOW BEET SALAD WITH WALNUT "PARM"

SERVES 4 TO 6 AS A SIDE

- **4 or 5 small red and yellow beets (12 ounces/340 g total), scrubbed**
- **5 ounces (140 g) arugula (about 5 cups)**
- **2 tablespoons extra-virgin olive oil**
- **¼ teaspoon kosher salt**
- **2 avocados, sliced**
- **2 oranges, peeled and thinly sliced into rounds**
- **3 tablespoons small fresh mint leaves**
- **2 tablespoons black or white chia seeds**
- **1 cup (120 g) Walnut "Parm" (recipe follows)**

Beets add eye-popping color and earthy sweetness to this beautiful, hearty salad. This root vegetable is one of just a few vegetables that provide betalains, the naturally occurring pigments responsible for their jewel-like yellow and red colors. If your beets come with greens attached, save them for another use, or sauté in olive oil until soft and add to the arugula before serving.

Instead of a dollop of goat cheese that so often tops a beet salad, a sprinkle of umami-rich Walnut "Parm" offers decadence without dairy.

1. Preheat the oven to 400°F (200°C).

2. Wrap the beets tightly with foil and place on a rimmed baking sheet. Bake for 20 to 25 minutes (for small beets) and up to an hour for large ones, or until a knife easily slips through the beets.

3. Once the beets are cool enough to handle (after about 5 minutes), slip off the skins using your hands, paper towels, or a vegetable peeler. Cut off the root end and slice the beets into ¼-inch (6 mm) rounds.

4. Place the arugula on a platter or in a large shallow bowl and toss with the oil and salt. Scatter the beet rounds, avocados, oranges, and mint on top. Sprinkle with the chia seeds and crumbles of "Parm" and serve.

continued

WALNUT "PARM"

MAKES 1 CUP (120 G)

- **1 cup (120 g) raw walnuts**
- **¼ cup (60 g) nutritional yeast**
- **2 tablespoons white miso paste**
- **1 small garlic clove**
- **1 teaspoon smoked salt, such as Maldon**

This crumbly topping has seduced hundreds of my Brain Health Kitchen students with its cheesy texture and flavor. Besides tossing this "Parm" on roasted beets, feel free to sprinkle it on salads, avocado toast, popcorn, roasted sweet potatoes, and any pasta dish where you would use Parmesan cheese.

1. Combine the walnuts, nutritional yeast, miso paste, garlic, and salt in the bowl of a food processor or blender. Pulse until the mixture forms small, uniform crumbles, like wet sand or coarsely grated Parmesan cheese.

2. Walnut "Parm" keeps in an airtight container in the refrigerator for up to 1 week.

SCIENCE BITE:

BEETS BOOST BLOOD FLOW TO THE BRAIN

Beets have long been studied for their ability to lower blood pressure, open up blood vessels, and allow blood to flow more freely to vital organs—like large muscle groups—during exercise. Now a study of older adults who consume beets an hour before exercise shows it can have the same beneficial effect on the brain. That's because the pigment in beets that makes them golden or red—betalain—is naturally packed with nitrates. These nitrates convert to nitrite and eventually nitric oxide in the body, resulting in a potent vasodilating effect, which means that it increases blood and oxygen flow, including flow to the brain.

Betalain may have a more direct effect on fending off Alzheimer's, though, by disrupting amyloid protein so that it is less likely to clump into a plaque, a hallmark feature of the disease.

Because beet juice is high in sugar, it is better to get your betalains through whole beets instead.

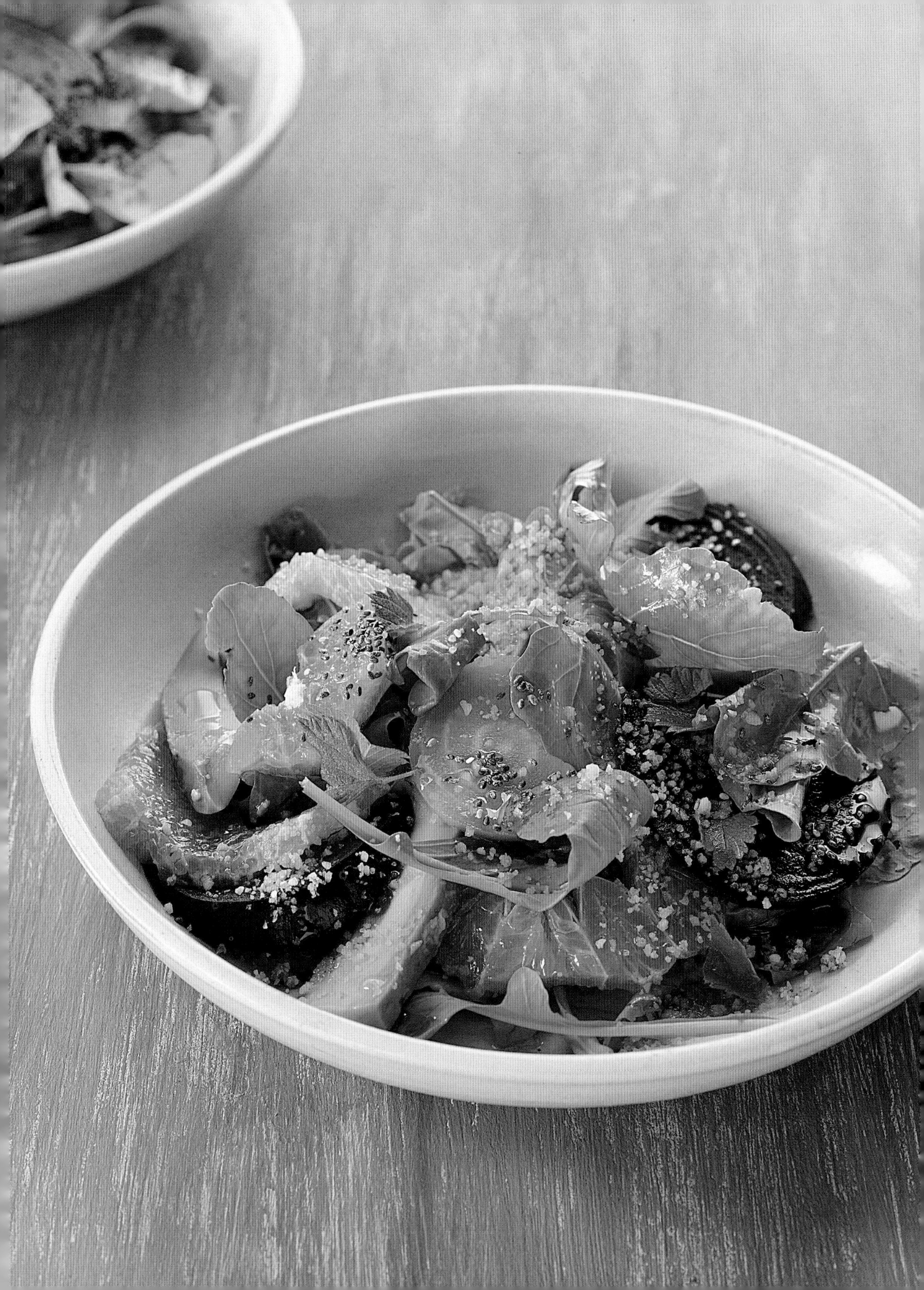

CREAMY CHESTNUT AND MUSHROOM SOUP

SERVES 4 AS AN APPETIZER

One 5- to 6-ounce (140 to 170 g) can or pouch cooked chestnuts, drained (see Tip)

2 tablespoons extra-virgin olive oil, plus more for drizzling

¾ teaspoon kosher salt

8 cups (1½ pounds/680 g) mixed mushrooms, trimmed and coarsely chopped, smaller ones left whole

1 medium yellow onion (10 ounces/285 g), diced

1 large garlic clove, coarsely chopped (about 1 teaspoon)

½ teaspoon freshly ground black pepper

Up to 4 cups (1 L) warm water

¼ cup (60 ml) Almost Instant Cashew Cream (page 370) or store-bought cashew cream (optional)

2 tablespoons poppy seeds

Fresh chives, finely chopped

A small amount of chestnuts goes a long way—adding lovely creaminess and subtle sweetness—in this plant-based mushroom soup. While you may think of chestnuts as a holiday food, this soup makes a case for keeping packets of cooked chestnuts in your pantry year-round. Not only do chestnuts provide a host of brain-healthy nutrients, they blend up silky smooth into a soup that is both rich and light.

Each bowl is topped with a sprinkling of omega-3-rich poppy seeds for a delightful crunch to each bite, along with toasted chestnuts and umami-rich mushrooms. Ordinary button mushrooms work well for the soup, or use a mix of different types like portobello, cremini, and shiitake for a nice contrast in the crispy mushroom topping. Serve this soup as a starter or double the recipe and make it a meal, and serve with a big green salad.

1. Finely chop ¼ cup (40 g) of the chestnuts. Heat 1 tablespoon of the oil in a large saucepan over medium-high heat. Add the chopped chestnuts and ¼ teaspoon of the salt and cook, stirring often, until golden brown, 3 to 5 minutes. Use a slotted spoon to transfer the chestnuts to a small bowl; set aside.

2. Add the remaining 1 tablespoon oil and the onion to the pan and cook over medium-high until soft and starting to brown, 5 to 7 minutes. Add the mushrooms, remaining whole chestnuts, plus the garlic, pepper, and remaining ½ teaspoon salt. Cook, stirring often, until the mushrooms release their water and the pan juices start to thicken, about 5 minutes. Add 3 cups (750 ml) water and bring to a boil, then reduce the heat to a gentle simmer and cook, uncovered, until the stock is slightly reduced, 15 to 20 minutes.

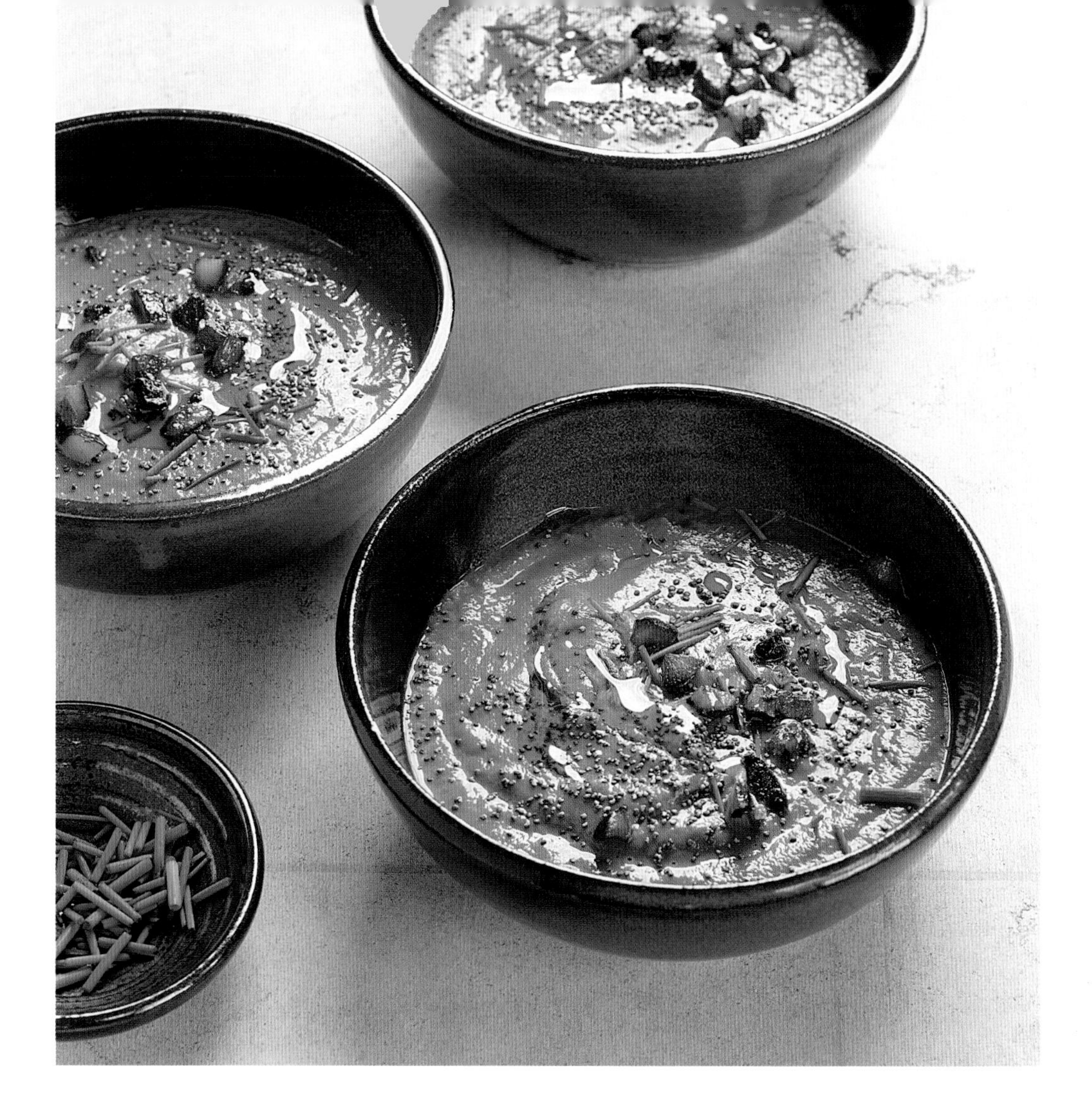

3. Carefully transfer the soup to a blender and puree, in batches if necessary, until completely smooth, 1 to 2 minutes, thinning with up to 1 cup (250 ml) of the remaining warm water until it is a creamy, pourable consistency.

4. To serve, divide the soup between bowls and top with a tablespoon of cashew cream (if using). Sprinkle with the poppy seeds, toasted chestnuts, and chives, then finish with a drizzle of oil.

TIP: *Look for chestnuts in cans or pouches in the baking aisle over the holidays and online the rest of the year.*

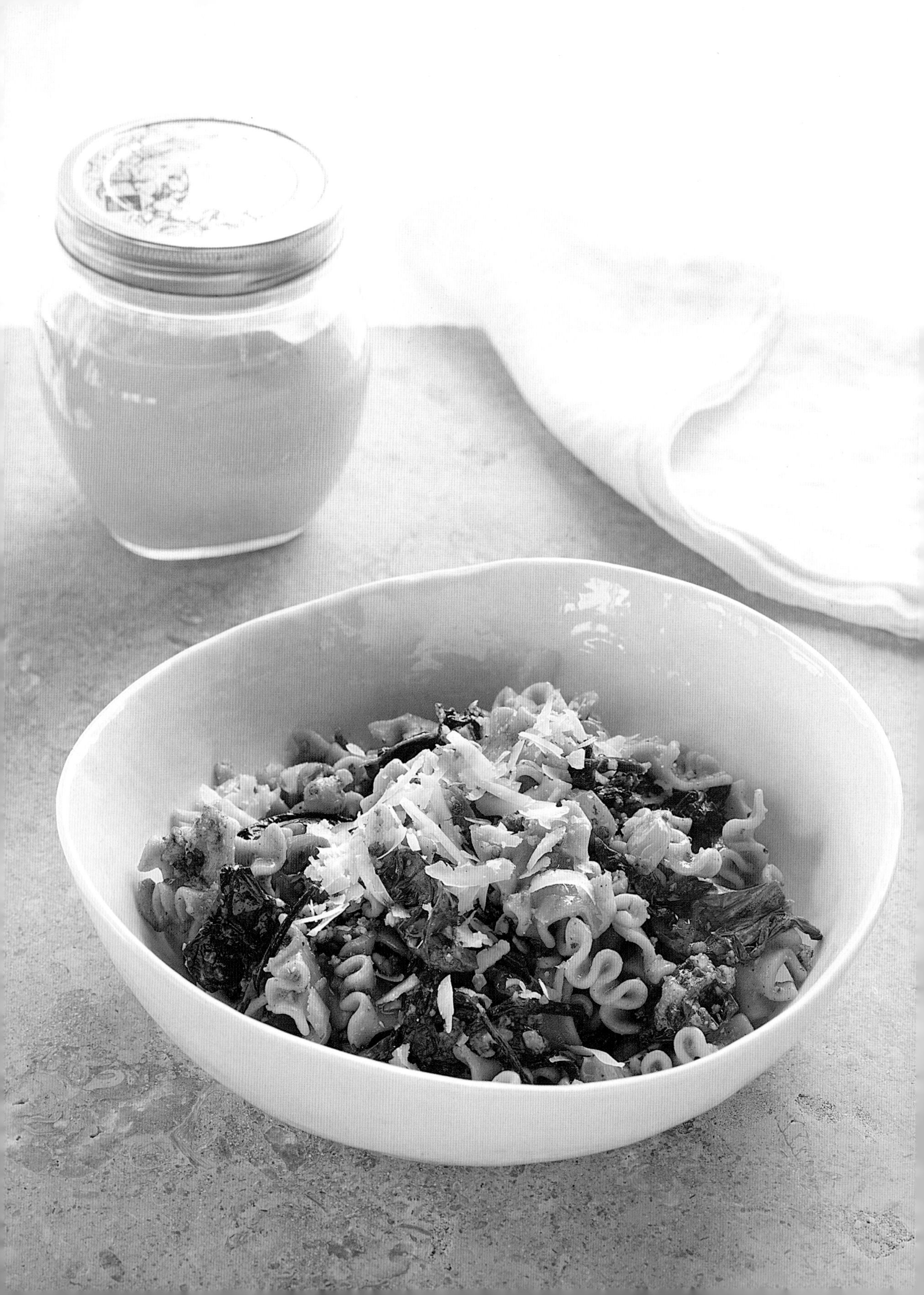

WHOLE-GRAIN PASTA WITH GOLDEN PESTO AND GREENS

SERVES 4

- **10 medium garlic cloves (2 ounces/60 g total) (see Tips)**
- **⅓ cup (55 g) shelled unsalted pistachios**
- **⅓ cup (55 g) pine nuts**
- **⅓ cup (40 g) raw walnuts**
- **1 teaspoon dried oregano**
- **½ teaspoon kosher salt**
- **⅛ teaspoon crushed red pepper flakes**
- **3 tablespoons extra-virgin olive oil**
- **⅓ cup (60 g) golden raisins**
- **1 bunch Swiss chard (7 ounces/200 g), stems finely chopped, leaves thinly sliced**
- **½ preserved lemon, peel finely chopped (about 2 tablespoons) (see Tips)**
- **12 ounces (340 g) whole-grain sturdy pasta (such as those shaped like trumpets, wagon wheels, bite-size shells, and shells)**
- **Grated Pecorino Romano cheese (optional)**
- **Freshly ground black pepper (optional)**

Eating for optimal brain health doesn't mean cutting out the dishes you have come to think of as comfort foods. Case in point: this elegant pasta recipe, which pairs a garlicky, nut-packed pesto with golden raisins and Swiss chard sautéed with briny preserved lemon. The pesto features three nuts—pistachios, walnuts, and pine nuts—because they all provide unique flavors and brain health virtues, too.

Pine nuts are buttery and delicious but can be difficult to find (not to mention expensive), so you could substitute almonds or pecans instead. Choose a whole-grain pasta with plenty of nooks and crannies (like trumpet or shell shapes) to capture the toasted nuts, golden nibs of garlic, and bits of salted lemon in each bite.

A double batch of the pesto keeps well in the fridge for up to ten days. Top it with a layer of olive oil to avoid discoloration, and scoop out spoonfuls to serve with crackers and white anchovies, toss into grain bowls, or dollop into a salad.

1. To make the pesto, coarsely chop the garlic in the bowl of a food processor. Add the pistachios, pine nuts, walnuts, oregano, salt, and red pepper flakes and pulse about 15 times, until all the nuts are smaller than a pine nut.

2. Heat 2 tablespoons of the oil in a large nonstick skillet over medium-low heat. Add the pesto and raisins and cook, stirring often, until the smallest pieces of nut start to brown, 5 to 7 minutes. Scrape the pesto into a small bowl and set aside.

3. Using the same skillet, heat the remaining 1 tablespoon oil over medium heat. Cook the chard stems and preserved

TIPS: *Preserved lemon peel adds a mellow, salty acidity to the dish. Look for jars in the condiments aisle of the grocery store. Or substitute 1 tablespoon lemon zest and ¼ teaspoon kosher salt.*

While I prefer fresh, high-quality garlic, using already peeled cloves of garlic from the grocery store is a real time-saver here.

lemon until soft and starting to brown, 3 to 4 minutes. Add the chard leaves and cook, stirring often, until the leaves are wilted but still vibrant, 5 to 6 minutes.

4. Bring a large pot of salted water to a boil. Stir in the pasta and cook until just al dente, usually 1 to 2 minutes less than the package directions. Reserve ½ cup (120 ml) of the pasta water, then drain the pasta in a colander. Return the pasta to the pot and add the pesto and chard. Toss well, drizzling with enough of the pasta water so the pesto and greens cling to the pasta.

5. To serve, scoop into shallow bowls. Top with grated cheese (if using), a drizzle of olive oil, and black pepper, if you like.

TOASTING NUTS AND SEEDS

Punch up the flavor and aroma of your nuts and seeds by briefly toasting them. This will make them more pleasantly crunchy and nut-brown as well as remove any slightly bitter flavors by releasing the tannins that reside in the skin. Those skins come off far easier after toasting; just rub between kitchen towels. Toasted nuts and seeds are better able to assert themselves when combined with other foods, too, pulling more than their weight in flavor.

Go for gentle toasting with the minimal temperature and time needed to achieve a nutty aroma and a slightly deeper color. While applying high heat over a longer period of time could damage their beneficial fats (like the omega-3 fatty acids), toasting in a low oven is not likely to change the nutritional value of your nuts and seeds significantly.

For best results, toast in the oven for an even application of heat (as opposed to using a skillet on the stove). Use a rimmed baking sheet lined with parchment paper; the contrast of the nuts and seeds against the paper will help you discern when they are toasted enough. Once cool, use the paper as a funnel to pour the nuts into airtight containers.

When a recipe calls for toasted nuts or seeds, cook up a big batch and freeze the rest for later. Frozen toasted nuts taste just as good as freshly toasted ones. With a stash of your favorites in the freezer, you'll be one step closer to making the Salted Chocolate and Olive Oil Gelato (page 337) and the tangerine-spiked gremolata that goes on the Grilled Shrimp Skewers with Asparagus and Quinoa-Pecan Pilaf (page 195).

NUT AND SEED TOASTING TIMES

Start with fresh, raw, unsalted nuts or seeds. Preheat the oven to 300°F (150°C). Place the nuts or seeds on a rimmed baking sheet lined with parchment paper and toast until just a shade darker, stirring halfway through the baking time to assure even cooking. Keep a close eye on them to avoid burning (your oven may cook faster than the times listed here). Cool completely before storing in airtight containers at room temperature (up to one week), in the refrigerator (up to three months), or in the freezer (up to six months). These storage times are about half that for whole, raw nuts. That's because toasting (or chopping) nuts releases their oils, causing them to oxidize faster.

WHOLE NUTS	
Almonds	16–18 minutes
Brazil nuts	12–14 minutes
Coconut, flaked	6–8 minutes
Coconut, shredded	4–6 minutes
Hazelnuts	15–20 minutes
Macadamia nuts	8–10 minutes
Peanuts (shelled)	15–20 minutes
Pecans	6–8 minutes
Pine nuts	8–10 minutes
Pistachios	6–8 minutes
Walnuts	6–8 minutes
SEEDS	
Pumpkin seeds (pepitas)	10 –12 minutes
Sesame seeds, black or white, unhulled	10–15 minutes
Sunflower seeds	15–20 minutes

PUMPKIN SEED-CRUSTED SALMON WITH GREEN TAHINI SAUCE

SERVES 4

½ cup (60 g) raw hulled pumpkin seeds (pepitas), toasted (see page 190) and coarsely chopped

1 teaspoon paprika

½ teaspoon ground cumin

½ teaspoon kosher salt

⅛ teaspoon cayenne (optional)

1 tablespoon extra-virgin olive oil

4 skin-on salmon fillets, 4 to 6 ounces (115 to 170 g) each, about 1 inch (2.5 cm) thick

⅓ cup (80 ml) water

¼ cup (60 ml) tahini

2 tablespoons fresh lemon juice

1 tablespoon hemp seeds, plus more to sprinkle on the finished dish

1 small garlic clove, crushed

1½ loosely packed cups (30 g) fresh flat-leaf parsley leaves and tender stems, roughly chopped, plus torn leaves for serving

Adding pumpkin seeds (aka pepitas) to this simple salmon dinner gives you both plant-based omega-3s as well as DHA and EPA from the salmon. By coating the fillets with toasted seeds, you also get a tasty crunchy coat on the salmon that keeps their beneficial fats from seeping out. Dollop the fillets with a quick hemp seed and tahini sauce, for a dish with layers of flavor that is jam-packed with nutritious seeds.

1. Preheat the oven to 350°F (180°C).

2. Stir together the pumpkin seeds, paprika, cumin, ¼ teaspoon of the salt, and cayenne (if using) in a small bowl.

3. Coat the bottom of a rimmed baking sheet with the oil. Place the salmon fillets, skin side down, on the pan and turn them over to coat the top and sides with oil. Press the seed mixture onto all sides of the fillets to form a crust, dividing evenly.

4. Bake for 10 to 12 minutes for medium-rare or 15 minutes for well done, until the salmon springs back a little when gently pressed with your fingers. (If using an instant-read thermometer, take the temperature in the thickest part of the fish: 120°F/48°C for rare, 125°F/50°C for medium-rare, and up to 140°F/60°C) for well done.)

5. Combine the water, tahini, lemon juice, hemp seeds, garlic, and remaining ¼ teaspoon salt in the bowl of a food processor or blender. Process until creamy, about 1 minute. Add the parsley and process on high speed, another 1 minute.

6. To serve, top each salmon fillet with about 3 tablespoons of tahini sauce and sprinkle with any pepitas from the baking pan and with more hemp seeds and parsley.

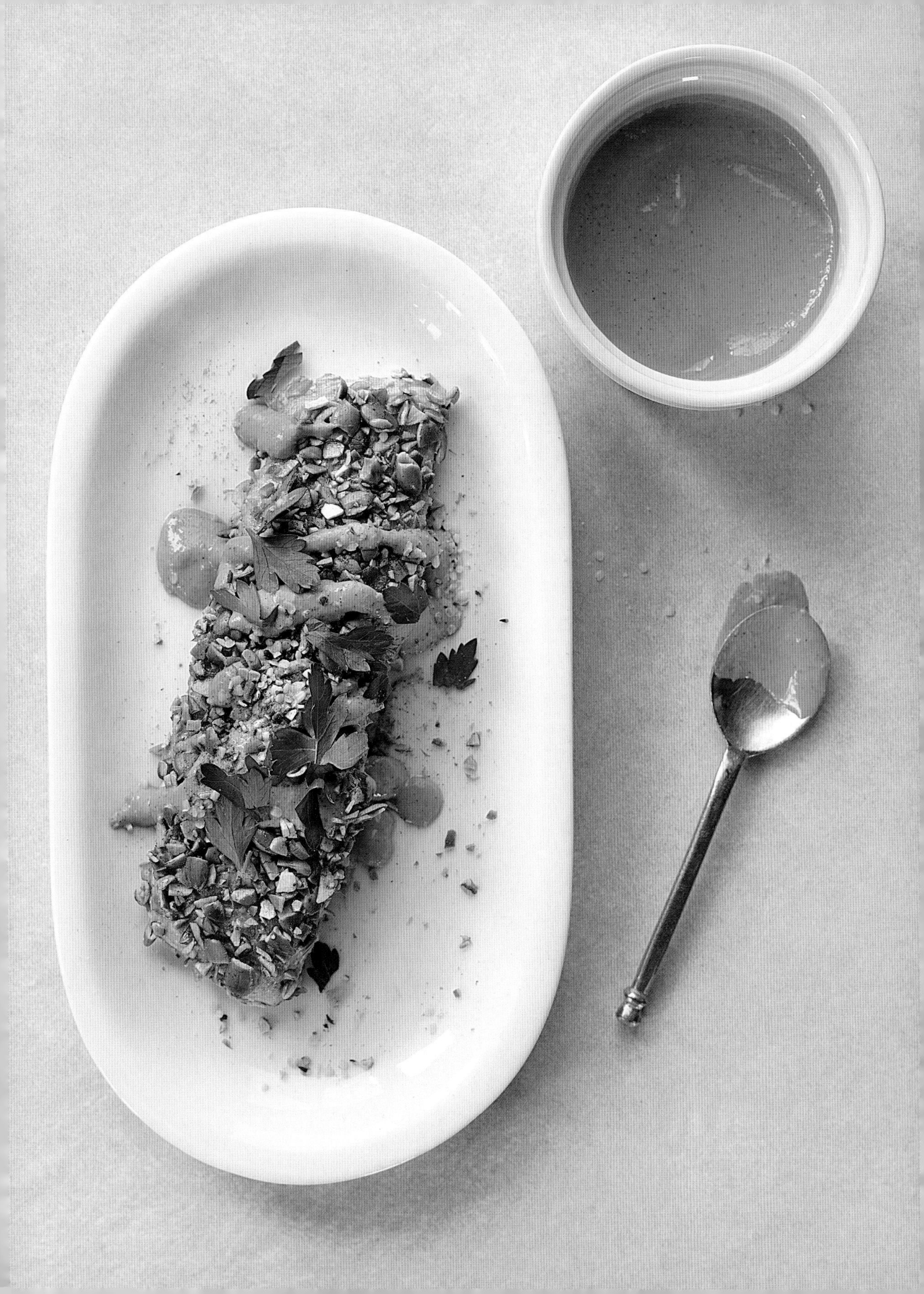

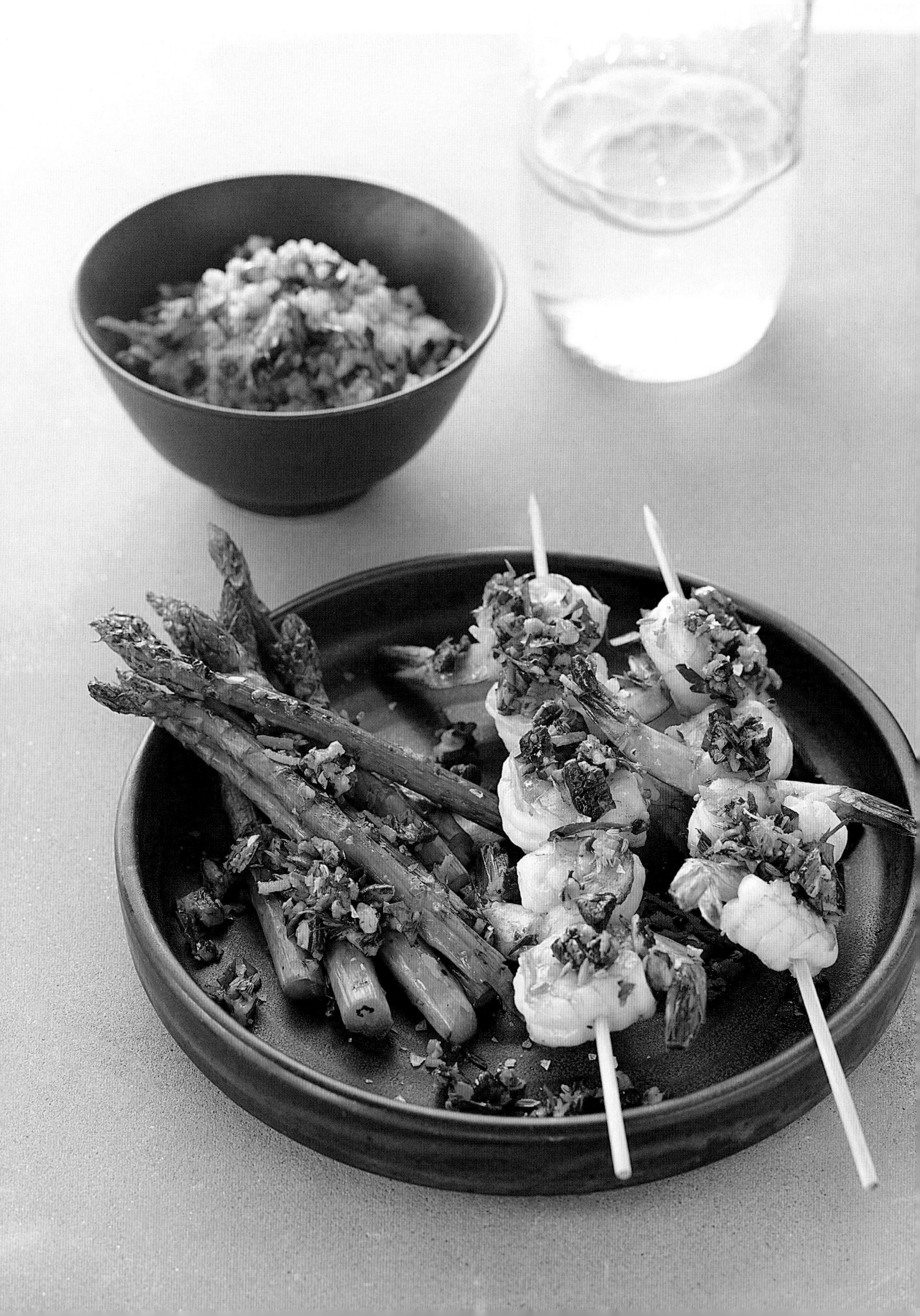

GRILLED SHRIMP SKEWERS WITH ASPARAGUS AND QUINOA-PECAN PILAF

SERVES 4

1 cup (200 g) quinoa, rinsed

2 cups (500 ml) water

1 teaspoon kosher salt

1 cup (115 g) pecans, toasted and coarsely chopped

½ loosely packed cup (10 g) fresh flat-leaf parsley leaves, finely chopped, plus a few torn leaves for serving

½ cup (120 ml) fresh tangerine or orange juice

2 tablespoons extra-virgin olive oil, plus more for brushing

1 tablespoon tangerine or orange zest

1 teaspoon fennel seeds, crushed

1 pound (455 g) peeled and deveined medium shrimp (about 30)

¼ teaspoon freshly ground black pepper

1 pound (455 g) slender asparagus, woody ends trimmed

Flaky salt (optional)

A nutty take on gremolata—a hand-chopped herb topping usually made with lemon and garlic—is an easy and delicious way to dress up simply prepared ingredients, like the shrimp and asparagus in this recipe. The pecans' high fat content adds a buttery flavor and a nice crunch to the quinoa (also a seed!), while crushed fennel seeds bring a warm, sweet flavor that goes well with shrimp. If you don't care for the subtle licorice taste of fennel, you can leave them out.

A grilling basket or mesh mat does double duty here: it protects the shrimp from the heat of the grill (see Tip) and keeps the asparagus from slipping between the grates. If you don't have either of these grilling tools, a metal cooling rack works just as well.

You'll need six to eight skewers for the shrimp; if using bamboo ones, soak them in water for at least fifteen minutes before threading the shrimp. And if you don't have a grill, cook the asparagus and shrimp under a broiler or in a grill pan, keeping an eye on the cooking time.

1. Warm a grill to medium-high (375°F/190°C). Alternatively, heat a grill pan over medium-high heat or turn the broiler to high.

2. Place the quinoa, water, and ¼ teaspoon of the kosher salt in a medium saucepan with a tight-fitting lid. Bring to a boil over medium-high heat, then reduce the heat to a gentle simmer. Cover and cook until the quinoa has absorbed almost all the water, 15 to 20 minutes. Remove from the heat, cover, and let the quinoa steam for at least 5 minutes or until you are ready to serve.

continued

3. To make the gremolata, stir together the pecans, parsley, 1 tablespoon of the tangerine juice, 1 tablespoon of the oil, the zest, fennel seeds, and ¼ teaspoon of the salt in a small bowl. Set aside.

4. Thread the shrimp on wooden or metal skewers, four or five per skewer—getting the skewer through both ends if possible. Place the asparagus on one side of a grill basket and the shrimp on the other. (If you don't have a grill basket or mesh mat, cover the grilling surface with foil or a metal cooling rack.) Brush with oil and sprinkle both sides with the pepper and ½ teaspoon of the kosher salt.

5. Grill the asparagus and shrimp until the shrimp are bright pink and opaque and the asparagus are starting to brown, about 5 minutes per side on the grill or 4 minutes per side under the broiler.

6. Use a fork to fluff the quinoa and toss with the remaining tangerine juice and half the gremolata. Divide the quinoa, asparagus, and shrimp skewers evenly between plates. Drizzle with oil and sprinkle with the remaining gremolata, some flaky salt (if using), and more pepper, if you like.

TIP: *Grilling over direct heat can create harmful AGEs (advanced glycation end products, page 280) in food, which is why you'll place the shrimp and asparagus on a grill pan or a mesh mat, which keeps their brain-healthy elements intact. If your asparagus spears are pencil thin, they'll be done at the same time as the shrimp. If you are using fatter asparagus, put them on the grill about 5 minutes before you start the shrimp.*

TOFU AND BABY BOK CHOY STIR-FRY WITH PEANUT SAUCE AND NOODLES

SERVES 4

One 12- to 14-ounce (340 to 450 g) block extra-firm tofu, drained and cut into 1-inch (2.5 cm) cubes

⅓ cup (80 g) smooth, no-sugar-added peanut butter

1½ tablespoons low-sodium soy sauce

1½ tablespoons rice vinegar

1 tablespoon sambal oelek (Indonesian fresh chili paste)

1 tablespoon honey

1 teaspoon sesame oil (toasted or dark)

1 teaspoon grated fresh ginger (from a ½-inch/1.25 cm piece)

1 large garlic clove

Up to ½ cup (120 ml) water

One 8-ounce (225 g) package udon noodles (see Tip)

1 tablespoon avocado oil

1 large red onion (12 ounces/ 340 g), cut into slices lengthwise

3 baby bok choy (10 ounces/ 285 g total), cored and sliced lengthwise (about 3 cups)

½ cup (70 g) raw or lightly toasted peanuts, coarsely chopped

This dish is all about the spicy peanut sauce and the crispy tofu. I even make a double batch of the tofu and the sauce just so I can snack on the golden-brown cubes dipped into the gingery sauce later in the week. I highly recommend making the entire recipe start to finish first, though, because this twist on a classic stir-fry comes together easily and features two vegetables—baby bok choy and red onion—making it a win for brain health.

Look for natural peanut butter with no added sugar or unhealthy oils (like refined palm, soybean, or hydrogenated oils). Allergic to peanuts? Use a creamy natural almond butter instead and serve toasted chopped almonds on top.

1. Line a rimmed baking sheet with a clean kitchen towel. Lay the tofu cubes in a single layer on half the towel. Fold the towel over to cover the tofu and press out as much water as possible. Top with a second baking sheet and weight it with something heavy, such as a cast-iron pan or two large cans of tomatoes. Let the tofu sit until drained of water, 20 to 30 minutes, or up to overnight, refrigerated. Pat dry with a clean towel.

2. Place the peanut butter, soy sauce, vinegar, sambal oelek, honey, sesame oil, ginger, and garlic in a blender and puree until completely smooth and creamy, adding water if needed by the tablespoon to make a smooth sauce. Set aside.

3. Bring a large pot of salted water to a boil and cook the noodles according to the package directions (usually between 8 and 12 minutes). Drain in a colander and toss with 1 teaspoon of the avocado oil to keep them from sticking.

continued

TIP: Udon noodles are sturdy wheat noodles that cook quickly and stand up well to being tossed into a stir-fry. Soba noodles are also a good choice here; some are made from all buckwheat (a gluten-free, grain-like seed) and others have a combination of buckwheat and wheat. Brown rice noodles are another good gluten-free option, too.

4. Heat 1 teaspoon of the avocado oil in a large nonstick skillet or wok over high heat. Add the tofu cubes to the pan and separate so they are not touching. Cook, undisturbed, until golden and crispy on one side, 3 to 4 minutes. Use long-handled tongs to turn the cubes over and cook until golden brown on the other side, for another 3 to 4 minutes. Transfer to a plate and keep warm near the stove.

5. Add the remaining 1 teaspoon avocado oil to the skillet and add the onion. Cook, stirring often, over medium-high heat, until starting to brown on the edges, 2 to 3 minutes. Add the bok choy and cook until the white stems are tender but the greens are still vibrant, 4 to 6 minutes.

6. Divide the noodles between shallow bowls and top with the vegetables. Drizzle with half the peanut sauce and toss to coat. Top with the tofu, remaining sauce, and peanuts.

NUT AND SEED BUTTERS

You can get your daily handful of nuts or seeds by enjoying a few tablespoons of delicious butters, albeit with less fiber. Smeared on sliced apples or whole-grain bread, they provide a satisfying snack. Look for butters without added sugar, flavorings, and inflammatory oils (such as soybean, palm, or hydrogenated oil). Buy only as much as you will use in the next few months, as these nut and seed butters are even more perishable than the little plants they come from.

There's a whole world of nut butters beyond peanut butter. Look for butters made from cashews, almonds, walnuts, pecans, and hazelnuts. Nut butters can add rich, buttery flavors and textures to your cooking, like the spicy sauce in the Tofu and Baby Bok Choy Stir-Fry with Peanut Sauce and Noodles (page 197).

Seed butters are a wonderful addition to your diet, even if you aren't allergic to nuts. Look for butters made from sunflower, hemp, pumpkin, and even poppy seeds. Tahini, made from sesame seeds, is not just for making hummus. In this chapter, tahini is folded into the batter of the Almond Butter–Tahini Blondies (page 201), replaces butter in the Chunky Whole-Grain Chocolate Chip Cookies (page 265), and becomes an easy green sauce to go with the Pumpkin Seed–Crusted Salmon (page 192).

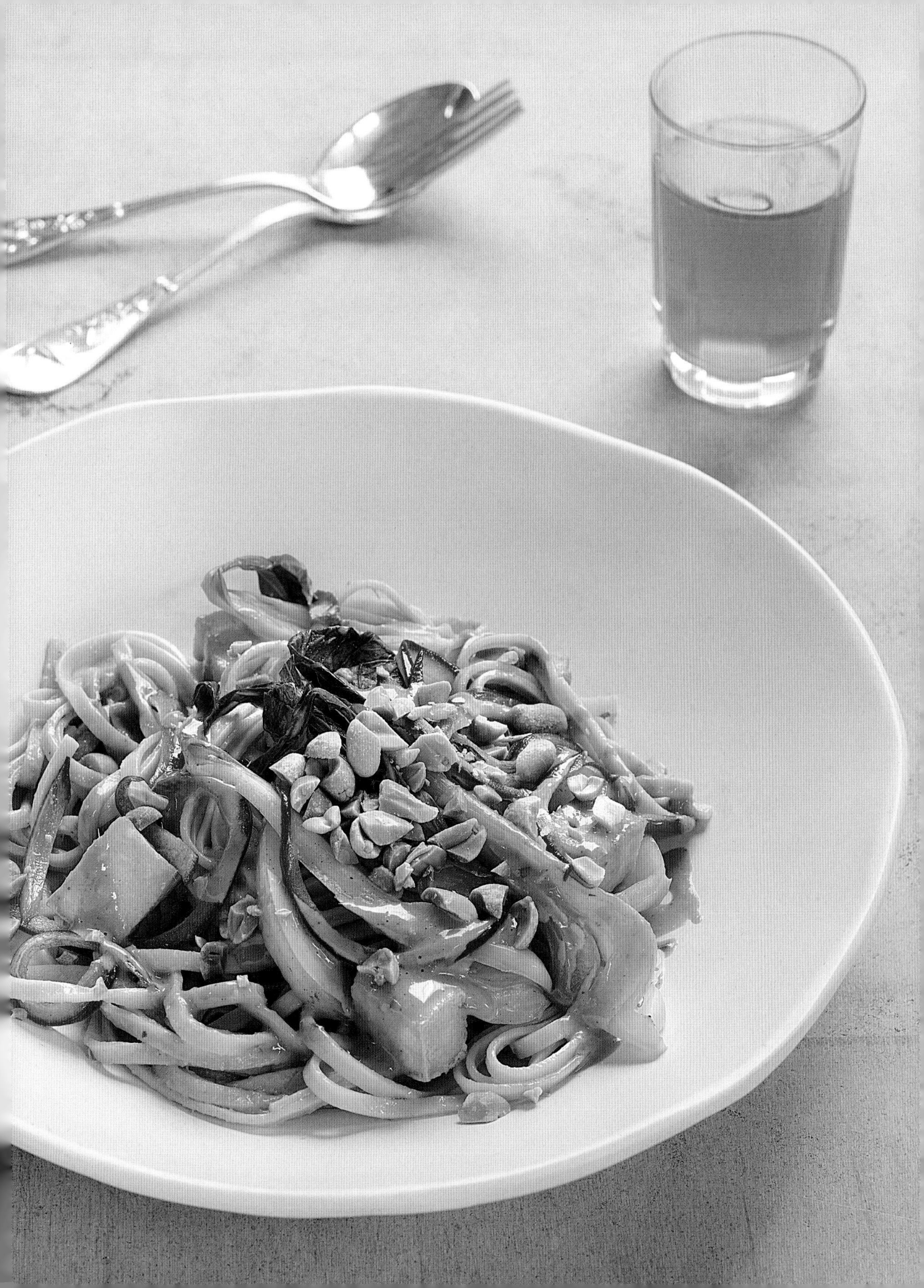

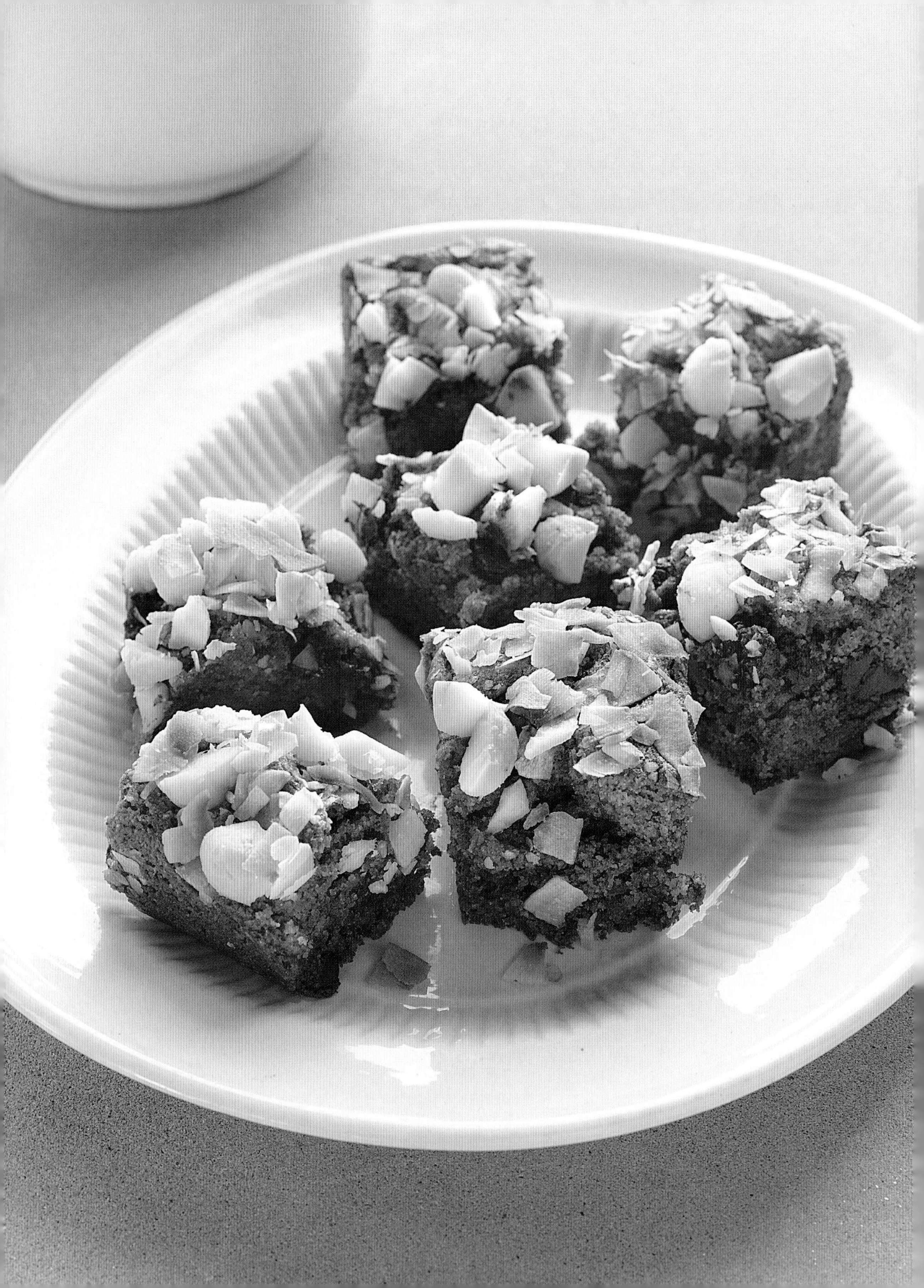

ALMOND BUTTER-TAHINI BLONDIES

MAKES 16

- ½ cup (120 ml) extra-virgin olive oil, plus more for greasing the pan
- ½ cup (85 g) coconut palm sugar
- ¼ cup (70 g) smooth almond butter, at room temperature
- ¼ cup (60 ml) tahini, well stirred and at room temperature
- 2 eggs, at room temperature
- 1 teaspoon pure vanilla extract
- ½ teaspoon almond extract
- 1½ cups (125 g) almond flour
- 1 teaspoon baking powder
- ½ teaspoon kosher salt
- 1 cup (170 g) dark chocolate chips (60% or more cacao)
- ½ cup (70 g) macadamia nuts, raw or roasted, coarsely chopped
- ½ cup (30 g) unsweetened coconut flakes (see Tip)

If you need to be convinced to add more nuts and seeds into your diet, then these blondies are the thing to do it. Decadent, chewy, and brownie-like, these satiating treats pack in nutrients from almonds, macadamia nuts, sesame seeds, and coconut. Incorporating high-quality chocolate chips made from 60 percent or more cacao (which is technically also a seed!), this recipe is a delicious example of how well different types of nuts and seeds work together.

Macadamia nuts are a buttery, big-flavor, high-fat nut, rich in the same oleic acid found in extra-virgin olive oil. Other soft nuts work well as a topping, too, such as whole cashews or pecans.

1. Set an oven rack in the center position and preheat the oven to 350°F (180°C). Grease a 9-inch (23 cm) square pan with oil and line with parchment so that the edges overhang.

2. Whisk together the oil, sugar, almond butter, tahini, eggs, vanilla, and almond extract in a large bowl until no lumps remain.

3. In a separate bowl, stir together the almond flour, baking powder, and salt. Fold the mixture into the wet ingredients until no streaks of flour remain. Fold in the chocolate chips.

4. Scrape the batter into the prepared baking pan and smooth with a spatula. Sprinkle the macadamia nuts and coconut evenly over the top. Gently press the toppings into the batter slightly.

5. Bake for 30 to 35 minutes, until the edges are brown and a tester inserted into the center comes out clean or with just

a few moist crumbs clinging to it. Cool completely before cutting into 2-inch (5 cm) squares.

6. To store, wrap tightly and keep in the refrigerator for up to 3 days or in the freezer for up to 3 months.

TIP: *Coconut flakes are thicker and wider than shredded coconut and have a more distinct coconut flavor. You can substitute unsweetened shredded coconut in this recipe, if you like, but add it in the last 15 minutes of cooking time to avoid burning.*

NUT AND SEED FLOURS

Nut-based flours (also called "meals" if more coarsely ground) can replace much of the all-purpose white flour in your baking, adding fiber, vitamin E, and healthy fats to cookies, cakes, and bars. Almond flour, sometimes labeled "superfine," is the most common type you'll find at the grocery store. Made from ground almonds that have been blanched and peeled, it has a light color and a fine texture, making it perfect for baked goods where you want a tender crumb, like in muffins and cookies. Almond meal is made with ground whole almonds that have not been peeled. It has a darker color and a coarser texture, making it a nice addition to rustic cakes. Sometimes you'll find toasted almond flour or meal made from toasted whole almonds (to boost color and flavor) instead of raw ones. Since nut-based flours are perishable, buy only as much as you'll use in a few months, and store in a cold, dark cupboard or in the refrigerator or freezer.

It's also easy to prepare your own. To make 1 cup (115 g) homemade almond flour or meal, pulse 1 cup (110 g) blanched almonds (for flour) or 1 cup (110 g) whole almonds (for meal) in the bowl of a food processor or powerful blender until powdery, being careful the nuts don't turn into almond butter. For toasted almond meal, toast the almonds first (page 190), then grind once they are cool. Use this same method with other nuts—walnuts, pecans, and hazelnuts (remove their papery skins first)—to create other types of fresh, delicious nut-based flours.

The selection of seed-based flours is ever-expanding. A boon for those allergic to tree nuts, look for flour made from coconut, sunflower seeds, quinoa (a grainlike seed), and buckwheat (a fruit seed related to rhubarb).

GLAZED CITRUS, ALMOND, AND OLIVE OIL CAKE

SERVES 12

- **⅔ cup (150 ml) fruity olive oil, plus more for the pan and the glaze**
- **1 small seedless orange (6 ounces/170 g), such as navel or Cara Cara**
- **1 small lemon (5 ounces/140 g), such as a Meyer lemon**
- **1½ cups (170 g) almond flour or meal**
- **1 cup (115 g) oat or quinoa flour**
- **1 tablespoon baking powder**
- **½ teaspoon kosher salt**
- **4 eggs, at room temperature**
- **1 cup (170 g) coconut palm sugar**
- **¼ cup (25 g) confectioners' sugar**
- **2 teaspoons warm water**
- **Fresh berries, for serving (optional)**

This cake makes a persuasive case for baking with almond flour, whether you are gluten-free or not. Olive oil adds peppery spice and amplifies flavors like orange and lemon better than butter does. The batter begins with a unique technique—you'll boil a whole orange and a lemon to puree into a marmalade-like spread. This gives the cake its citrusy intensity and helps keep it moist for days. Using the whole fruit not only studs the cake with chewy bits of orange and lemon, it contributes a good dose of fiber and beneficial flavonoids from the peel.

You can use almond flour or meal interchangeably here with good results, with the meal resulting in a more rustic, nubby texture. Toasted and ground whole almonds work, too (see the sidebar). To reduce the amount of sugar, omit the glaze.

1. Preheat the oven to 350°F (180°C). Brush a nonstick 9-inch (23 cm) springform pan with oil.

2. Place the orange and lemon in a saucepan and cover with water. Bring to a boil, then reduce to a simmer. Cook until you can easily insert the tip of a knife into the peel easily, about 30 minutes. Drain and set aside until cool enough to handle.

3. Combine the almond flour, oat flour, baking powder, and salt in a medium bowl; set aside.

4. Cut the lemon and orange in half through the equator. Scoop out the pulp and seeds from the lemon and discard, then scoop out just the seeds from the orange, keeping the pulp. Place the lemon rind and the deseeded orange in the bowl of a food processor. Pulse until it resembles a thick marmalade. Scrape into a measuring cup; you should have about 1 cup (250 g).

continued

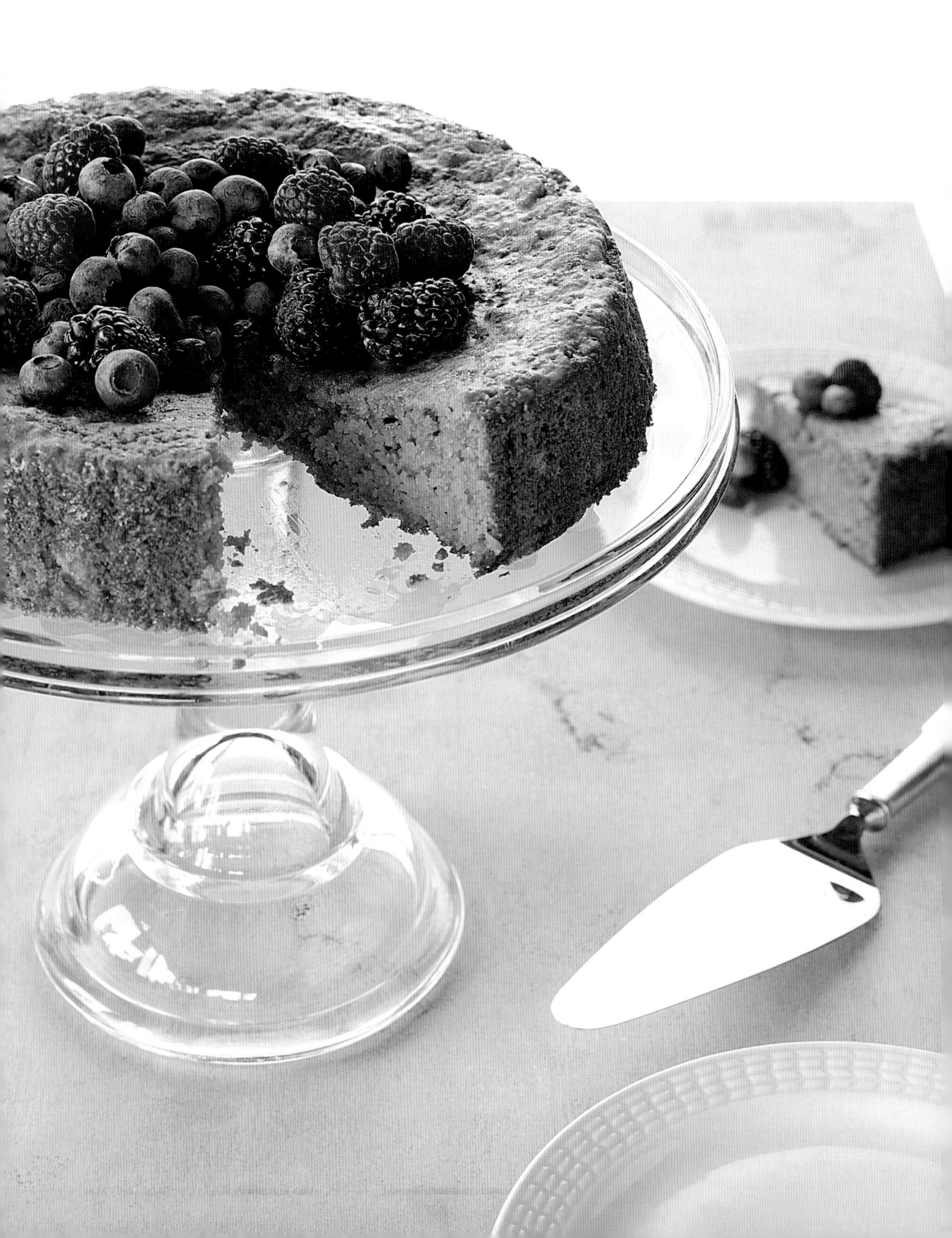

5. Combine the eggs and coconut sugar in the food processor and process until frothy, about 1 minute. With the machine running, pour the oil through the top of the feed tube and process for another 1 minute until smooth. Scrape the egg mixture into the flour mixture and combine by hand until no streaks of flour remain. Fold in the marmalade until evenly distributed.

6. Pour the batter into the prepared springform pan and bake for 40 to 50 minutes, until the edges pull away from the sides and a tester inserted into the center comes out clean. Set aside to cool completely.

7. To make the glaze, stir together the confectioners' sugar and 2 teaspoons of the warm water until no lumps remain. Add up to 2 teaspoons oil until smooth and glossy.

8. Run a flexible metal spatula or a knife between the edge of the pan and the cake, then release the sides. Pour the glaze over top and spread to the edges in an even layer with the back of a spoon or an offset spatula.

9. When the glaze has set, cut the cake into wedges and serve with fresh berries (if using).

10. To store, cover tightly and refrigerate for up to 5 days. Or wrap each wedge individually and store in the freezer for up to 3 months.

PEAR AND FIG BREAKFAST CRISP

SERVES 4 TO 6

3 tablespoons pure maple syrup

3 tablespoons extra-virgin olive oil

1 tablespoon fresh lemon juice

1 teaspoon pure vanilla extract

½ teaspoon ground ginger

½ teaspoon kosher salt

3 ripe but firm red or green Anjou or Bosc pears (1½ pounds/680 g), cored and sliced ¼ inch (6 mm) thick

½ cup (90 g) dried figs, sliced ¼ inch (6 mm) thick

1 cup (100 g) rolled oats

½ cup (45 g) sliced almonds

2 tablespoons hemp seeds

2 tablespoons hulled pumpkin seeds (pepitas)

Plain, unsweetened yogurt (coconut, whole milk, or nut-based)

If you have ever had a piece of fruit pie for breakfast and wished it was a little less sweet and more, well, breakfasty, this pear and fig crisp is for you. The granola-like topping provides you with your daily dose of nuts and seeds—crunchy toasted almonds, chewy hemp seeds, and cheery green pepitas—all clustered with maple syrup–coated oats. Pears and figs together evoke thoughts of crisp fall mornings, but you can make this breakfast crisp year-round as long as you have ripe but firm pears.

While berries are the fruit with the most solid evidence for protecting your brain health, pears and figs, in my opinion, are a close second. Both provide impressive amounts of fiber, potassium, and flavonoids. Pears, especially, provide the type of flavonol linked to a reduced risk of Alzheimer's.

1. Preheat the oven to 375°F (190°C).

2. Whisk together 1 tablespoon each of the maple syrup and oil, the lemon juice, ½ teaspoon of the vanilla, the ginger, and ¼ teaspoon of the salt in a large bowl. Fold in the pears and figs. Transfer to a 9-inch (23 cm) square baking dish.

3. Using the same bowl, stir together the oats, almonds, hemp seeds, pumpkin seeds, the remaining 2 tablespoons each maple syrup and oil, the remaining ½ teaspoon vanilla, and the remaining ¼ teaspoon salt. Toss well to combine and sprinkle evenly over the pears.

4. Cover tightly with foil and bake for 30 minutes. Remove the foil and bake for another 15 to 18 minutes, until the filling is thick and bubbling and the crisp topping is golden brown.

5. Serve warm, at room temperature, or cold scooped into bowls. Top with a dollop of yogurt.

TIP: *You can assemble the crisp the day before, refrigerate it overnight (tightly covered), and pop it in the oven in the morning.*

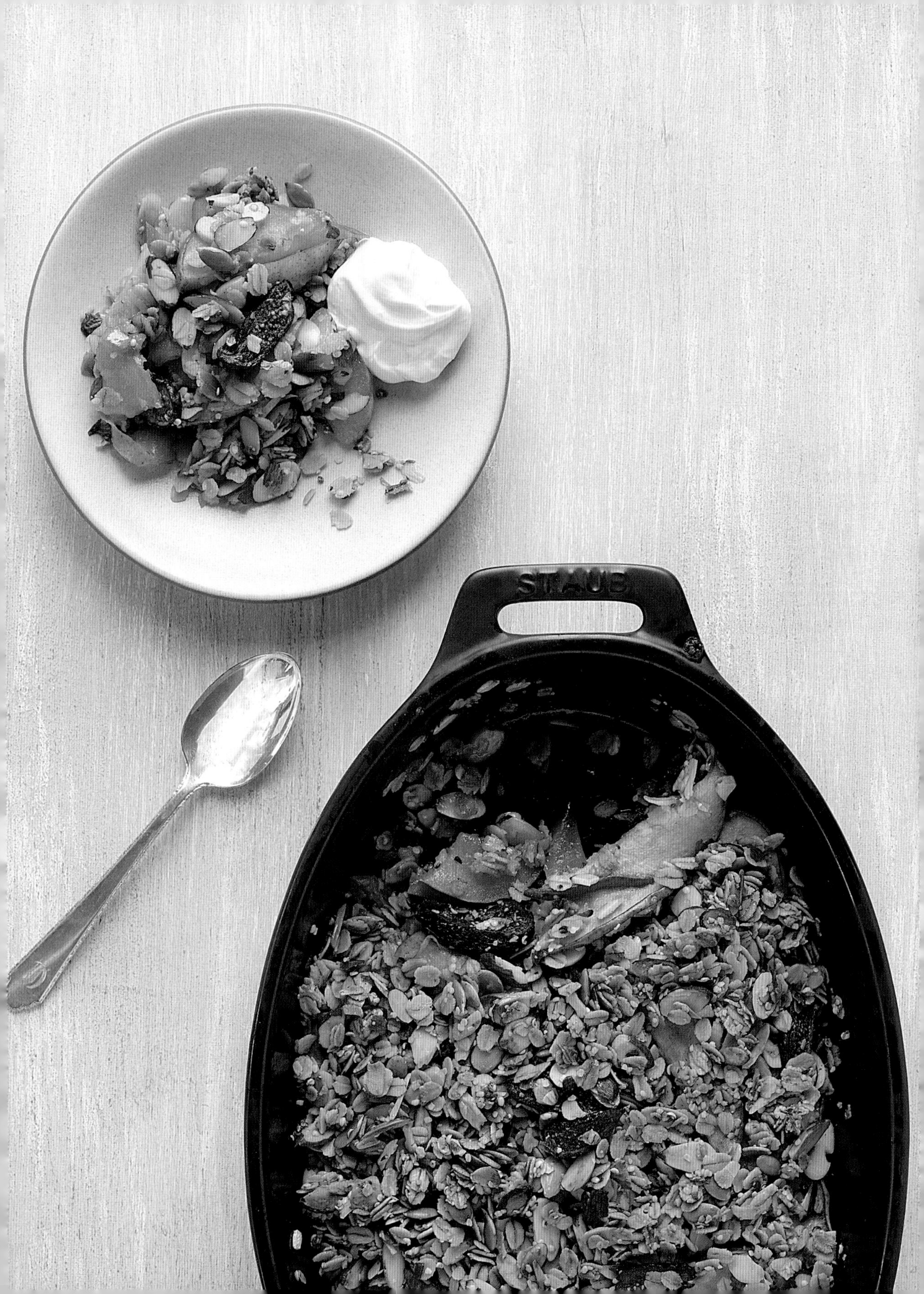
STAUB

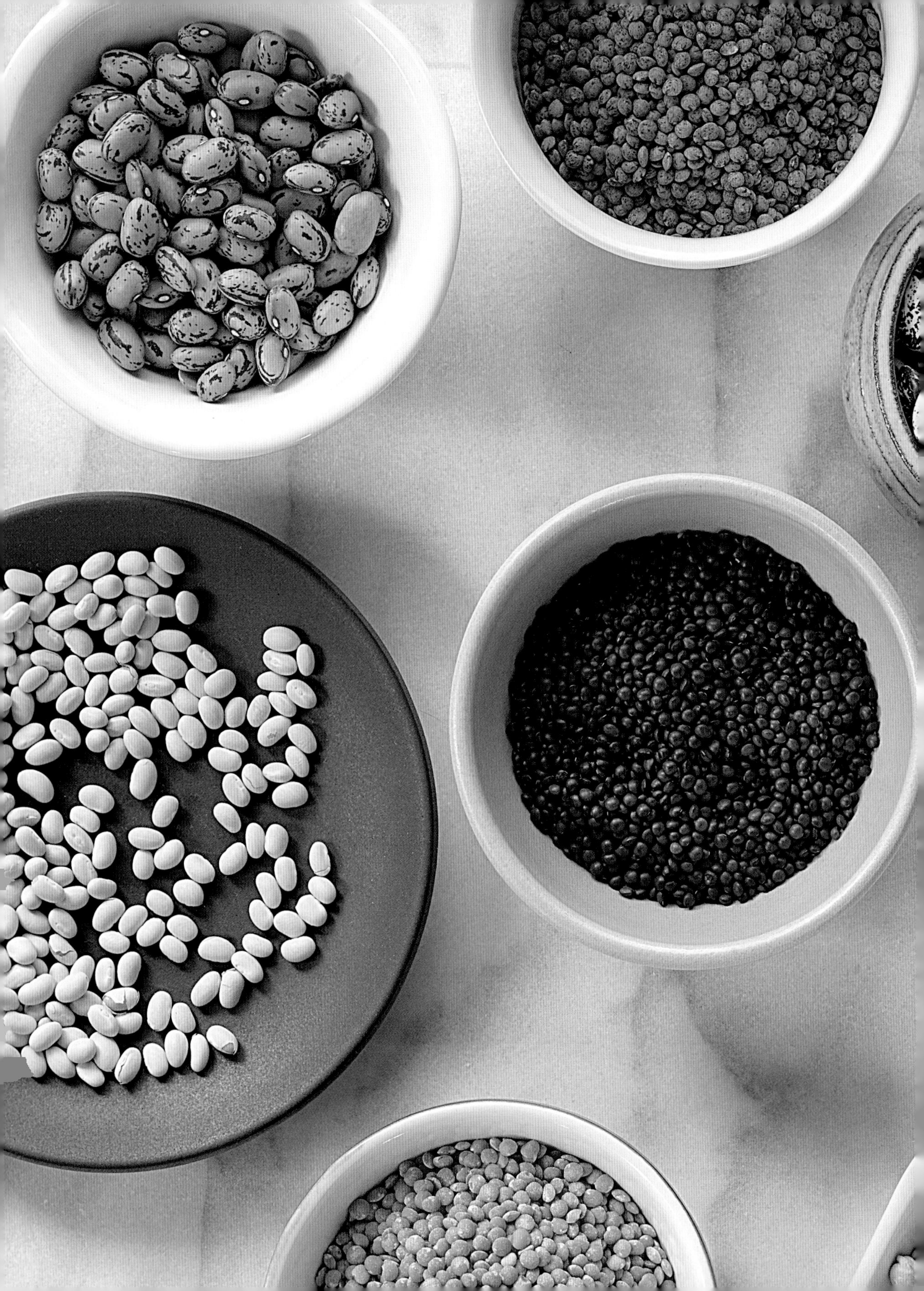

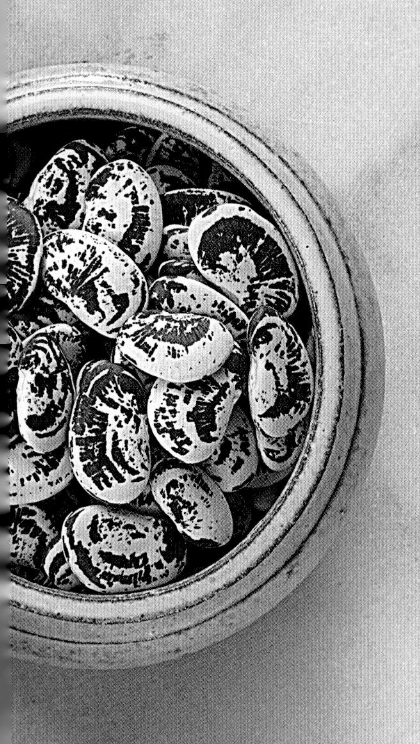

BEANS AND LENTILS

Brain-healthy eating means celebrating beans and lentils for the pantry heroes they are. These tiny plants have big personalities and are ready to slip into any number of versatile roles in your cooking. Beans and lentils are members of the legume family, along with peas (both fresh field peas and dried black-eyed ones) and peanuts, an honorary nut (as you may recall from page 181). With names like Black Beluga, Christmas lima, and Appaloosa (because they resemble spotted ponies), legumes can be delightfully colorful, too. Not to mention economical: even the priciest specialty beans cost less than a dollar per serving.

Wherever you find dementia-free, long-living people, beans are on the menu. Whether it's the Japanese making meals from soybeans, the Costa Ricans topping a bowl of black beans with plantains for breakfast, or the Italians enjoying minestrone for lunch, legumes are an important source of protein and a daily staple around the globe.

Eating beans will help you live longer, but what can they do for your brain? First, beans are rich in many of the nutrients a brain needs to thrive, like the flavonoids that come from their pigments and many of the B vitamins. Second, they provide soluble fiber, important for lowering harmful blood cholesterol and fortifying gut health, particularly through enabling the creation of brain-boosting short-chain fatty acids (page 232). Third, bean eaters are slimmer, on average, than people who don't eat beans, and obesity is a known risk factor for Alzheimer's. Eating legumes has metabolic benefits, too, like keeping blood sugar and insulin levels from spiking (see Science Bite: The Lentil Effect, page 225). It could be that legumes are so satiating (because of their fiber and protein content, not to mention their deliciousness) that when you eat more beans, you consume fewer of the brain-unhealthy foods.

Cooking up a pot of homemade beans (page 215) is a wonderful way to prepare heirloom varieties—uniquely delicious beans grown from seeds that have been cultivated for generations, though it works just as well with standard dried beans, too. With cranberry beans and stock ready to go, for example, you are halfway to a hearty bowl of old-school minestrone soup (page 229) using tricks I learned in my grandmother's kitchen. Or you could fold those same beans into a breakfast bowl with greens and eggs poached right in the bean stock (page 106). A pot of black beans can show up for dinner as part of the spicy butternut squash filling for stuffed poblano peppers (page 237).

My affection for the humble chickpea, aka garbanzo bean, finds inspiration in both the whole and flour form. You can turn a batch of hummus into a family-style meal (page 235) with caramelized onions, spiced meat, and even more chickpeas on top. Chickpea flour becomes a filling pancake (page 127) and a surprising ingredient in cookies (page 240).

Lentils are the tiniest legumes, smaller than a pea and lens-shaped, yet packing in more protein than even beans. Their petite size makes them a pantry MVP, cooking up quicker than beans and without the need for soaking first. Just like beans, lentils come in a variety of colors, the different pigments each with its own array of antioxidants. Some lentils are more starchy than others, such as the red lentil, which collapses as it cooks, making it well suited to lending creaminess to a soup (page 226) or a dip (page 221). Others, like the

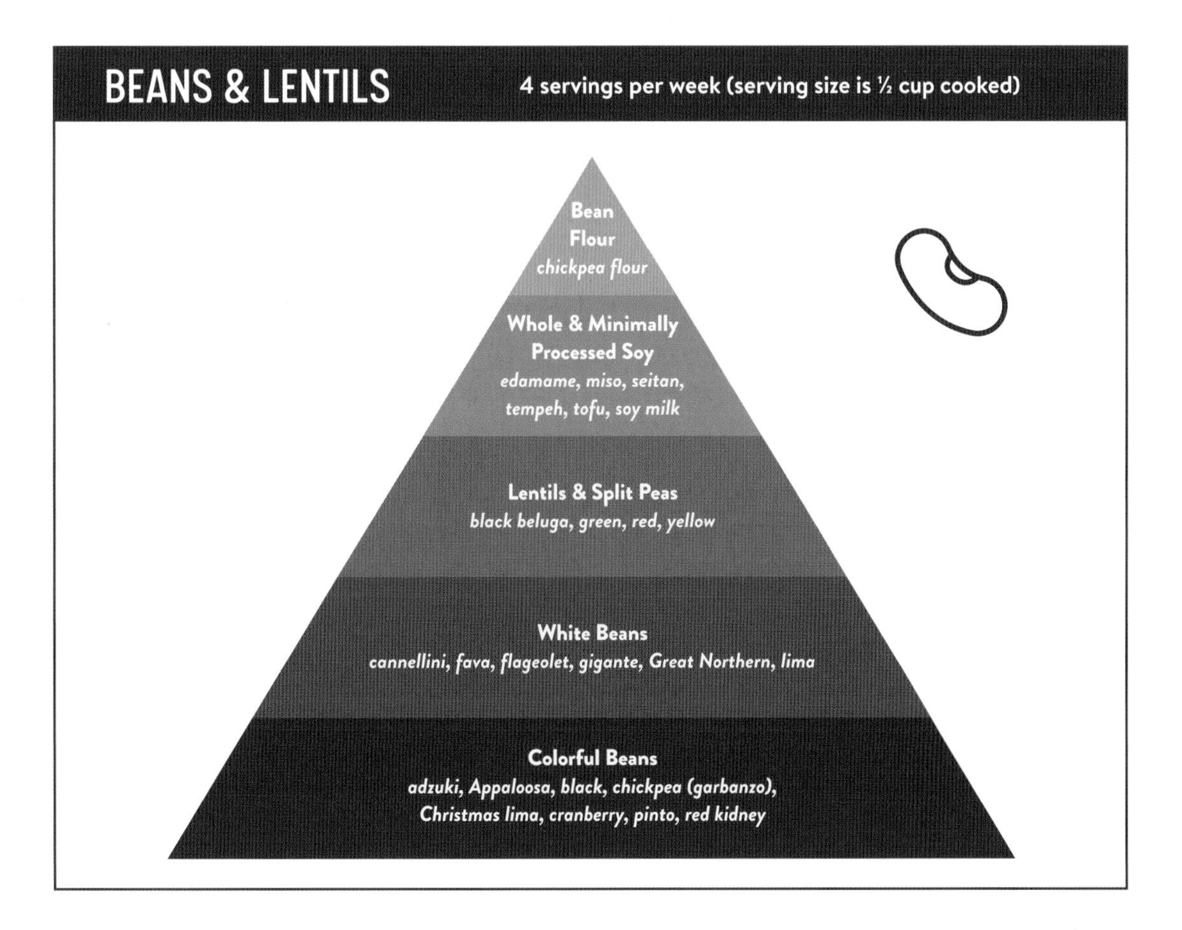

Black Beluga and the French green lentil (aka lentilles du Puy), keep their shape after cooking with a pleasing toothsome bite. Puy lentils are ideal for making a lentil salad, like the zippy grapefruit and bitter greens one (page 224).

SHOPPING FOR BEANS

Whether you are stocking up on dried and canned beans from the grocery store or hunting down a specialty type, you are bound to have a wide variety to choose from. As a bonus, beans are some of the most economical of all the brain-healthy foods.

Every grocery store has a good selection of beans and lentils, both canned and dried. These include black, pinto, kidney, and white beans (the latter available in many varieties, such as Great Northern, navy, cannellini, and white kidney beans). Even the most humble bag of brown or green lentils can transform into a nourishing soup. Keep your cupboards stocked with all the lentils—red, yellow, brown, green, and black—and use them liberally in your cooking. Look for specialty beans, too, like Ayocote and Eye of the Goat. These heirloom varieties are grown from seeds that have been handed down through generations. They may be prized for their distinctive markings, like the mahogany scribbles on Borlotti, or for a unique flavor, like the Christmas lima that tastes like toasted chestnuts. See Resources (page 390) for heirloom bean purveyors.

Head over to the produce aisle and you may spot vacuum-packed pouches of cooked lentils, a convenient and high-quality choice. And don't forget that soybeans are beans, too (see page 230). Find them in tofu and tempeh or as frozen edamame beans, both shelled or still in their pods. While in the freezer section, look for frozen green peas and sometimes fava beans that have been frozen from fresh.

Undeniably convenient, canned beans have been pressure cooked right in the can, and they're ready to use without further prep. While canned beans are slightly more expensive than buying dried legumes and cooking them yourself, they will always be consistently tender and creamy. The downside to canned beans is that sometimes they are too tender, turning to mush when you add them to dishes. That makes canned beans a good choice when you plan to puree them into a dish anyways, such as for making a creamy white bean soup or black bean dip. But when the toothsome and creamy texture of the beans adds to the enjoyment of a dish, like in bean salad, freshly cooked are best.

Another potential pitfall of canned beans is their sodium content. Salt is essential for building flavor when cooking beans (see page 220), but too much salt is not part of a brain-healthy diet, especially if you have high blood pressure. Read the label before you buy: look for "no salt added" on the label or a sodium content under 1 percent in the nutrition facts. If you can't find low-sodium beans, be sure to rinse well before using. That bean liquid, however, in low-sodium brands, can be a tasty addition to your cooking. This is especially true for canned chickpeas, since their cooking liquid—called aquafaba, Latin for "bean water"—can add flavor and body to foods, such as soups, stews, and hummus.

There are scientific concerns over the hormone-disrupting effects of chemicals used to line cans, such as bisphenol A (BPA), bisphenol S (BPS), and other phthalate compounds. Whenever possible, look for brands that say BPA-, BPS-, and phthalate-free. (This is especially important if you will be consuming the bean liquid.) If seeking out phthalate-free cans is not an option, be sure to rinse the beans well. Or avoid cans altogether by purchasing cooked beans in glass jars (such as lupinis that come from Italy, pickled and ready for snacking), paper boxes, or BPA-free pouches.

Rest assured that canned beans are just as nutritious as those you cook from scratch. That's because all legumes are so incredibly nutrient-dense, they can afford to lose a few of those nutrients during processing. There are key differences, however, in flavor and texture between brands. Pay attention to which ones you prefer. If you stock your cupboards with different varieties of canned beans and lentils that you really love, they will become trusted pantry staples. (See Resources, page 390, for my favorites.)

ORGANIC OR NOT?

Even though organic is the best choice here, the wide-reaching health benefits of boosting your bean intake far outweigh any concerns of pesticide exposure. Organically grown brands, however, tend to be packaged in phthalate-free cans and are lower in sodium, too.

EASY WAYS TO EAT YOUR LEGUMES

There are so many easy ways to get legumes into your day-to-day diet, and the recipes in this chapter barely scratch the surface. Sometimes the best recipe for eating beans isn't a recipe at all—it's a throw-together meal that doesn't take much time, or effort, to be great. Here are ten nonrecipe recipes that start with already cooked beans or lentils, whether homemade or from a can, jar, or packet.

1. Toss rinsed cannellini beans with pesto (store-bought or homemade, page 105) and toasted pine nuts. Serve warm or cold, on its own or atop greens.

2. For a plant-based curried chickpea salad, warm chickpeas in a skillet with olive oil and curry powder. Smash half with a fork, then stir in yogurt or vegan mayo, chopped apple, celery, raisins, and salt to taste.

3. For a chopped salad, rinse Great Northern beans, shake dry, and toss with olive oil, halved cherry tomatoes, pitted olives, and cucumbers. Finish with a squeeze of lemon juice, salt, and pepper.

4. Add a can of drained navy beans to oil-packed tuna with some oil from the tin. Finish with lots of parsley and lemon.

5. For a black bean salsa, stir together rinsed black beans, fresh or frozen and thawed corn kernels, and chopped roasted red peppers. Add a squeeze of lime juice, salt, and pepper.

6. For a creamy bean dip, simmer together pinto beans, garlic, canned green chiles, and enough almond milk, water, or bean liquid to make a chunky sauce. Blend until smooth and bake until bubbling hot.

7. Warm gigante beans and their liquid, garlic, salt, and pepper in a small saucepan. Mash half the beans to make a chunky sauce, then serve on toast drizzled with olive oil.

8. For a springtime soup, simmer lima beans in vegetable or chicken stock (or use the bean liquid plus water) until hot. Add slivered asparagus, frozen peas, and the juice of one lemon, then finish with salt, pepper, and whatever fresh herbs you have.

9. For a creamy black bean soup, simmer black beans and their liquid, garlic, cumin, and chili powder in a saucepan. Puree, adding just enough water to make a thin soup. Finish with avocado slices and chopped tomatoes.

10. For a quick lentil soup, simmer lentils and their liquid, chopped carrots, and celery in a saucepan, adding more water if needed to make it soupy. Finish with a spoonful of sherry vinegar or lemon juice, salt, and pepper.

A VERY GOOD POT OF BEANS

MAKES 5 TO 6 CUPS (900 G TO 1.08 KG) COOKED BEANS AND 2 TO 3 CUPS (480 TO 720 ML) BROTH

1 tablespoon extra-virgin olive oil

2 medium carrots (8 ounces/230 g), scrubbed and finely chopped (about 1 cup)

1 small yellow onion (5 ounces/140 g), finely chopped

1 large garlic clove, crushed with the side of knife (optional)

2½ teaspoons kosher salt

2 cups (1 pound/455 g) dried beans, rinsed and picked over for debris

One 3-by-5-inch (7.5 by 13 cm) piece kombu (dried seaweed)

This one recipe for cooking a pot of beans can be used with three different methods. Employ the stovetop method when you have the time to be present while your beans cook, and you'll be rewarded with poofs of their comforting aroma each time you check the pot. If you have a slow cooker, it will provide you with a nearly foolproof hands-off method, freeing you up to do other things while your beans transform from raw to cooked. A pressure cooker or multicooker, such as the Instant Pot, gets the job done in record time.

STOVETOP METHOD

This method is generally a hands-off process, since for the bulk of the cooking time, you only need to check on your beans about every half hour to make sure they are covered with ample water.

1. Heat the oil in a large saucepan or Dutch oven over medium heat until shimmering. Add the carrots, onion, garlic (if using), and ½ teaspoon of the salt and cook, stirring often, until soft, 4 to 5 minutes.

2. Add the beans and kombu to the pot and enough water to cover by 2 inches (5 cm) for soaked beans, 3 inches (7.5 cm) for unsoaked ones. Bring to a boil over high heat, then reduce the heat to a lively simmer, stirring occasionally, for about 10 minutes. Reduce the heat to its lowest setting, cover the pot, and cook until the beans are tender but still have a firm bite, 1 to 1½ hours. Remove and discard the kombu and stir in the remaining 2 teaspoons salt. Return to a gentle simmer with the lid off until the bean broth has reduced slightly and the beans are very tender, 10 to 20 minutes. Let cool completely.

continued

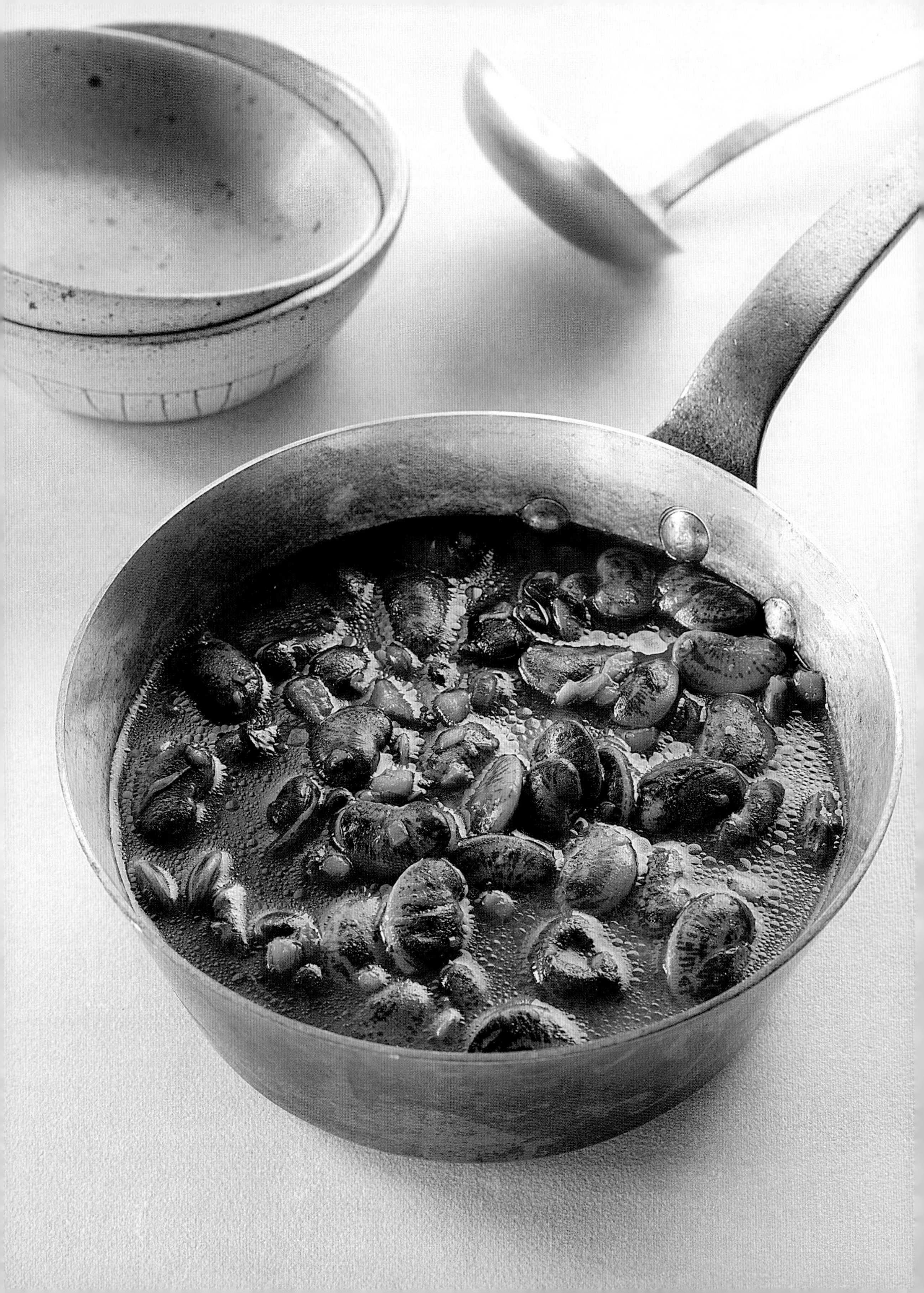

TIP: If you misjudge the timing and your beans are underdone, you have two options. Push the Sauté button and simmer with the lid off, tasting as you go to check for doneness. Or if they are very firm, pressure-cook for an additional 5 minutes. Push the Cancel/End button to turn off the machine, then push Beans/Chili or High Pressure and set the time manually for 5 minutes. Allow the machine to release pressure naturally (which takes 10 to 15 minutes) before removing the lid.

3. To store, pour the beans and their broth into airtight containers, such as quart mason jars, and keep in the refrigerator for up to 1 week. Or pour into zip-top freezer bags or plastic airtight containers and freeze for up to 3 months.

INSTANT POT METHOD

Pressure-cooking your beans in a multicooker, such as an Instant Pot, is a fast, convenient method for getting exceptionally creamy beans. The bean cooking time chart (page 219) is essential here, especially with heirloom beans that come in different shapes and sizes.

1. Using the Sauté setting, warm the oil until it shimmers. Stir in the carrots, onion, garlic (if using), and ½ teaspoon of the salt. Cook, stirring often, until soft, 4 to 5 minutes.

2. Add the beans, kombu, and 6 cups (1.4 L) water to the pot. Depending on your Instant Pot model, push either the Beans/Chili button or the High Pressure button and set the time manually according to the chart on page 219. Manually release the pressure (by carefully turning the valve with the end of a wooden spoon) and switch back to the Sauté setting. Remove the kombu (set aside to use later or discard) and stir in the remaining 2 teaspoons salt. Cook until the beans are tender but still hold their shape and are well seasoned, about 10 minutes. Serve right away or cool completely before storing.

3. To store, pour the beans and their broth into airtight containers, such as quart-size glass mason jars, and keep in the refrigerator for up to 1 week. Or pour into zip-top freezer bags or plastic airtight containers and freeze for up to 3 months.

SLOW COOKER METHOD

A slow cooker lets you cook a perfect pot of beans without having to tend to them. If possible, check the beans about every hour to be sure there is enough water to cover. If you plan to be gone, just add an extra ½ cup (120 ml) water when you set up the slow cooker.

1. If your slow cooker has a sauté feature, warm the oil until shimmering then stir in the carrots, onion, garlic (if using), and ½ teaspoon of the salt. If not, just add everything to the pot at the same time with the beans, with enough water to cover by 2 inches (5 cm) for soaked beans or 3 inches (7.5 cm) for unsoaked ones. Cover and cook on high for 3 to 4 hours (soaked) or 4 to 5 hours (unsoaked), checking after 3 hours for doneness.

2. When the beans are tender but still firm, remove and discard the kombu, and stir in the remaining 2 teaspoons salt. Reduce the heat to low and simmer, uncovered, until the liquid has reduced slightly and the beans are very tender, 10 to 20 minutes. Let cool completely.

3. To store, pour the beans and their broth into airtight containers, such as quart-size glass mason jars, and keep in the refrigerator for up to 1 week. To freeze, pour into zip-top freezer bags or plastic airtight containers for up to 3 months.

KOMBU:

THE MAGIC INGREDIENT

Adding kombu—a type of dried seaweed—to the pot does wonders for your beans. It's a powerful flavor enhancer, thanks to its glutamate content (the same nutrient that imparts umami flavor in foods like Parmesan cheese and mushrooms). It also tenderizes (to the same degree as if the beans had been soaked) by swapping sodium and potassium ions with the beans. In doing so, it provides a saltiness that can take the place of actual salt needed to season the beans. Kombu also makes beans more digestible by breaking down the carbohydrates that sometimes lead to flatulence. The kombu will plump up and become very soft as the beans cook; be sure to pluck it from the pot before the final simmering stage or it will turn to shreds. You can chop it up and add it to your dish if you like.

INSTANT POT BEAN COOKING TIMES

Bean cooking times vary tremendously based on the freshness of the beans, whether or not you've given them a soak, and the altitude. Use the cooking time ranges here for soaked and unsoaked beans as a guide. For the freshest dried beans, such as high-quality heirloom beans, start with the shortest time. For beans that have been in your pantry for more than six months, a presoak and/or a longer cooking time will ensure a creamier result.

Beans cook more slowly at higher altitudes. For best results, increase the cooking time by 5 percent for each 1,000 feet (300 m) you go up in altitude above 2,000 feet (600 m).

TYPE OF BEAN	COOKING TIME IN MINUTES (SOAKED/UNSOAKED)
Appaloosa	10–15/20–25
Ayocote	12–15/35–40
Black	10–15/20–25
Black-eyed peas	10–15/20–25
Cannellini (white kidney)	20–25/35–40
Chickpea (garbanzo)	20–25/35–40
Christmas lima	8–10/18–22
Cranberry	8–10/23–27
Eye of the Goat	9–13/23–26
Flageolet	10–15/20–25
Pinto	20–25/25–30
Red kidney	20–25/25–30
Royal Corona/gigante	20–25/25–30
White kidney/Great Northern	20–25/25–30

A FEW RULES OF THUMB FOR THE PERFECT POT OF BEANS

If you get in the habit of regularly making a pot of beans, you'll be rewarded with the backbone for quick meals and substantial snacks to last for days. Pick one of the three cooking methods (page 215), depending on your time and equipment, and follow these simple rules.

TIMING. Cooking times vary depending on the size, shape, and freshness of your beans. Freshly dried beans will cook up faster than those more than a year old. And some older beans may never cook up tender, no matter how long you simmer them. Start checking for doneness in the last stage of cooking—just spoon a few beans from the pot and taste. They should be very creamy on the inside but still hold their shape. Once you are in the habit of cooking beans on a regular basis, replenish your cupboards with the freshest beans you can find.

BUILDING FLAVOR. Adding aromatics to the pot infuses your beans with flavor you just can't get from a can. Keeping the aromatics simple—just onions, carrots, and garlic—adds just enough vegetables to coax out the delicate, nutty nuances from the beans without asserting their own flavors. This will make your beans versatile enough to slip into different roles in your cooking. But if you want more boldly flavored beans, change up the aromatics. Add more garlic, a bay leaf, peppercorns, warm spices (like cumin and cayenne), and fresh or dried chiles, but avoid highly acidic ingredients (like tomatoes or vinegar) because they could make the beans tough.

USING JUST ENOUGH WATER. You want enough water to cook the beans, but adding too much will dilute the rich stock. With the stovetop and slow cooker methods, it's smart to check your beans every half hour and add more boiling water if the level dips below the beans. This serves to concentrate the stock, making it more deeply flavored. For the Instant Pot method, add the exact amount of water called for. You can adjust the water content later, once the beans are fully cooked, by simmering them in the pot with the lid off.

SAVVY SALTING. Adding a small amount of salt to the beans helps bring out their flavors. No matter which method you choose, save most of your salting for the last stage of cooking, since adding it earlier could toughen the beans and impede how they absorb other flavors. These instructions will give you a well-seasoned, medium salty pot of beans; feel free to adjust the degree of saltiness before adding salt in the last step.

NOTE: *One of the perks of cooking beans from scratch is the rich broth that ends up in the pot. You can use the bean broth as you would stock to give dishes a rich foundation of flavor. Whenever you use the stock as part of another dish, be sure to taste first and adjust with seasonings as you like.*

GARLICKY WHITE BEAN DIP WITH SWEET POTATO FRIES

MAKES 1½ CUPS (220 G)

- **1 large head garlic (3 ounces/85 g)**
- **¼ cup (60 ml) extra-virgin olive oil, plus more for drizzling**
- **4 cups (285g) frozen sweet potato fries, store-bought and preferably waffle-cut (about half of one 20-ounce/567 g bag)**
- **1½ cups (265 g) cooked white beans (page 215) or one 15-ounce (425 g) can, drained**
- **2 tablespoons to ¼ cup (60 ml) fresh lemon juice**
- **1 teaspoon Dijon mustard**
- **½ teaspoon kosher salt**
- **¼ teaspoon freshly ground black pepper**
- **Sumac, paprika, or cayenne pepper**
- **Flaky salt (optional)**
- **2 tablespoons za'atar (see Tip)**

Roast a whole head of garlic doused in olive oil and you'll quickly wonder why you don't do so more often. The garlic cloves lose their bite and collapse inside their skins, becoming butter soft. Blended into a white bean dip, the result tastes decadent.

Tossing good-quality, store-bought sweet potato fries with extra-virgin olive oil and za'atar after baking gives them a brain-healthy upgrade.

1. Set an oven rack in the center position and preheat the oven to 425°F (220°C). Line a rimmed baking sheet with parchment paper.

2. Remove any loose papery skins from the garlic and cut off about ½ inch (1.5 cm) of the top. Place on a square of parchment paper or foil and drizzle with 2 tablespoons of the oil. Seal tightly and place on one side of the prepared baking sheet. Roast for about 15 minutes, then scatter the frozen sweet potato fries on the other side of the baking sheet in a single layer. Bake for 15 to 20 minutes, or according to the directions on the package, until the fries are golden and crispy. By then the garlic should be buttery soft when pierced with a knife.

3. Remove the garlic packet. Reduce the oven temperature to 250°F (120°C) and keep the fries warm in the oven while you make the dip.

4. When the garlic is cool enough to handle, squeeze the roasted garlic from each clove into the bowl of a food processor, saving the oil left behind to drizzle on the finished dip. Add the beans, 2 tablespoons of the lemon juice, and the

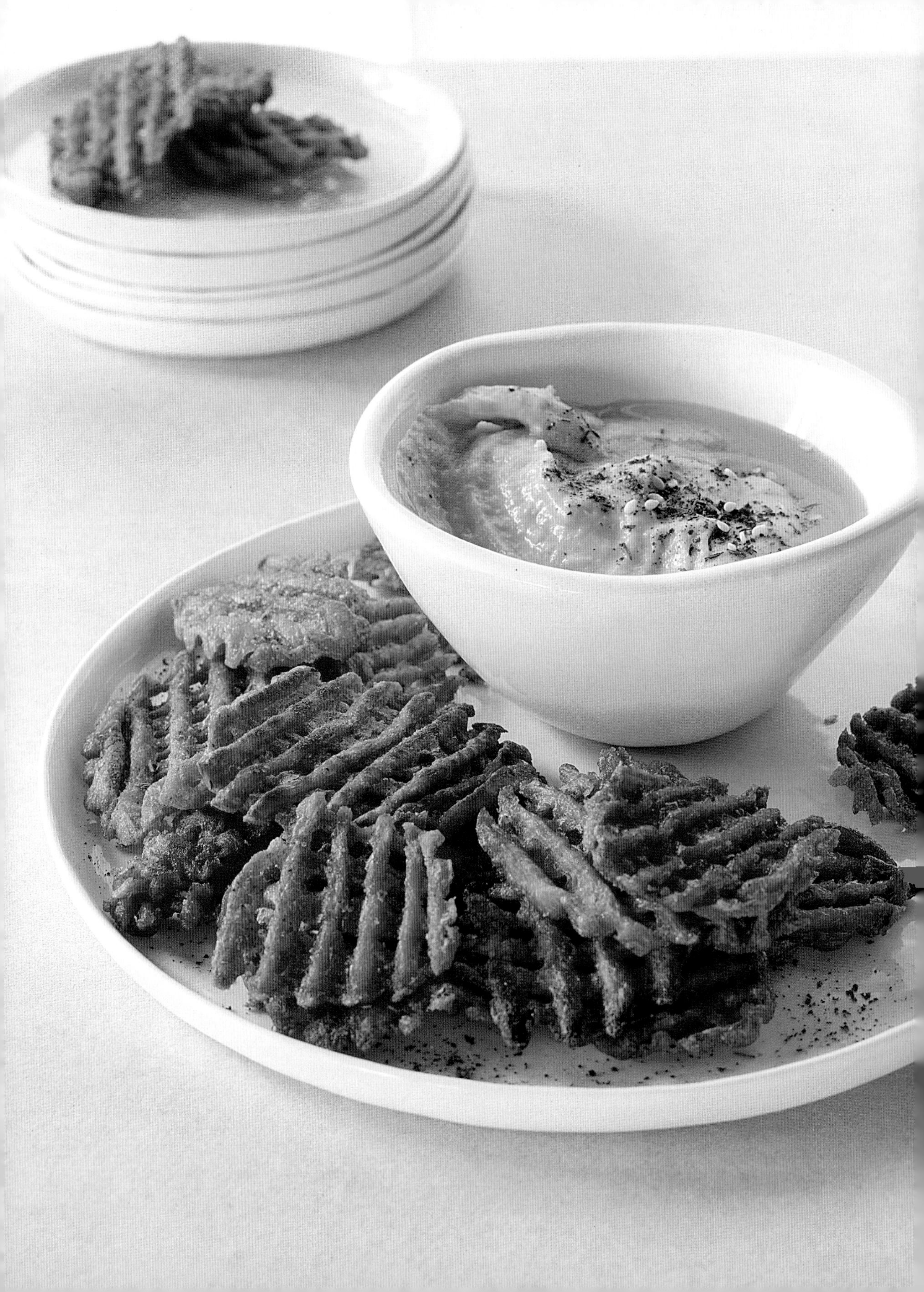

mustard, kosher salt, and black pepper. Process on high speed until smooth and creamy, about 1 minute, scraping down the sides of the bowl halfway through. With the machine running, pour the remaining 2 tablespoons oil through the feed tube in a slow stream until you have a smooth sauce that is the consistency of warm hummus. Season to taste with up to 2 more tablespoons of the remaining lemon juice, if you like.

5. Spoon the dip into a small bowl, drizzle with the remaining garlic oil, and sprinkle with sumac and flaky salt (if using). Toss the hot sweet potato fries with a drizzle of olive oil and sprinkle evenly with the za'atar, tossing again to coat. Serve immediately with the dip.

TIP: *There are hundreds of regional variations for za'atar throughout the Mediterranean. Sesame seeds and sumac are almost always included, plus an assertive dried herb, such as thyme, marjoram, or hyssop. In addition to Middle Eastern and specialty food shops, many grocery stores in the United States carry za'atar, but if you can't find it, it's easy to make a simple version. Stir together one part sumac, one part dried oregano, and two parts toasted sesame seeds.*

SCIENCE BITE:

ZA'ATAR: A MIX OF THREE BRAIN-BOOSTING FOODS

Za'atar, a staple of the Mediterranean diet, has been referred to as a brain-boosting food for centuries. That may be because three of its classic ingredients have each been found to have neuroprotective properties. Sumac (see the Science Bite on page 57) is actually a berry, rich in flavonoids. Sesame seeds provide sesamol, a nutrient found to reduce amyloid plaque formation in the brain. And oregano, which has long been studied for its enhancement of cognitive function, provides carvacrol, a nutrient of interest for Alzheimer's researchers. Small amounts, as you would get from using oregano as a culinary herb, seem to boost the production of neurotransmitters, like serotonin and dopamine. Further study in humans is needed to determine if carvacrol's neuroprotective properties can be used to treat those with Alzheimer's.

WARM LENTIL, GRAPEFRUIT, AND BITTER GREENS SALAD

SERVES 4 TO 6 AS A SIDE

- 1 cup (200 g) du Puy, green, or brown lentils, rinsed (see Tip)
- 1 large grapefruit
- 4 anchovy fillets, finely chopped, or 1 teaspoon anchovy paste
- 1 large garlic clove, minced
- 3 tablespoons extra-virgin olive oil, plus more for drizzling
- 2 teaspoons Dijon mustard
- ½ teaspoon kosher salt
- ¼ teaspoon crushed red pepper flakes
- 1 small head radicchio (7 ounces/200 g), cored and thinly sliced (about 4 cups)
- 1 medium head endive (4 ounces/115 g), thinly sliced lengthwise
- ½ cup (80 g) almonds, toasted (page 190) and coarsely chopped
- Freshly ground black pepper
- Flaky salt (optional)

TIP: *Other green or brown lentils work well here, too, though they usually have shorter cooking times.*

The tiny French green lentil, sometimes called du Puy for the region in which they are grown, is pleasantly peppery and holds its shape after boiling. Tossing the lentils with the vinaigrette while still warm helps them soak up all the bold flavors going on in this salad, from the anchovies to the garlic to the grapefruit. Warm lentils also mellow the sharpness of the bitter greens. Serve as a side dish with simply prepared fish, chicken, or shrimp.

1. Bring a medium pot of salted water to a boil and add the lentils. Reduce the heat to a gentle simmer, cover, and cook until the lentils are soft but still hold their shape, 20 to 25 minutes. Drain in a colander and transfer back to the pot.

2. While the lentils cook, cut off the stem ends of the grapefruit, then cut off the peel. Slice between the white pith and the flesh to remove the segments. Squeeze any juice left from the peels into a small cup. (You should have 1 to 2 tablespoons.) Discard the peels.

3. In a large serving bowl, use a fork to mash together the anchovies and garlic until you have a paste. Whisk in the oil, 1 tablespoon of the grapefruit juice, and the mustard, kosher salt, and red pepper flakes. Add the warm lentils and toss to combine. Fold in the radicchio and endive, then top with the grapefruit segments and almonds. Drizzle with any remaining grapefruit juice and more oil, then season with black pepper and flaky salt (if using).

TIP: *For a creamy version of the vinaigrette, double the ingredients, use lemon instead of grapefruit juice, and blend until smooth. Store in the fridge, tightly covered, for up to 5 days.*

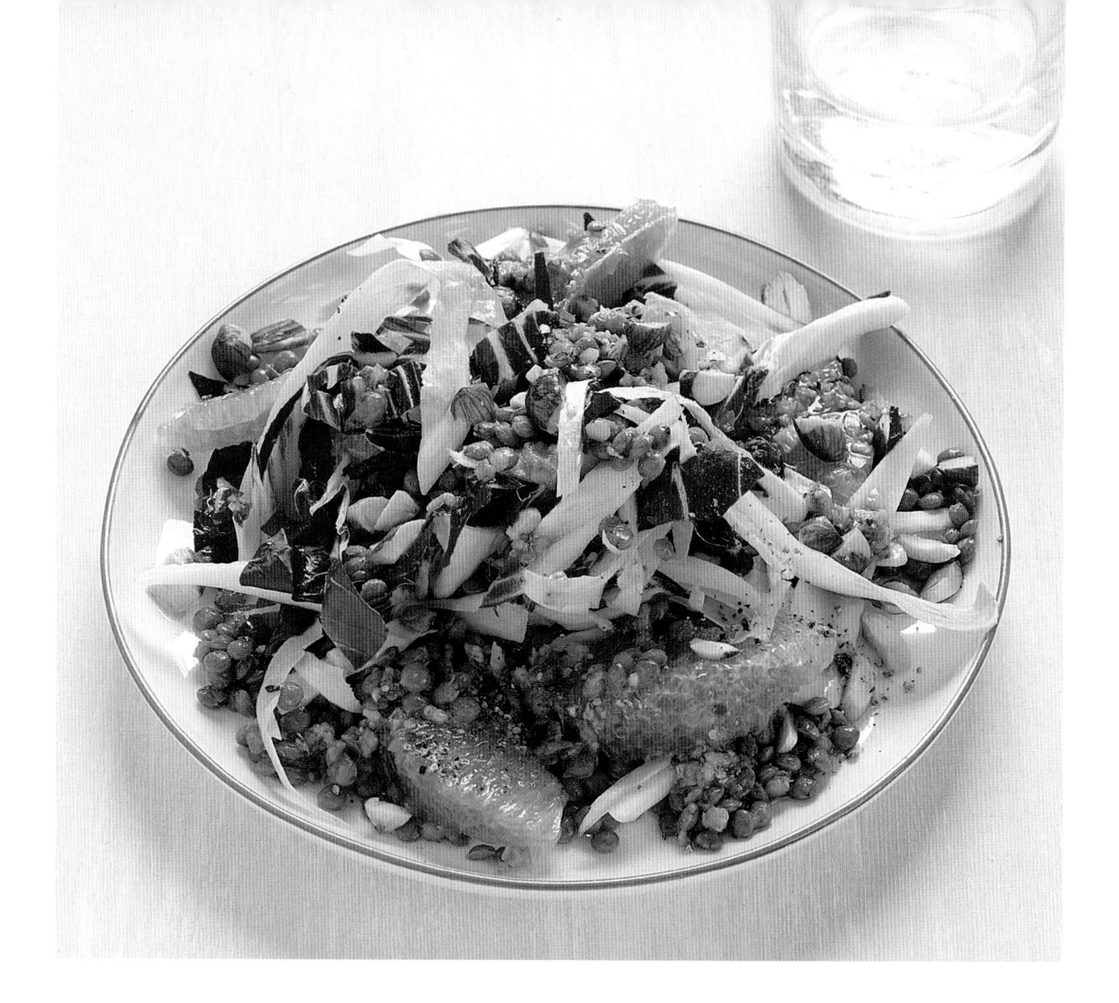

SCIENCE BITE:

THE LENTIL EFFECT

When you eat a legume-rich meal, your body absorbs sugar more slowly hours, even a day, later. Is it magic? No, just the amazing impact of your gut microbiota. Lentils and other legumes provide soluble fiber—the type your gut microbiota love. You get an initial blunting of blood sugar just after eating beans, like you would from any fiber-rich food. Then, hours later, after your gut microbiota have had a chance to feast, they produce propionate, a beneficial compound that relaxes the stomach muscle, serving to slow down absorption of sugar into the bloodstream after the next few meals you enjoy. This may also explain why legumes are thought to have an appetite-suppressing effect, and why people who eat legumes tend to be slimmer than those who don't. Which is a roundabout way of explaining: eating legumes improves your metabolic health, which serves to protect your brain from Alzheimer's.

CREAMY CANNELLINI BEAN SOUP WITH FRIZZLED SAGE AND BREADCRUMBS

SERVES 4

4½ cups (795 g) cannellini beans, freshly cooked (page 215; see Tips to use canned beans)

2 cups (480 ml) bean broth from A Very Good Pot of Beans (page 215)

1 large garlic clove

10 to 12 fresh sage leaves

3 tablespoons extra-virgin olive oil

1 cup (65 g) homemade breadcrumbs (see Tips) or store-bought panko

1 cup (240 ml) unsweetened almond milk or vegetable or chicken stock (page 376)

Up to 1 teaspoon kosher salt

Freshly ground black pepper

Flaky salt (optional)

Cannellini beans are classic in this brain-healthy take on Tuscan white bean soup, but you could use any white bean, such as the Royal Corona, Great Northern, or flageolet. Almond milk adds a touch of natural sweetness, creating a nice contrast to the sage—an herb with brain health benefits.

1. Combine the beans, broth, and garlic in a medium saucepan over high heat. Bring to a boil, then reduce the heat to a very low simmer. Set the lid ajar and let the beans simmer, stirring occasionally, while you cook the sage and breadcrumbs.

2. Gently press the sage leaves with your hands to make them lie flat, leaving the stem long for easier grasping. Warm the oil in a large skillet over medium heat. When the oil shimmers, add the sage leaves and cook, undisturbed, until they frizzle and curl, about 5 seconds, then use tongs to flip and cook on the other side, another few seconds. Transfer to a paper towel–lined plate. Pour the sage-infused oil into a heatproof measuring cup.

3. Add the breadcrumbs to the skillet and cook over medium heat, stirring often, until golden, 3 to 5 minutes. Transfer to a small bowl.

4. Carefully transfer the hot beans, broth, and garlic to a blender. Blend on low speed until pureed, about 1 minute, then increase the speed to high until creamy and velvety smooth, another 2 minutes. (Alternatively, use an immersion blender to puree the beans right in the pot.) Add the milk and blend until fully incorporated, another 30 seconds. Return the bean soup to the pot and simmer over medium heat until warm. Taste; add up to 1 teaspoon kosher salt, if you like.

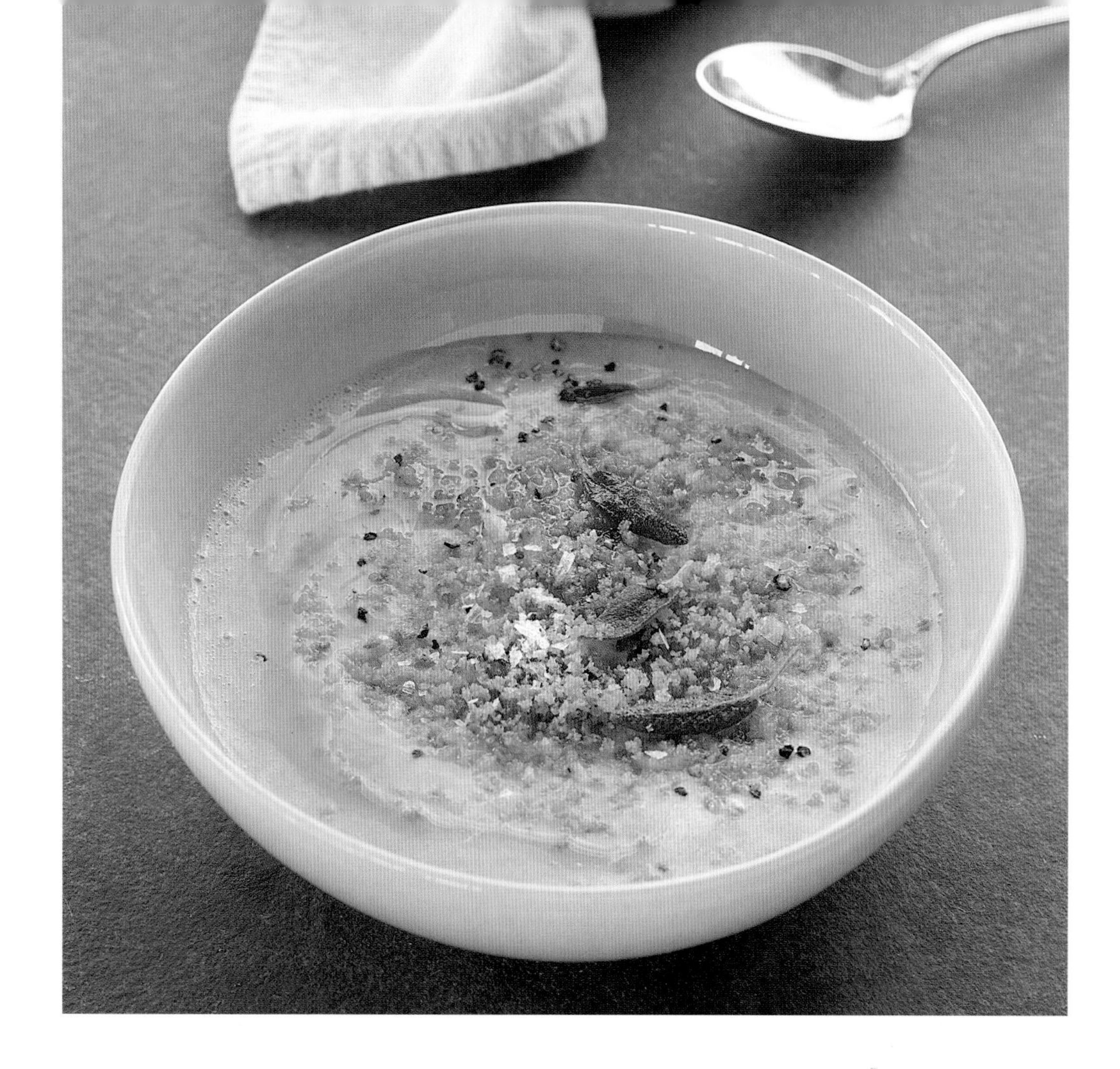

5. To serve, divide the soup evenly between bowls. Top with some breadcrumbs and sage and season with pepper and flaky salt, if using. Finish with a drizzle of the reserved sage-infused oil.

TIPS: *For homemade breadcrumbs, cut and discard the crust from two thick slices of slightly stale, whole-grain bread. Pulse in the bowl of a food processor or blender until you have pebbly crumbs, the largest ones no bigger than a lentil.*

To make this recipe using canned beans, pour the liquid from three 15-ounce (425 g) cans into a measuring cup and top off with water, chicken stock, or vegetable stock to measure 2 cups (480 ml) total. Use this liquid and the beans in the recipe above.

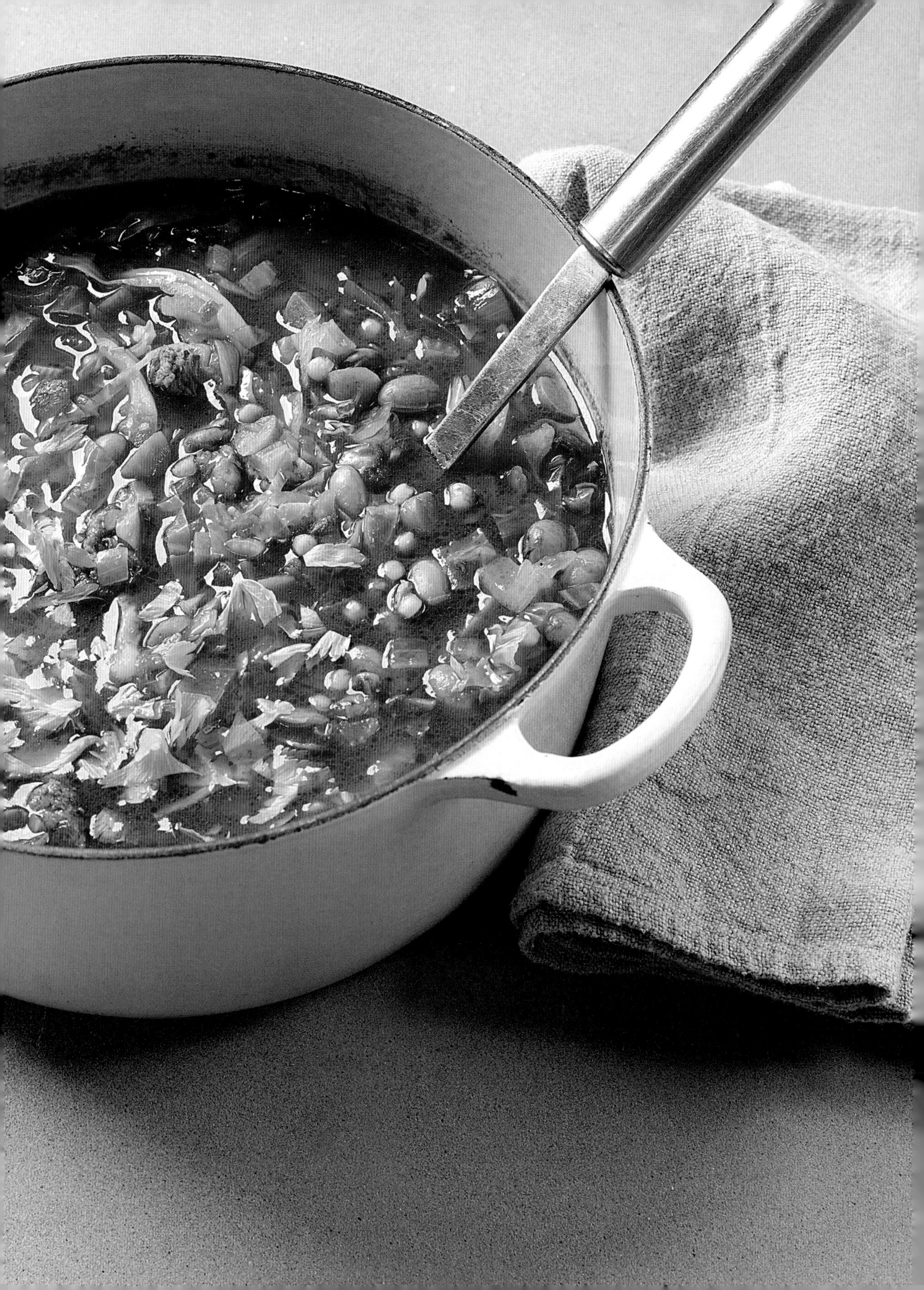

CRANBERRY BEAN AND SAUSAGE STEW

SERVES 4 TO 6

¼ cup (60 ml) extra-virgin olive oil, plus more for drizzling

½ pound (225 g) bulk turkey or chicken sausage

4 medium-size celery stalks (7 ounces/200 g), finely chopped, leaves coarsely chopped and reserved

3 medium carrots (12 ounces/340 g), scrubbed and coarsely chopped (about 1½ cups)

1 medium yellow onion (10 ounces/285 g), finely chopped (about 2 cups)

½ small green cabbage (1¾ pounds/790 g), thinly sliced (about 4 cups)

1 teaspoon kosher salt

¼ teaspoon black pepper, plus more for serving

6 cups (1.4 L) chicken or vegetable stock (page 374) or bean broth (page 215)

3 cups (575 g) cooked cranberry beans (page 215) or two 15.5-ounce (440 g) cans, rinsed

1½ cups (360 ml) marinara sauce, homemade (page 379) or store-bought

¼ cup (60 g) small whole-grain pasta, such as fregola sarda or orzo

One 2-inch (5 cm) piece Parmesan cheese rind

Freshly grated Parmesan cheese (optional)

This hearty stew is an ideal way to create a meal from a pot of beans. It's a spin-off of my grandmother's minestrone—an all-day simmer of vegetable scraps, canned tomatoes, and freshly cooked beans. Her secret ingredient was the spent end piece of a Parmesan wedge, which she saved in a coffee can in the back of the fridge for adding body and rich, salty flavor to soups and stews. In the final stretch of cooking, she threw in a handful each of barley, rice, and a tiny pasta, like orzo or stars.

This streamlined version keeps the old-school minestrone vibes, like the Parmesan rind and the chewy bits of pasta, but swaps in a few pantry staples to speed up the cooking time. Use freshly cooked beans if you have them, or choose another large, creamy bean from a can, such as gigante beans or Great Northerns. Good marinara sauce from a jar is a real time-saver. Look for high-quality lean turkey or chicken sausage at better grocery stores or farmers' markets.

1. Warm 1 teaspoon of the oil in a large saucepan over medium heat. Add the sausage and cook, stirring to break into crumbles, until no pink remains. Transfer with a slotted spoon to a plate. Pour off any fat from the pan into a heatproof container and discard once cool. Warm the remaining oil over medium heat. Add the celery, carrots, onion, cabbage, ½ teaspoon of the salt, and the pepper. Cook, stirring often, until the onion is translucent and the vegetables are starting to soften, 10 to 12 minutes.

2. Add the sausage, stock, beans, marinara, pasta, Parmesan rind, and the remaining ½ teaspoon salt to the pot. Bring to a boil over high heat, then reduce the heat to a gentle simmer. Cook, stirring often to make sure nothing sticks to the bottom of the pot, until the pasta is tender, 10 to 15 minutes. Discard the Parmesan rind.

continued

3. To serve, ladle into bowls, top with grated Parmesan (if using), celery leaves, and more pepper, then drizzle with olive oil.

4. To store, keep in an airtight container in the refrigerator for up to 2 days or in the freezer for up to 3 months. The soup thickens with time, so thin with water or stock when reheating.

TIP: *The celery has a dual function here—as part of the aromatic base for the stock and as a fresh leafy green garnish for the finished dish—so look for celery with plenty of tender leaves.*

SOY FOODS ARE LEGUMES, TOO

Whole foods made from soybeans are part of your legume intake. This includes enjoying actual soybeans, such as those found in pods as edamame, or soy-derived tofu, tempeh, miso, and unsweetened soy milk. Soybeans provide a unique polyphenol family of compounds called isoflavones shown to have far-reaching beneficial heart and brain health actions, including lowering harmful blood cholesterol, maintaining strong bones, reducing menopausal symptoms, and preventing the buildup of inflammatory plaques inside blood vessels that lead to heart attack and stroke.

Decades ago physicians were hesitant to recommend eating soy. That's because some studies (mostly in petri dishes and animals) hinted that one of soy's isoflavones acted like estrogen in the body and could induce estrogen-dependent cancers, like breast cancer. Now we know these phytoestrogens, as they are called, are completely different from the hormone estrogen your body makes. In fact, one of the isoflavones, genistein, has been shown to reduce the incidence of age-related cognitive decline in elderly Japanese women. Other studies point to the gut microbiome as a key mediator in boosting isoflavones into molecules like equol that act directly on brain cells to combat aging. As the research builds, soy foods are becoming an increasingly crucial part of a brain-healthy diet. Just be sure to buy whole-food forms of soy, preferably non-GMO (for less pesticide exposure), and avoid the processed soy (like the soy protein isolate) found in many snack bars and protein powders.

RED LENTIL FALAFEL BURGERS WITH LEMONY TAHINI SAUCE

SERVES 4

- **1 cup (200 g) dry split red lentils, soaked in water for 20 minutes**
- **2 loosely packed cups (40 g) fresh flat-leaf parsley leaves and tender stems**
- **1 small red onion (7 ounces/200 g), finely chopped (about 1 cup)**
- **3 medium garlic cloves**
- **2 tablespoons tahini, well stirred and at room temperature**
- **1 tablespoon extra-virgin olive oil**
- **1 teaspoon ground cumin**
- **1 teaspoon ground coriander**
- **1 teaspoon kosher salt**
- **3 tablespoons chickpea flour**
- **Olive oil cooking spray**
- **4 whole-grain buns or four 6-inch (15 cm) pita bread rounds, cut in half to form pockets**
- **4 thick tomato slices**
- **Romaine or butter lettuce, torn into large pieces**
- **½ cup (120 ml) Lemony Tahini Sauce (recipe follows)**

There's much to love about falafel—the Middle Eastern staple starring the humble chickpea. Usually, these crispy herb and bean fritters are fried then nestled into a pita sandwich with cucumbers and pickled onions, all drizzled in a garlicky white sauce. Here they're baked—it's better for brain health to avoid eating deep-fried foods—and eaten as a burger.

A few things will help you make perfectly textured patties: Avoid overzealous mixing in the food processor—just pulse until the ingredients start to bind. Then, when forming the patties, don't press too hard. Compress them just enough so that they hold together. Finally, spraying with olive oil before baking creates a crisp exterior, not quite as crisp as deep-fried, but with a brain-healthier fat profile.

Serve on a burger bun or stuff them into pita pockets. Or skip the bread altogether and serve these on top of a bed of greens with chopped tomatoes and use the Lemony Tahini Sauce as a dressing.

1. Drain the lentils and discard the soaking water. Place them in the bowl of a food processor with the parsley and pulse about 10 times, until coarsely ground. Add the onion and garlic, then pulse another 10 times. Add the tahini, oil, cumin, coriander, and salt. Blend until you have a mostly smooth mixture that still has some whole lentils throughout, 30 to 45 seconds. Scrape into a medium bowl and add the chickpea flour. Mix with a wooden spoon until evenly combined. Cover the bowl and refrigerate for at least 30 minutes and up to overnight.

2. Set an oven rack in the center position and preheat the oven to 375°F (190°C). Line a rimmed baking sheet with parchment paper.

continued

3. Using your hands, scoop up ½ cup (130 g) of the lentil mixture and form into a patty about 1 inch (2.5 cm) thick. Compress just enough that it holds together, but not too much. Place on the prepared baking sheet and repeat for a total of four patties. Coat generously on both sides with cooking spray and bake for 25 to 35 minutes, until golden brown. In the last 10 minutes of baking, wrap the buns in foil and place them directly on the oven rack.

4. To serve, top each bottom bun with a patty, 1 tomato slice, 2 or 3 lettuce leaves, and 2 tablespoons Lemony Tahini Sauce. Serve open-faced or top with the rest of the bun.

LEMONY TAHINI SAUCE

MAKES ABOUT ½ CUP (120 ML)

¼ cup (60 ml) tahini, well stirred and at room temperature

2 tablespoons fresh lemon juice

1 tablespoon extra-virgin olive oil

¼ teaspoon kosher salt

Up to 2 tablespoons warm water

Whisk together the tahini, lemon juice, oil, and salt in a small bowl. Add warm water by the teaspoon, if needed, to make a smooth sauce.

SCIENCE BITE:

HOW LENTILS STACK UP WHEN IT COMES TO FIBER

While all lentils are good for you, black belugas provide about twice as much fiber as the green, brown, and red ones. Just one serving of black belugas (about 1 cup/170 g cooked) provides a whopping 9 grams of fiber, or about one-third of the recommended daily fiber intake. Named for their striking resemblance to black beluga caviar, these tiny purplish black pulses also provide a good dose of anthocyanins, the same flavonoid pigment that makes blueberries so good for your brain.

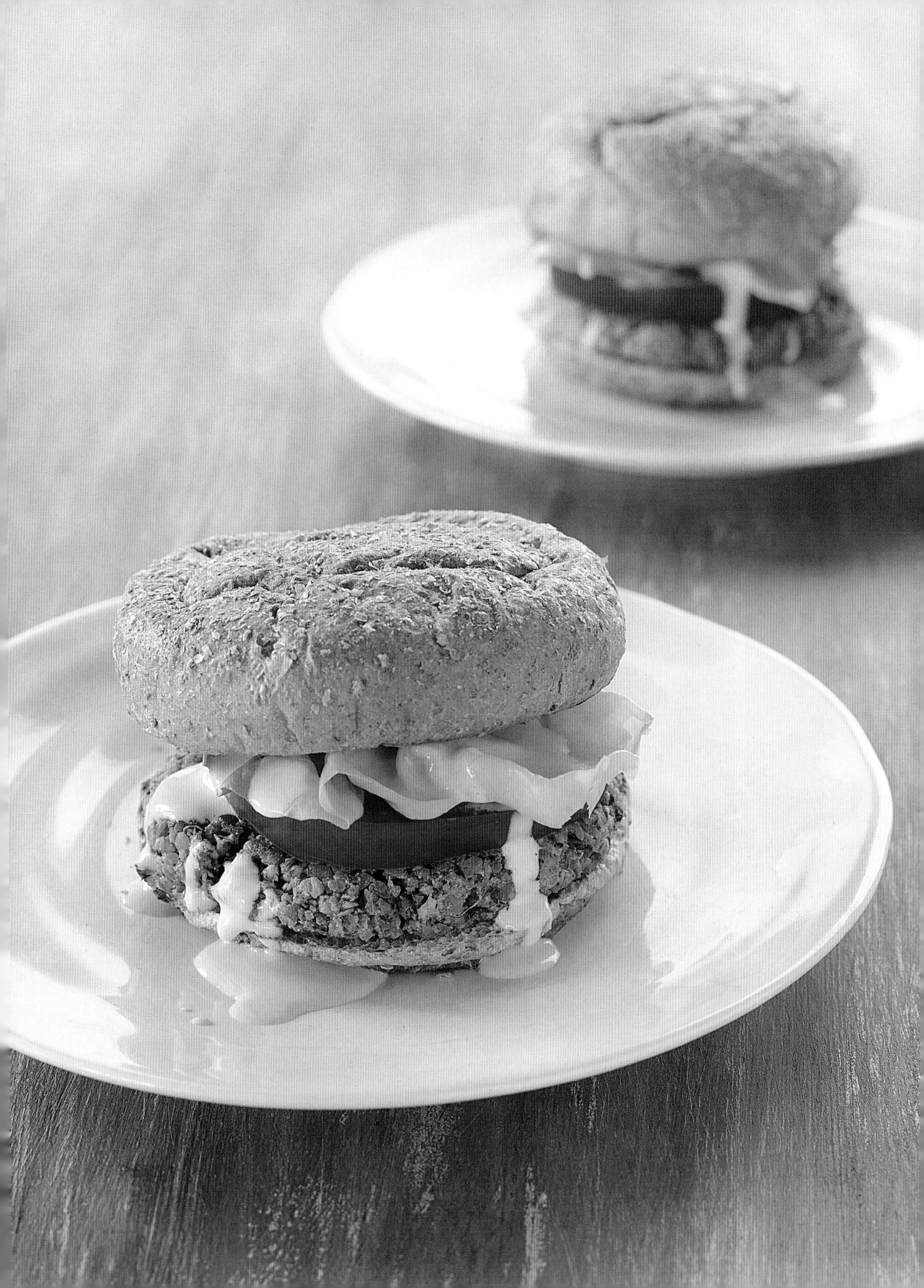

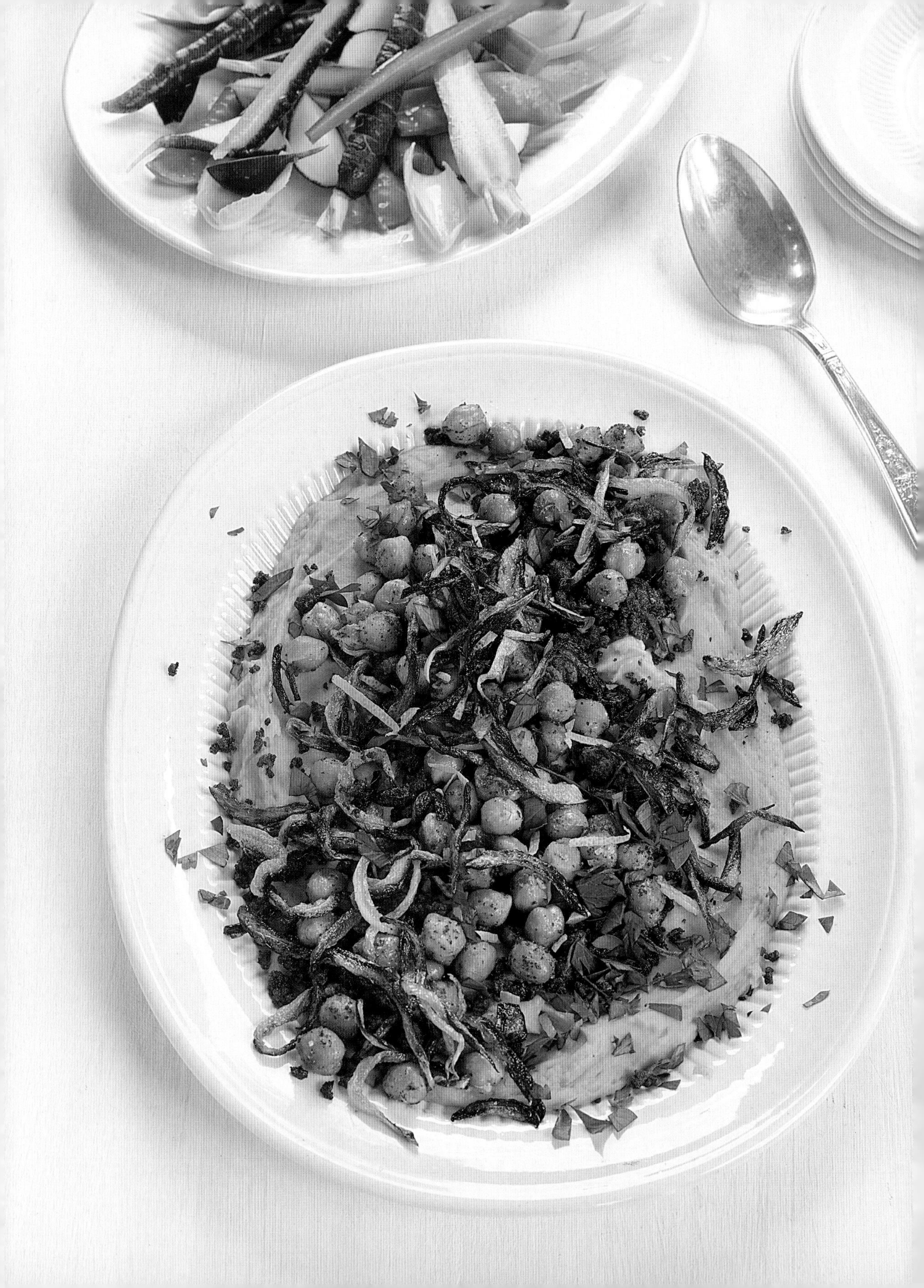

FAMILY-STYLE HUMMUS WITH CARAMELIZED ONIONS AND CRISPY BEEF

SERVES 4 TO 6

3 tablespoons extra-virgin olive oil, plus more for drizzling

3 cups (720 g) hummus (from two 17-ounce/480 g store-bought containers)

Four to six 6-inch (15 cm) pita rounds, cut into sixths

Olive oil cooking spray

1½ cups (260 g) cooked chickpeas (page 215) or one 15-ounce (425 g) can

½ teaspoon ground cumin

½ teaspoon sumac, plus more for garnish

1½ teaspoons kosher salt

1 large yellow onion (12 ounces/340 g), thinly sliced (about 2 cups)

½ pound (225 g) ground grass-fed beef, bison, or turkey

½ teaspoon ground allspice

¼ teaspoon freshly ground black pepper

½ loosely packed cup (10 g) fresh flat-leaf parsley leaves, coarsely chopped

1 tablespoon lemon zest (optional)

Generous portions of carrot sticks, endive leaves, radish slices, and sugar snap peas

Have you ever hungrily tucked into a tub of hummus, eaten more than anticipated, and found your appetite ruined? That's one way to have "hummus for dinner." Here's a better way: make hummus—homemade or store-bought—the anchor for a family-style meal. Hummus is packed with good-for-you ingredients, like chickpeas, tahini, olive oil, and warm spices, making it an excellent choice for a brain-healthy snack. This dinner rendition adds spiced ground meat and chickpeas, inspired by the Lebanese dish hummus kawarma, a lamb-topped dish served as one small plate among many, mezze-style.

The meat plays a supporting role here, much like it does in meals throughout the Mediterranean. While the Western diet puts meat at the center of the plate, the Mediterranean lifestyle features the plant-based elements as the main event, with meat as a garnish. To make this dish vegetarian or vegan, replace the meat with 3 cups (285 g) sliced mushrooms and follow the directions below, or top each serving with roasted vegetables (like cauliflower florets or sliced carrots) instead.

1. Preheat the oven to 250°F (120°C).

2. Coat the bottom of a large shallow ovenproof bowl or platter with 1 tablespoon of the oil. Spread the hummus in an even layer, cover tightly with foil, and place in the oven to warm. Place the pitas on a rimmed baking sheet and spread out in a single layer. Spray with oil and place in the oven while you prepare the rest of the dish.

3. Heat the chickpeas in a large nonstick skillet over medium heat until dry, 1 to 2 minutes. Add the cumin,

continued

sumac, 1 tablespoon of the oil, and ½ teaspoon of the salt. Cook, stirring occasionally, until golden, 5 to 7 minutes. Transfer to a shallow baking dish or pie plate and keep warm in the oven.

4. Using the same skillet, heat the remaining 1 tablespoon oil over medium heat. Add the onion and ½ teaspoon of the salt. Cook, stirring often, until the onion is very tender and a deep golden brown, 10 to 12 minutes. Use a slotted spoon to transfer the onion to the hummus, scattering the onion evenly atop, leaving any remaining oil behind in the skillet. Cover the hummus again with the foil and return to the oven.

5. Return the skillet to medium heat and add the beef, allspice, pepper, and the remaining ½ teaspoon salt. Cook, stirring often to break the meat into crumbles, until crispy and brown, 5 to 7 minutes. Use a slotted spoon to transfer the mixture to the hummus, leaving behind any fat. Top with the chickpeas, parsley, lemon zest (if using), and more sumac. Drizzle with oil. Serve with the warm pitas and vegetables.

TIP: *If you don't have allspice, mix together equal parts cinnamon, nutmeg, and cloves.*

CHEESY BLACK BEAN AND BUTTERNUT SQUASH-STUFFED POBLANOS

SERVES 4 TO 6

2 cups (½-inch/1.25 cm) butternut squash cubes (8 ounces/225 g), fresh or frozen

2 tablespoons water

1½ cups (225 g) corn kernels, fresh or frozen

1½ cups (240 g) cooked black beans (page 215) or one 15-ounce (425 g) can, drained

2 cups (480 ml) green enchilada sauce from a jar or a can (see Tips)

1 teaspoon chili powder

1 teaspoon kosher salt

4 medium poblano peppers (1 pound/455 g), cut in half lengthwise from stem to tip, and deseeded (see Tips)

2 ounces (about ¼ cup/ 60 g) goat cheese, feta cheese, or queso blanco

Fresh cilantro leaves

½ cup (60 g) hulled pumpkin seeds (pepitas), toasted (page 190)

Quick-Pickled Pomegranate Red Onions (page 383, optional)

The dark green poblano pepper has a delightfully earthy flavor that falls somewhere between a sweet bell pepper and a jalapeño on the heat scale. Poblanos are brain health superstars thanks to their high amounts of capsaicin, fiber, vitamin A, and the flavonoid quercetin.

This vegetarian main comes together quickly if you employ store-bought enchilada sauce and frozen squash and corn. Canned black beans work fine here, too, but if you have time, it's worth cooking up a pot of dried beans (see page 215). Try this with an heirloom variety of black or red beans, such as Pinquitos, Rio Zapes, or Vaqueros. For a full meal, serve these stuffed poblanos with brown, black, or red rice. For dairy-free stuffed peppers, omit the cheese and top with sliced avocado instead.

1. Set an oven rack in the center position and preheat the oven to 375°F (190°C).

2. Place the butternut squash and water in a large microwaveable bowl. Cover tightly with a silicone lid or a plate and microwave on high until you can easily insert a knife into the largest cube, 3 to 5 minutes. Set aside to cool slightly, then mash about half of the squash into a rough paste, keeping the other cubes intact. Stir in the corn, beans, ¼ cup (60 ml) of the enchilada sauce, the chili powder, and salt. Set aside.

3. Spread the remaining 1¾ cups (420 ml) enchilada sauce evenly over the bottom of a 9-by-13-inch (23 by 33 cm) baking dish. Place the poblanos, cut side up, on the sauce.

continued

Divide the squash and black bean filling between the peppers (about ½ cup/150 g per pepper), being sure to include the heart-shaped pockets near the stem. Use your hands or a fork to break the cheese into large crumbles and press into the filling. Cover tightly with foil and bake for 40 to 50 minutes, until you can easily insert the tip of a knife into the peppers and the cheese is melted and bubbling.

4. Just before serving, sprinkle the peppers with cilantro, pumpkin seeds, and pickled onions, if using, and spoon sauce from the pan over top.

TIPS: *Look for green enchilada sauce in packets, cans, and jars in the Latin American food section of the grocery store. The ingredient list should be short: just chiles and/or tomatillos, onion, spices, and vinegar. Avoid brands with added sugar and unhealthy oils like refined palm and soybean.* *(See Resources, page 390.)*

When shopping for fresh poblanos, look for fat peppers that are all about the same size. The long, skinny ones will be harder to stuff.

While the poblanos themselves fall low on the spiciness scale, their seeds are very spicy. You may want to wear gloves to remove the seeds and be careful not to touch your face or eyes.

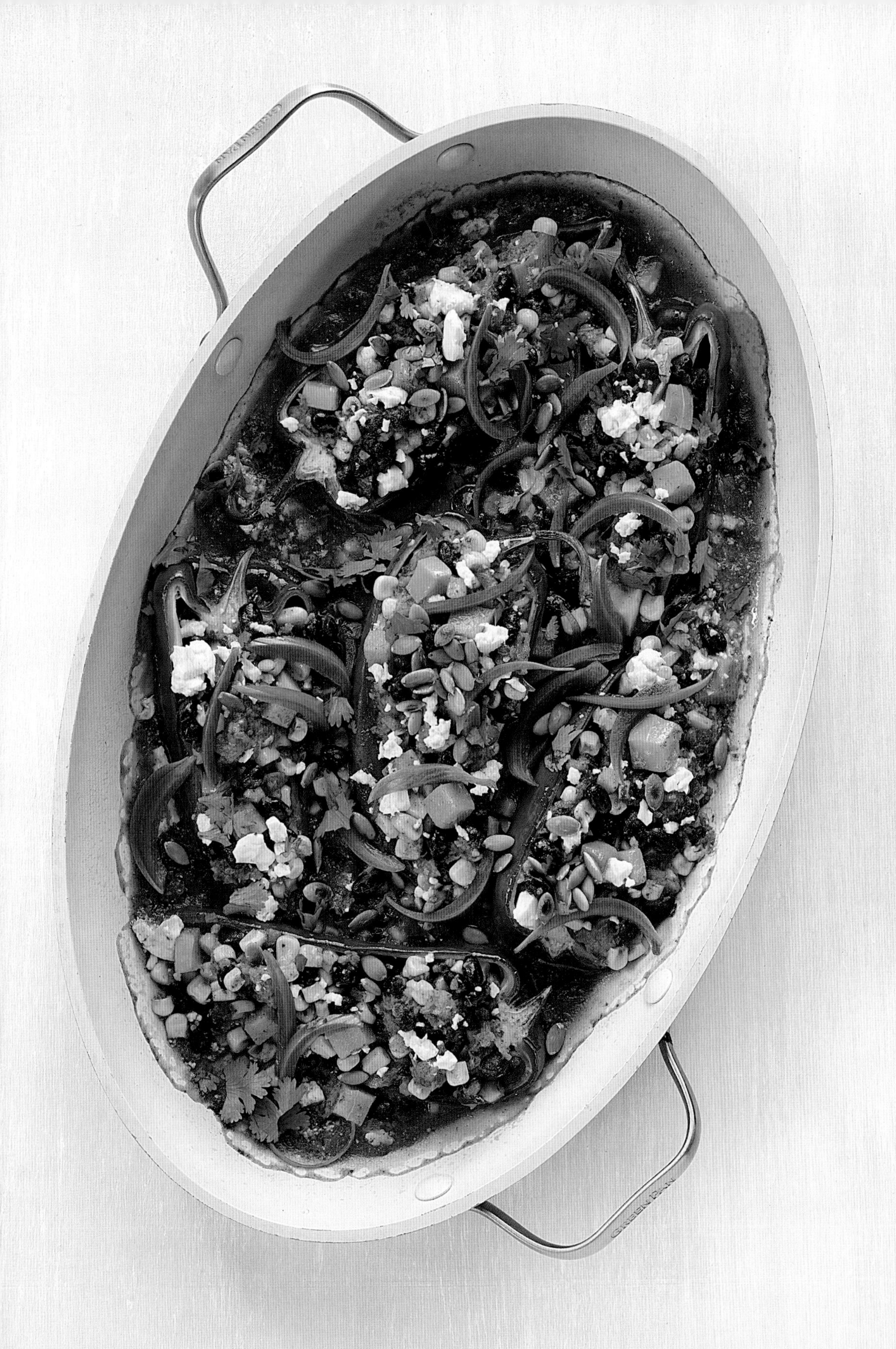

CHEWY CHAI-SPICED CHICKPEA COOKIES

MAKES 12 COOKIES

Olive oil cooking spray

1 cup (115 g) chickpea flour

¾ cup (90 g) oat flour

1 tablespoon ground cinnamon

1 tablespoon ground ginger

2 teaspoons ground cardamom

½ teaspoon baking powder

½ teaspoon baking soda

½ teaspoon kosher salt

¼ teaspoon finely ground black pepper

⅓ cup (80 ml) pure maple syrup

6 tablespoons (90 ml) extra-virgin olive oil

2 eggs

1 teaspoon pure vanilla extract

2 tablespoons candied ginger, finely chopped

Think of these cookies as a cross between a warming chai latte and a soft spice cookie—with an emphasis on *spice*. Just like a good cup of chai, they blend comforting cinnamon, ginger, and cardamom notes with a nice kick from the black pepper. Incorporating chickpea flour, these cookies have a decidedly adult flavor.

That being said, most people will have a hard time pegging chickpea as the primary flour here. It tastes like a much more subtle version of the chickpea itself—nutty and a tiny bit beany, but in a good way that lets the spices shine. Chickpea flour also makes these cookies a nutrient-dense treat. The flour is rich in protein, has a low glycemic index, and provides brain health nutrients like folate, potassium, zinc, and magnesium. These cookies are lower in sugar than most and, thanks to the olive oil, rich in brain-friendly fats, too.

1. Set an oven rack in the center position and preheat the oven to 350°F (180°C). Line a rimmed baking sheet with parchment paper and coat with cooking spray.

2. Whisk together the chickpea flour, oat flour, cinnamon, ground ginger, cardamom, baking powder, baking soda, salt, and pepper in a large bowl.

3. Combine the maple syrup, oil, eggs, and vanilla in a large mixing bowl. Using a stand or handheld mixer, beat on medium speed until well combined, about 2 minutes, scraping down the sides of the bowl a few times. Add the flour mixture and beat on low speed until thoroughly combined.

4. Divide the dough into twelve equal-size balls, about scant 3 tablespoons each. Place on the prepared baking sheet leaving 2 inches (5 cm) between cookies. Sprinkle each

TIP: *Look for chickpea flour (also called garbanzo bean flour) in the gluten-free section of the grocery store (see Resources, page 390). Garbanzo/fava flour can be used interchangeably here, as can gram, a similar, legume-based flour made from split chickpeas, aka yellow gram lentils. If the gram flour is toasted, which brings out its nutty flavors, it's called besan. All of these variations on chickpea flour are delicious, nutrient-dense additions to your cooking.*

cookie with about ½ teaspoon candied ginger, pressing gently into the dough, along with any of the ginger sugar from the cutting board.

5. Bake for 8 to 9 minutes, until the edges are set, the bottoms are starting to brown, and the centers of the cookies are still soft. Transfer to a rack to cool.

6. These cookies are best enjoyed the same day as or the day after baking. Cookie dough freezes well in an airtight container for up to 3 months.

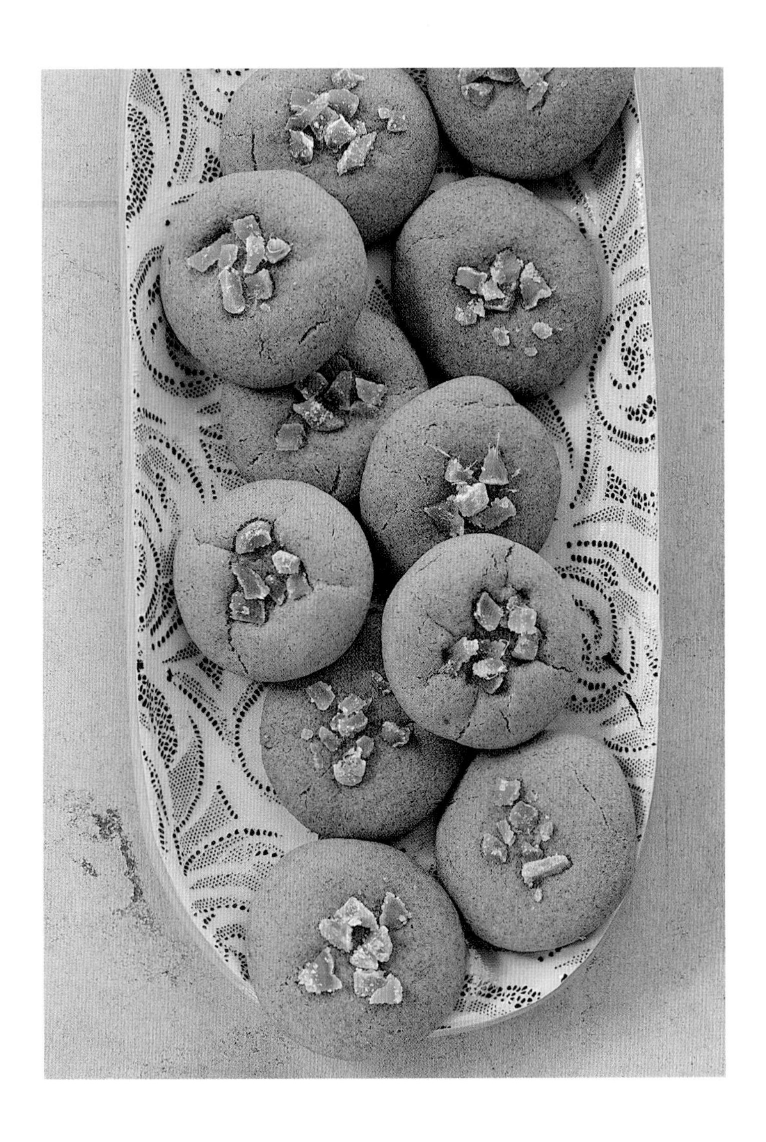

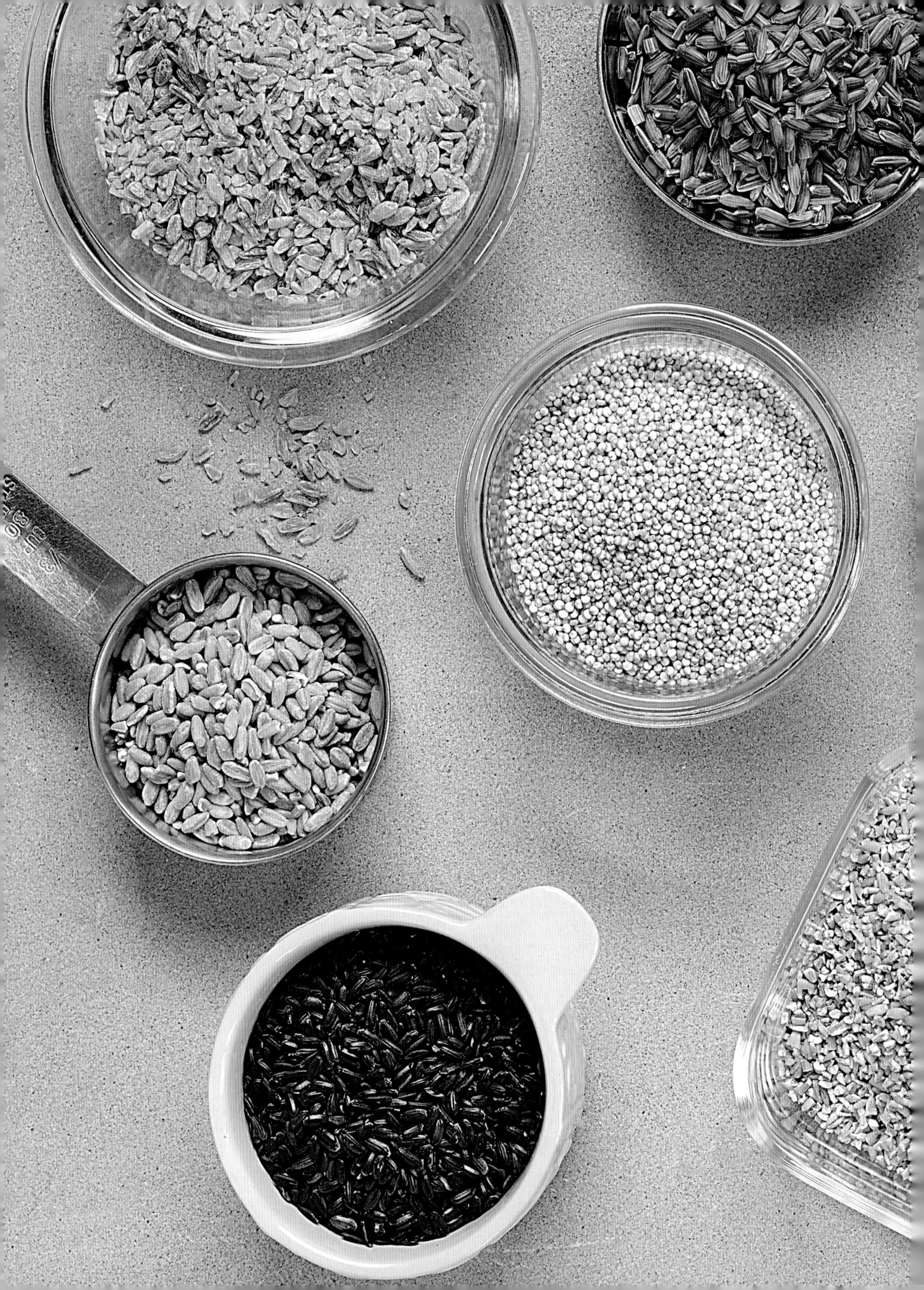

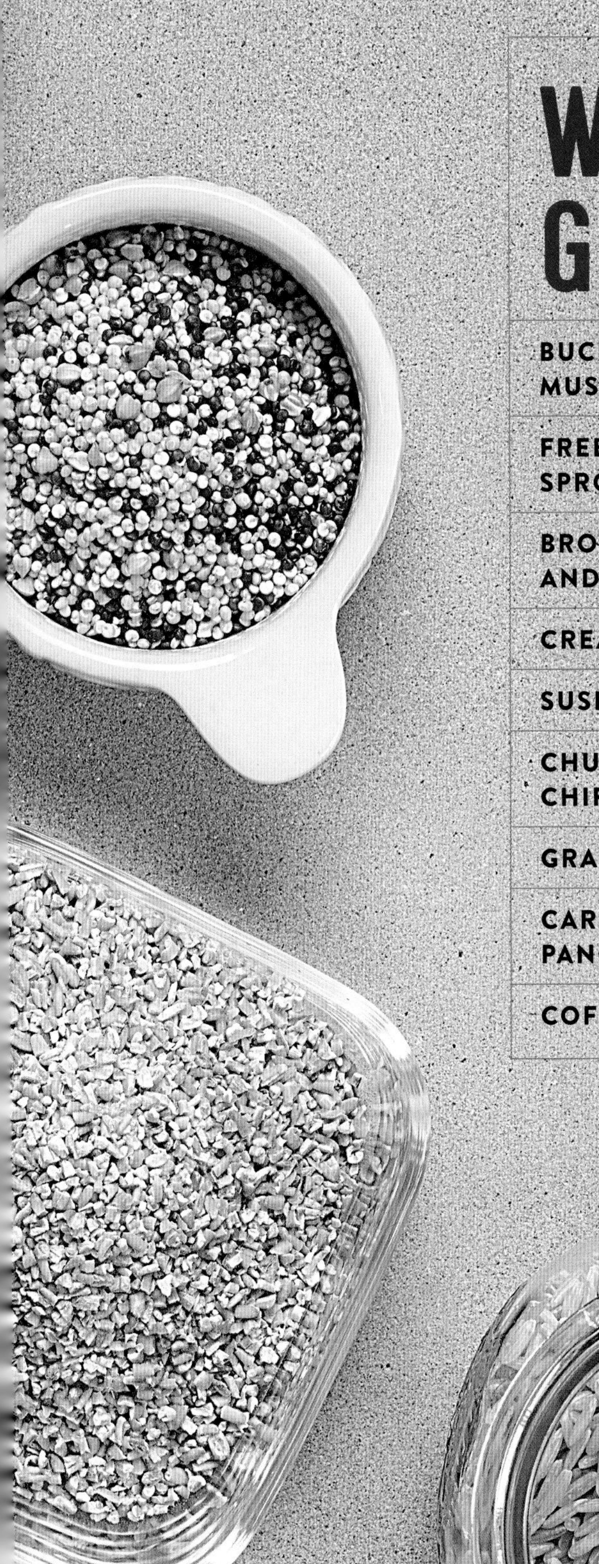

WHOLE GRAINS

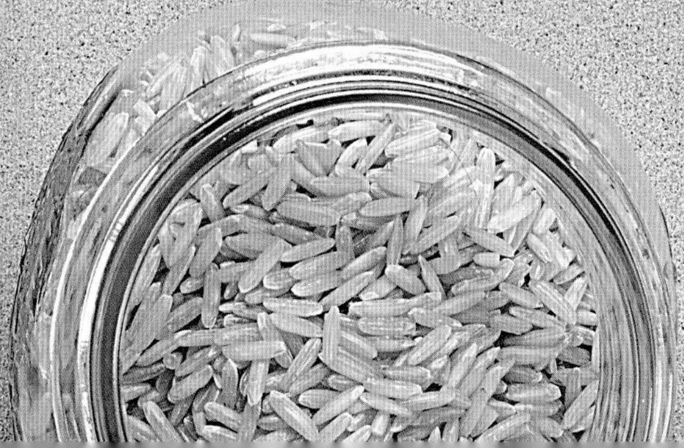

Whole grains are one of the brain-healthy food groups in the MIND diet study. They are integral to the Mediterranean style of eating and a staple food in all the Blue Zones (page 19). While the research on grains so far is not as specific to brain health as it is with berries and their impressive anthocyanins or DHA-rich seafood, whole grains play an important role in your neuroprotective diet. Not only are they nutrient-dense in their own right, but whole grains also amplify the nutrition of whatever you pair them with.

The health benefits of whole grains have often been attributed to their fiber content, but that's just part of the story. While fiber—with its ability to lower harmful cholesterol and cultivate good gut bugs—is key for brain health, new research shows that whole grains also provide flavonoids, phytonutrients that combat oxidative stress in the brain. Rolled oats, for example, are rich in avenanthramides, an antioxidant that releases nitric oxide into the bloodstream, opening up small blood vessels and increasing blood flow to the brain. The combination of fiber and flavonoids is so powerful because these beneficial molecules piggyback onto the fiber as it travels through your digestive tract, enhancing absorption throughout.

A grain is considered whole when it keeps all three of its original parts intact: bran, germ, and endosperm. The bran is the outer husk of the grain. It contains brain-healthy B vitamins, the potent antioxidant vitamin E, and the bulk of the grain's fiber. The germ is the seed of the grain, which provides B vitamins, minerals, protein, and healthy fats. The endosperm is a spongy layer that sits between the germ and the bran, and it supplies protein, minerals, and antioxidants. A whole grain can be cracked, rolled, ground, among other preparations, and still be considered whole grain. For instance, if the bran, germ, and endosperm are still in the same proportions after being cracked, it is considered a whole grain.

Refined grains start out whole with all their elements intact. But instead of being minimally processed (gently chafed to remove the inedible outer husk, cracked, or rolled), highly processed refined grains become thoroughly stripped. During this process, a refined grain loses about half of its protein, two-thirds of its nutrients, and almost all of its fiber. The naked grain is mostly starch and a useful product for companies. The fact that they are mild tasting, easier to cook, and able to last a long time on the supermarket shelf makes refined grains amenable for use in a wide variety of processed foods, such as conventional pizza, boxed cereal, bread, and packaged baked goods. Sadly, these are the grains that fill the typical American diet and the reason grains, in general, have been vilified. (See Grain-Free Diets and the Brain, page 250.) Because they're broken down into simple starches, these refined grains can spur inflammation, decrease insulin sensitivity, and contribute to poor brain health.

There is no need to eliminate whole grains from your diet unless it is medically necessary. Whole grains are delicious, inexpensive, and versatile. They are proven to reduce the risk of diseases that shorten your life. More than fifty-seven studies have examined the health outcomes of eating a diet that includes whole grains, and the results are clear: eating whole grains reduces chronic disease, whether it be heart disease, diabetes, or even cancer. PREDIMED, the same study that documented the health benefits of a

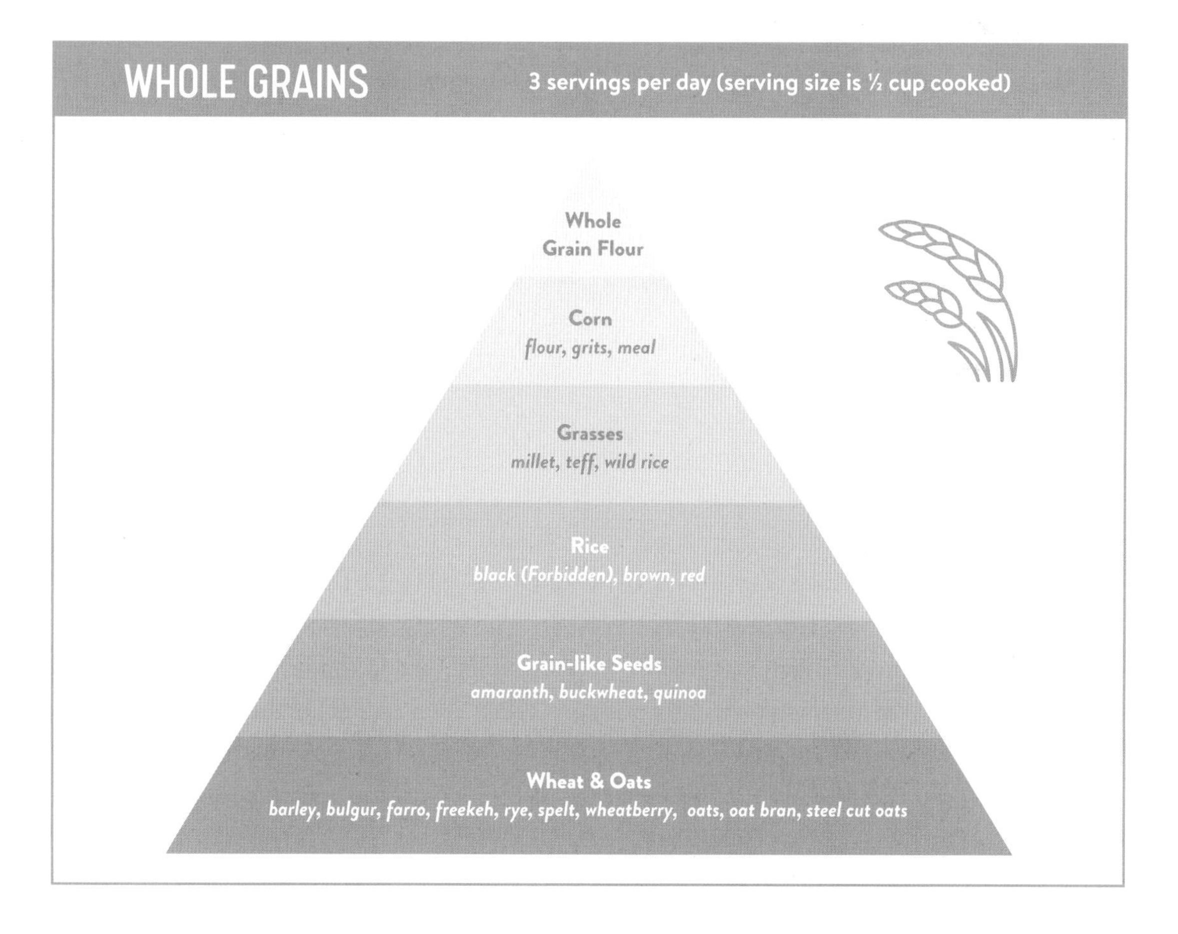

IS IT REALLY "WHOLE GRAIN"?

Food labels can be especially misleading when shopping for grains. The term "whole grain" has become a marketing ploy to make a packaged food appear more healthful than it is. When a loaf of bread is labeled "whole grain," for example, it could still be mostly refined grains. Ignore words like *multigrain* and *enriched* on the package and look at the ingredient list. If the first ingredient contains the word *whole*, such as whole-wheat flour or whole oats, that is a good sign. Be aware, however, that even if the second ingredient is listed as "whole," that ingredient could be as little as 1 percent of the total.

Food companies often use the term "whole grain" on packages to make a refined grain look better for you than it really is. How do you tell the difference? All it takes is a simple math trick. When researchers at the Harvard School of Public Health evaluated more than five hundred food products to discern which contained the highest amount of whole grains, they discovered a formula you can easily do in your head. First, find the total number of carbohydrates on the nutrition label. Divide that by ten. Now compare that number to the number of grams of fiber on the label. If the fiber content is higher than a tenth of the total carbohydrates, your bread is mostly whole grain. The Harvard researchers also found that when a food fits this criterion, it is more likely to have less added sugar, sodium, and unhealthy fats.

Another way to find high-quality whole-grain foods is to look for the gold leaf logo of the Whole Grain Stamp on packages. This means the product is certified by the Whole Grains Council, a nonprofit consumer advocacy group, and it tells you how much whole grain is actually in the food—100 percent, 50 percent, or a lesser amount per serving. Visit the council's website for more information and as an evidence-based resource about buying grains (see Resources, page 390).

Mediterranean diet, found that when people eat whole grains regularly, they have 30 percent less incidence of cardiovascular events, such as heart attack and stroke. There were cognitive benefits, too. When participants were given cognitive tests, those who ate three or more servings of whole grains each day outperformed those who were in the control group. While refined grains can incite inflammation in the body and the brain, whole grains are proven to be anti-inflammatory. In other words, the more whole grains participants consumed, the less inflammation they had, an effect that persisted for years after the study was completed.

Fortunately, it is quite easy to attain the recommended three ½ cup (about 50 g) servings of cooked whole grains per day. This could be a piece of (truly) whole-grain bread, a small bowl of oatmeal, and a scoop of freekeh in your salad. In this chapter, there are recipes for making grains the basis for a meal, such as the brown rice paella on page 257 and the grain bowls on page 263. Breakfast is a great time for whole grains, too, whether it's a quick breakfast bowl (page 206) or a scoop of granola with berries and yogurt (page 268).

SHOPPING FOR WHOLE GRAINS

Find packaged grains, such as quinoa, buckwheat, and different rice varieties, on supermarket shelves near the rice. The bulk section is a good place to locate specialty grains like rye berries, oat groats, and spelt. Freshness is key, so be sure to shop at a store with high turnover.

Ancient and heirloom grains like spelt and buckwheat groats are worth seeking out at natural food stores, specialty stores, or online. Many of these grains are grown on small, family-owned farms using seeds handed down through generations. In contrast to modern grains, these are bred for flavor, not supermarket shelf life. As these high-quality grains grow in popularity, you are likely to find more intriguing choices like Kamut (khorasan wheat), teff, amaranth, and einkorn edging their way onto supermarket shelves.

Part of the grass family, whole-grain forms of wheat include wheat berries, farro, rye, spelt, and barley. Bulgur is a whole-grain wheat that is cracked to form a fluffy pilaf, like you find in the Levantine salad tabbouleh. Freekeh has a unique flavor that comes from how it is harvested—cracked open while still green and roasted to get to the wheat kernel.

When shopping for whole-wheat flour, look for "100% whole wheat" on the label. You may also see white whole-wheat flour (the "white" here referring to a type of whole wheat), a fiber-rich swap for refined all-purpose white flour that can be easily substituted in recipes.

Many varieties of rice can be a wonderful component of your brain-healthy diet. Just like wheat, rice retains more of its fiber and nutrients if not overly processed. Brown, Forbidden (black), and red rice are all whole grains that retain their fiber-rich outer coating along with phytonutrients, many of which are the plant pigments that give them their color. White rice, on the other hand, is brown rice stripped of its husk, bran, and germ. Brown rice is always a brain-healthier choice than white, which is low in fiber and has a high glycemic index (the ability to make blood sugar spike after a meal). When you do eat white rice (such as when enjoying sushi at a restaurant), be sure to pair it with lots of vegetables.

Buckwheat, amaranth, and quinoa are considered honorary grains, aka pseudograins, because they are cooked and enjoyed similarly to grains. Though buckwheat sounds like a type of wheat, it is actually a gluten-free plant most closely related to rhubarb and sorrel. Its whole form is a groat, which can be cooked into a pilaf or porridge; the toasted form is called kasha. Buckwheat is also milled into a deliciously nutty and slightly bitter flour. It enhances the flavors of dark chocolate, as in the chocolate chip cookies on page 265, and forms the base of classic Breton galettes (page 251).

Amaranth and quinoa are seeds that cook up fluffy and tender with toasted nut flavors. Both can be milled into flour, too. Quinoa is especially rich in nutrients: like a full complement of essential amino acids and a whopping 6 grams of protein and 2.5 grams of fiber in each serving. Quinoa flour gives Caramelized Apple and Quinoa Pancakes (page 273) a delicious, toasted-nut flavor.

Besides wheat, the most common whole-grain grasses are millet, wild rice, and teff. Wild rice is a colorful, chewy addition to pilafs and soups, like the turkey soup on page 289. Teff, the world's tiniest grain, originates from Ethiopia where it is an important staple. Ground into flour, teff adds a hint of hazelnuts and chocolate to baked goods, along with a good dose of protein and iron. To bake with it, substitute teff flour for about 25 percent of the white flour in a recipe.

Corn on the cob is a vegetable, of course, but the actual corn kernel, when dried and milled into cornmeal, is considered a grain. Whole-grain corn is a brain-healthy addition to your diet. Look for coarse or medium cornmeal for making polenta or finely ground cornmeal for baked goods, like the berry cornbread on page 68. And don't forget popcorn—these kernels make an excellent snack. Try them drizzled with olive oil and sprinkled with nutritional yeast.

Oats are a nutrient-dense staple food in many cultures. Famous for their fiber content and cholesterol-lowering ability, oats come in many whole-grain forms. Oat groats are the kernels of the oat, aka the most whole form of the grain. When oat groats are processed into rolled oats, the inedible outer husk is chafed off to make them more cookable, but they are still considered whole because they retain another husk, the oat bran, plus the germ and endosperm. Steel-cut oats (aka pinhead or Irish oats) retain a bit more of both husks and thus have a chewier texture than rolled oats. They also take longer to cook and benefit from an overnight soak in water to speed up the cooking time.

Oat bran is the fiber-rich portion of the groat. High in both soluble and insoluble fiber with well-studied cholesterol-lowering effects (page 267), oat bran is a worthy addition to your brain-healthy pantry. Cook into a porridge or use it to boost the fiber and nutrition of other foods. In this chapter, it adds a hearty touch to chocolate chip cookies (page 265).

Oat flour is a nutrient-dense flour that adds nubby texture and nutty flavors to baked goods. It's easy to make yourself in a food processor or blender. (Learn how on page 132.) Swap it in for some of the white flour in a recipe to increase the fiber and nutrients (about ¼ cup/30 g oat flour for 1 cup/120 g of white flour).

Instant oats are rolled oats that are cut into smaller pieces so they can be cooked up quickly in a microwave or on the stove. While undeniably convenient, many brands add sugar and artificial flavorings, so read the nutrition label carefully.

EASY WAYS TO ADD A SERVING OF WHOLE GRAINS

A big batch of whole grains like brown rice or barley is great to have on hand throughout the week. Refrigerate in an airtight container for up to five days or freeze cooked grains in single-serving zip-top bags for later use.

1. For a simple breakfast bowl, warm 1 cup (100 g) cooked whole grains with plant-based milk and top with things like fruit, nut butter, and seeds.
2. Stir ½ cup (50 g) cooked whole grains into any soup.
3. Fold ½ cup (50 g) cooked brown rice into pancake batter.
4. Toast grains (like oat and quinoa) with olive oil and spices to serve as a crouton-like salad topping.
5. Add a scoop of cooked whole grains to a vegetable frittata before baking.

GRAIN-FREE DIETS AND THE BRAIN

Giving up or severely limiting grains is a feature of two popular diets—the paleolithic diet (aka paleo) and the ketogenic diet (aka keto). The premise of the paleo diet is simple: if the cavemen didn't eat it, you shouldn't either, according to the diet's founders. All grains (a consequence of the agricultural revolution) are off-limits under this plan. Even quinoa, which has been consumed by highland people of South America since the Neolithic age (around 4000 BCE), is considered a modern food. On the plus side, paleo cuts out many brain-harming foods, such as those full of refined sugar and simple carbohydrates. But there are no studies that scientifically evaluate the benefits of paleo in reducing Alzheimer's or other types of dementia, or for reducing related conditions like diabetes and cardiovascular diseases. The problem with paleo is that it categorically eliminates entire food groups proven beneficial for reducing Alzheimer's, such as legumes and whole grains. And it is much higher in saturated fat than recommended for a brain-protective diet.

The goal of the ketogenic diet is to shift the body into ketosis, a metabolic state in which your body utilizes ketone bodies instead of glucose for fuel. The diet combines high-fat foods and a strict limit on carbohydrates (20 milligrams or less per day, depending on the keto variation) with fasting to spur your body into starvation mode. Keto has been proven to be beneficial for weight loss, although long-term studies—evaluating whether people can keep the weight off—are mixed.

You may have read that the keto diet can reverse the symptoms of Alzheimer's. At first glance, this makes sense because the brain of someone with Alzheimer's can no longer utilize glucose for energy. Instead, the Alzheimer's brain responds to ketone bodies, what it would normally use during states of starvation when no food is available. There have been promising, although inconsistent, results when Alzheimer's patients are switched to a keto diet—their brains can finally use energy and symptoms may improve. This is far from being the standard of care, however, as more comprehensive studies need to be done. The sad truth is that once Alzheimer's has reached a certain stage, reversing the disease is just no longer possible.

No data suggests that keto is a good idea for preventing Alzheimer's. There are some elements of keto that are good for the brain, however, like intermittent fasting and avoiding refined sugars and simple carbohydrates. But the keto diet is too restrictive in the foods known to be neuroprotective, such as legumes and whole grains, and too plentiful in foods known to accelerate brain aging, like foods high in saturated fat. The problem with putting your body into starvation mode long term is that it also starves the brain of the nutrients it needs to thrive and age well.

BUCKWHEAT GALETTES WITH MUSHROOMS AND LEEKS

SERVES 4

3 eggs

1 cup (240 ml) water

4 tablespoons extra-virgin olive oil, plus more for the pan and for drizzling

1¼ cups (150 g) buckwheat flour

¾ teaspoon kosher salt

4 tablespoons extra-virgin olive oil

3 large leeks (1 pound/455 g), white and tender green parts thinly sliced

4 cups (¾ pound/340 g) mixed mushrooms, trimmed and thinly sliced

¼ teaspoon freshly ground black pepper, plus more for serving

½ cup (4 ounces/115 g) grated cheese, such as Gruyère, smoked Gouda, or crumbled Lemony Cashew Ricotta (page 373)

1 avocado, sliced

4 loosely packed cups (160 g) tender lettuces, such as butter, Bibb, or baby lettuces

Flaky salt (optional)

Buckwheat shines in these savory French pancakes. This gluten-free flour is nutty and has a pleasant bitter note (a hint to its flavonoid content). While buckwheat galettes can be a blank canvas for any topping you like, they go especially well with other earthy plant foods, as here with mushrooms and leeks.

Though the batter benefits from resting for at least four hours, you can also just let it sit at room temperature while you prepare the rest of the recipe. The recipe makes enough batter for you to mess up the first galette (I always do!).

These veggie-packed galettes are best served right from the pan. If you want to serve all at the same time, keep them warm in a 300°F (150°C) oven and add the avocado just before serving.

1. Whisk together the eggs, water, and 3 tablespoons of the oil in a large bowl until frothy and pale yellow. Whisk in the buckwheat flour and ¼ teaspoon of the kosher salt until you have a very smooth batter. Set aside or cover and refrigerate for at least 4 hours and up to overnight.

2. When you're ready to cook the galettes and you'd like to serve them all together, set an oven rack in the center position and preheat the oven to 300°F (150°C).

3. Heat 2 teaspoons of the oil in a large nonstick skillet over medium-high heat. Add the leeks and sprinkle with ¼ teaspoon of the kosher salt. Cook, stirring often, until soft and starting to brown, 6 to 8 minutes. Transfer to a small bowl.

continued

4. Using the same skillet, pour in the remaining 1 teaspoon oil. Add the mushrooms, sprinkle with the pepper and the remaining ¼ teaspoon kosher salt, and cook, stirring often, until the edges are crispy and brown, 6 to 8 minutes. Transfer to the bowl with the leeks and toss together.

5. To make the galettes, place a 9- to 10-inch (23 to 25 cm) nonstick skillet or crêpe pan over medium heat and add a few drops of oil. Whisk the batter briefly, then pour ½ cup (120 ml) in a thin stream over the pan, swirling to evenly cover. Cook until bubbles start to form on the surface, 30 seconds to 1 minute.

6. Reduce the heat to low and sprinkle with 2 tablespoons of the cheese and a heaping ½ cup (about 70 g) of the leek and mushroom mixture. Top with one-quarter of the avocado (if serving right away) and fold the galette over like a quesadilla. Slide onto a plate and serve immediately. (If keeping the galettes warm in the oven, add the avocado just before serving.) Repeat with remaining ingredients.

7. To serve, top each galette with 1 cup (40 g) of the greens, drizzle with oil, and sprinkle with flaky salt (if using) and more pepper, if you like.

TIPS: *When shopping for buckwheat flour, look for the freshest product you can find. High-quality buckwheat flour has a sandy color with lots of flecks of dark brown—an indication that much of the fiber-rich hull was included when the seeds were milled into flour.*

Save the leek tops for making stock (page 376). They'll keep in a zip-top bag or other airtight container for up to 3 months in the freezer.

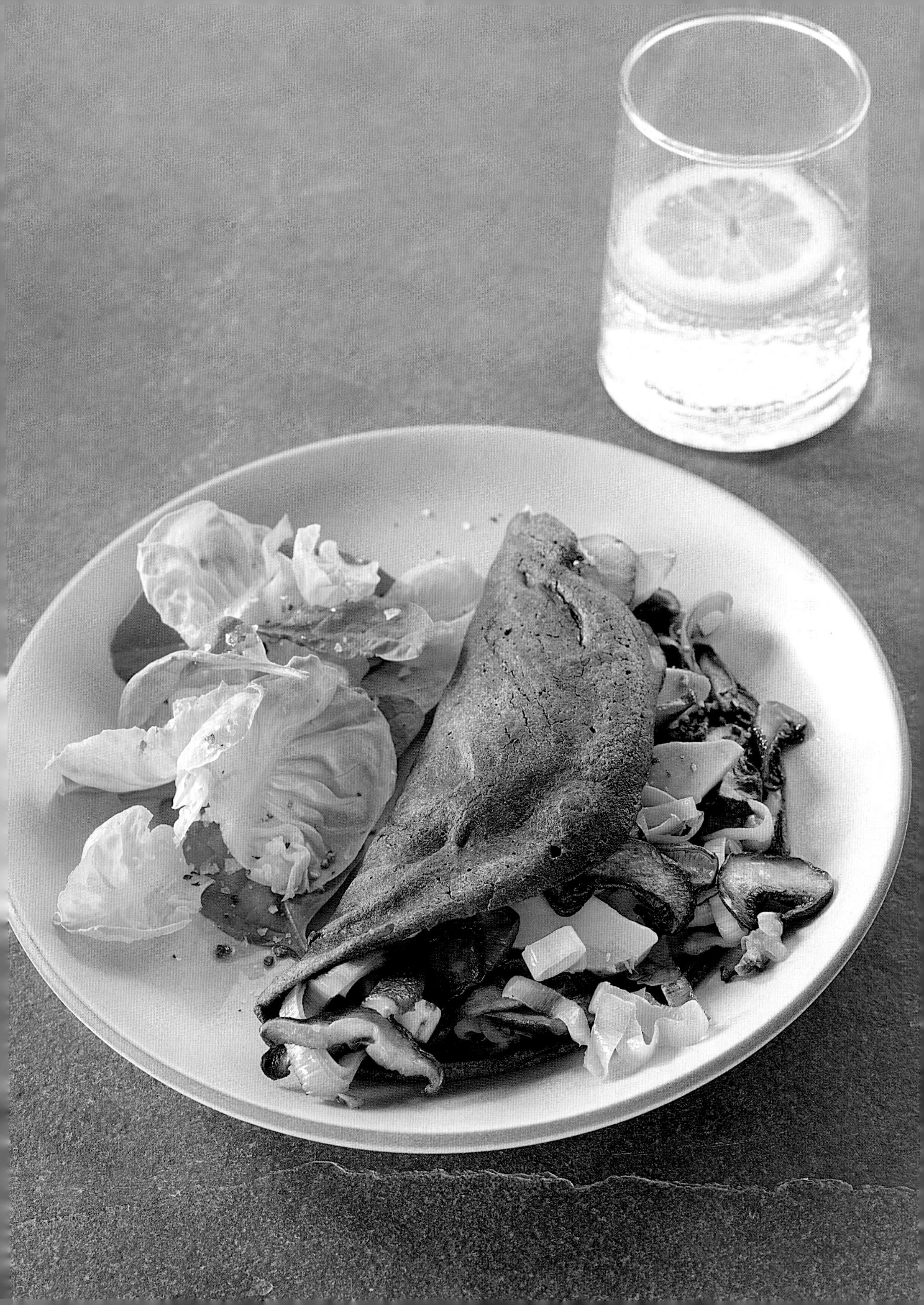

FREEKEH SALAD WITH BRUSSELS SPROUTS AND CRISPY CAPERS

SERVES 4 TO 6 AS A SIDE

1½ cups (300 g) freekeh

¼ cup (60 ml) extra-virgin olive oil, plus more for drizzling

1 teaspoon kosher salt

½ cup (120 g) capers (salt- or olive oil packed), drained and patted dry

2 large garlic cloves, thinly sliced

1½ pounds (680 g) Brussels sprouts, trimmed and thinly sliced

½ teaspoon freshly ground black pepper

½ loosely packed cup (10 g) fresh flat-leaf parsley, finely chopped

1 cup (145 g) unsalted blanched hazelnuts, toasted (page 190) and coarsely chopped

2 tablespoons white wine vinegar

1 ounce (30 g) pecorino cheese, shaved into long strips

Flaky salt (optional)

Freekeh is one of the most nutrient-dense types of wheat. It's high in fiber, protein, and two brain-specific carotenoids, lutein and zeaxanthin. Its unique grassy, slightly smoky flavor pairs especially well with acidic foods like vinegar and lemon. Here it joins shredded Brussels sprouts and crispy capers in a grain salad that's perfect on its own or alongside a main dish like roasted salmon. Other sturdy whole grains work well in this grain salad, like farro, barley, and brown rice.

1. Bring a medium saucepan of salted water to a boil over high heat. Stir in the freekeh, reduce the heat to a gentle simmer, and cook, stirring occasionally, until tender but still chewy, 15 to 25 minutes or according to the package directions. Drain and transfer to a large shallow serving bowl. Toss with 1 tablespoon of the oil and ½ teaspoon of the kosher salt; set aside.

2. Meanwhile, heat 1 tablespoon of the oil in a large nonstick skillet over medium-high heat. Add the capers and cook, stirring often, until crispy and golden brown, about 4 minutes for small capers and 6 minutes for large ones. Use a slotted spoon to transfer to a paper towel–lined plate, leaving any oil behind.

3. Add the garlic to the pan and cook over medium heat until just barely golden, about 30 seconds. Transfer to the plate with the capers.

4. In the same skillet, add 1 tablespoon of the oil, the Brussels sprouts, pepper, and the remaining ½ teaspoon kosher salt. Cook over medium heat, stirring occasionally, until wilted, 2 to 3 minutes.

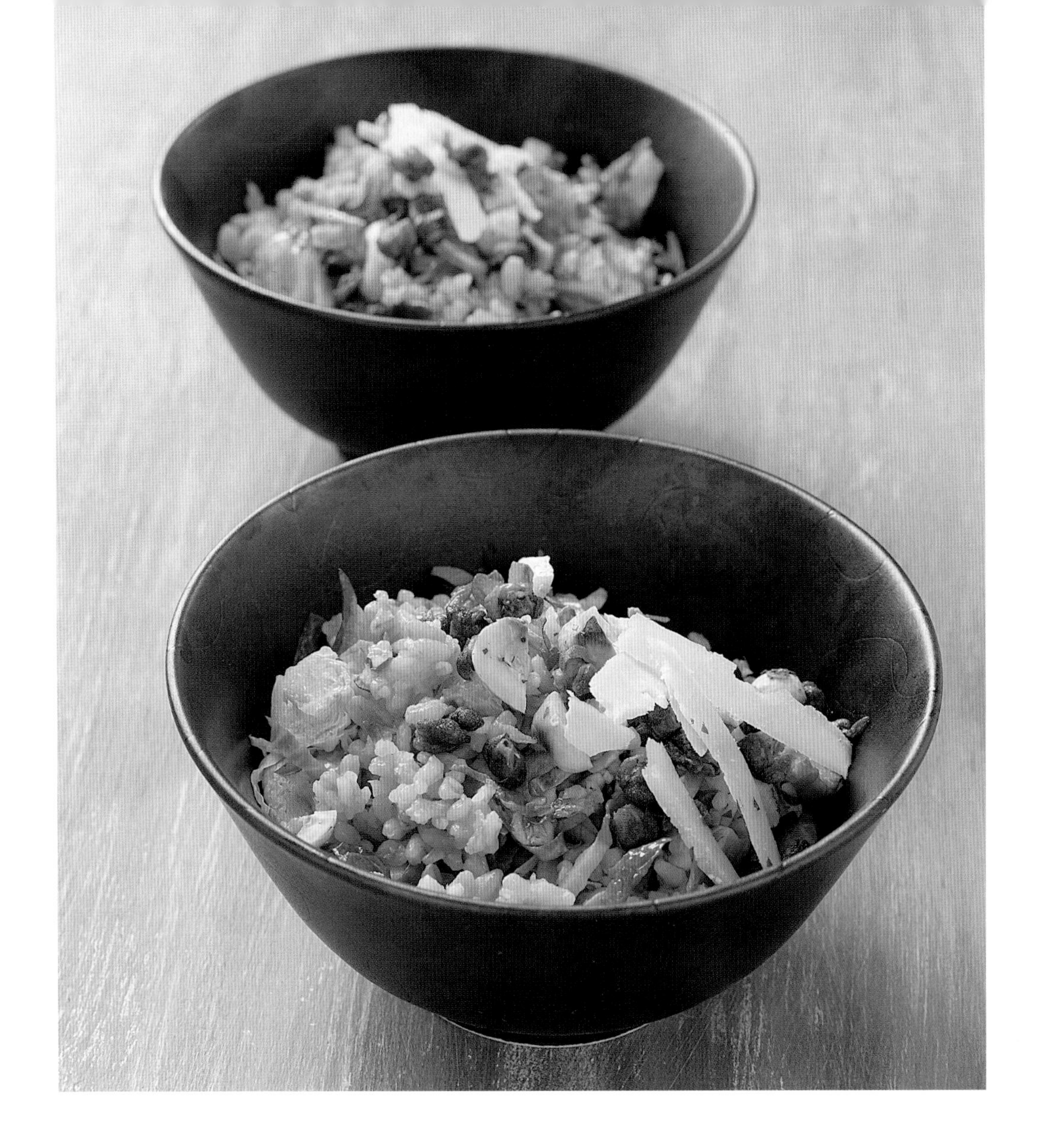

5. Add the Brussels sprouts and parsley to the freekeh and toss to combine. Add the garlic, hazelnuts, vinegar, and the remaining 2 tablespoons oil; toss again. Top with the capers, pecorino, a drizzle of olive oil, and a sprinkle of flaky salt, if you like.

TIP: *To quickly slice the Brussels sprouts, use a food processor fitted with a large slicing blade.*

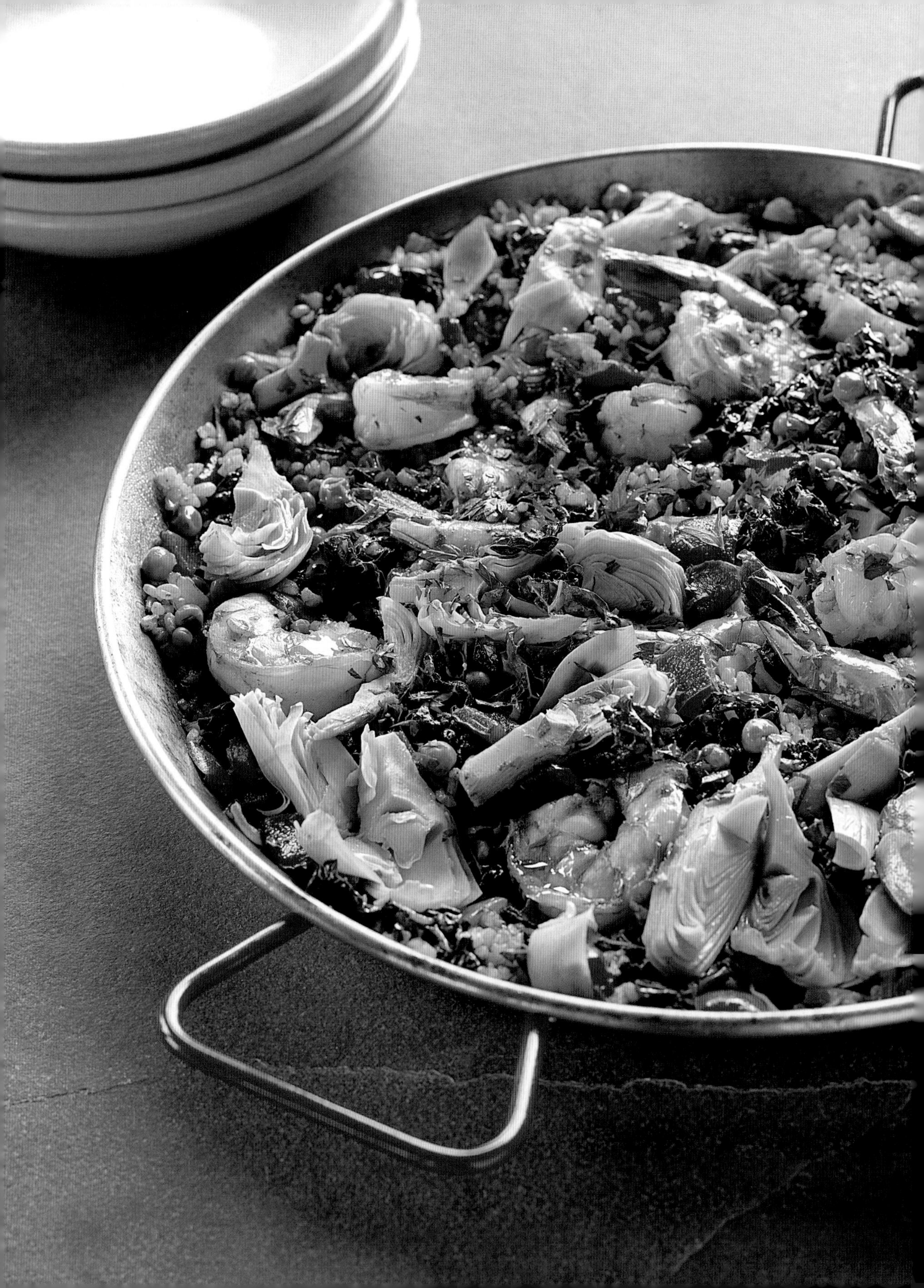

BROWN RICE PAELLA WITH SHRIMP AND ARTICHOKES

SERVES 4 TO 6

6 cups (1.4 L) chicken or vegetable stock

1 teaspoon saffron threads

¼ cup (60 ml) extra-virgin olive oil, plus more for drizzling

1 large yellow onion (12 ounces/340 g), finely chopped (about 2 cups)

2 large red bell peppers (12 ounces/340 g total), diced (about 2 cups)

1 teaspoon kosher salt

3 medium garlic cloves, minced (about 1½ teaspoons)

2 cups (165 g) shredded frozen kale

2 cups (430 g) long-grain brown rice, rinsed

Up to ¼ cup (60 ml) water (optional)

1 cup (145 g) peas, fresh or frozen

1 pound (455 g) large shrimp (about 12), peeled and deveined

One 13.75-ounce (240 g) can water-packed quartered artichoke hearts, drained

½ loosely packed cup (10 g) fresh flat-leaf parsley, finely chopped

Freshly ground black pepper (optional)

Lemon wedges

I learned how to make paella from my Spanish host mother, Pilar, as a sixteen-year-old exchange student in Villafañe. She introduced me to Manzanilla olives and gazpacho and taught me how to cook traditional dishes like tortilla and torta. Pilar cooked her paella over an open fire at a leisurely pace; it was always the centerpiece of a party. Though I imagine she never used brown rice or kale in paella, I think she'd agree it's delicious.

Paella is an inherently brain-healthy dish because of saffron, a food of interest to Alzheimer's researchers (see the Science Bite on page 258) that also gives the rice a distinctive golden yellow color and floral flavor. This version swaps in fiber-rich whole-grain brown rice for the traditional short-grain white rice. In the name of brain health, it packs in more vegetables, too.

While this paella remains festive and special enough to serve guests at a party, the streamlined method transforms it into a dish worthy of your weekly dinner rotation.

1. Bring the stock to a boil in a medium saucepan over high heat. Reduce the heat to low, stir in the saffron, and keep warm on the stove.

2. Heat the oil in a 15-inch (38 cm) paella pan or a large skillet over medium-high heat. Add the onion, bell peppers, and ½ teaspoon of the salt. Cook, stirring often, until the vegetables are fragrant and soft, 7 to 9 minutes. Reduce the heat to medium-low, stir in the garlic, and cook, stirring often, another 1 minute.

continued

3. Stir in the kale, rice, stock, saffron, and remaining ½ teaspoon salt. Bring to a boil, then reduce the heat until the mixture bubbles gently. Cover and cook until the stock is almost fully absorbed and the rice is tender, 55 to 65 minutes. If the rice needs more time, pour up to ¼ cup (60 ml) water over the surface, cover, and check for doneness in 5 minutes.

4. Scatter the peas over the surface of the dish, then nestle the shrimp and artichoke hearts into the rice. Cover and cook over medium-low heat until the shrimp is pink and opaque throughout, 6 to 8 minutes.

5. Just before serving, drizzle with oil, sprinkle with parsley, and finish with black pepper, if you like. Serve with lemon wedges.

TIP: *A paella pan is a round, shallow pan with handles that sometimes comes with a lid. If your paella pan doesn't have a lid, cover with another large skillet or a tightly fitted piece of foil. If you don't have a paella pan, use a large skillet or Dutch oven instead.*

SCIENCE BITE:

SAFFRON AS A MEMORY-ENHANCING THERAPY

Prized as a brain food in ancient Persia, saffron is now being studied by Alzheimer's researchers for its memory-enhancing effects. Saffron may support brain health by blocking amyloid clumping and boosting acetylcholinesterase levels, a key brain neurotransmitter.

When researchers compared saffron head-to-head against the FDA-approved Alzheimer's drug donazepil, the results were surprising. Thirty milligrams of saffron (equivalent to one pinch of saffron threads) blocked just as much acetylcholinesterase as the drug and was just as effective in improving cognitive function. Eating saffron every day isn't practical—it's touted as the world's most expensive spice—but ongoing studies are likely to determine if saffron will be part of the toolbox for treating Alzheimer's.

CREAMY CARROT FARROTTO

SERVES 4 TO 6

- **¾ pound (340 g) slender carrots with tops attached, scrubbed well, cut into 4-inch (10 cm) pieces**
- **2 tablespoons extra-virgin olive oil**
- **1 teaspoon kosher salt**
- **2 cups (500 ml) carrot juice**
- **4 cups (1 L) vegetable stock, homemade (page 374) or store-bought (low-sodium, if possible)**
- **1 large shallot (5 ounces/ 140 g), finely chopped (about ½ cup)**
- **2 large garlic cloves, finely chopped (about 2 teaspoons)**
- **1½ cups (300 g) semi-pearled or pearled farro (see Tip)**
- **½ cup (60 g) Walnut "Parm" (page 184) or freshly grated Parmesan cheese**
- **1 tablespoon white wine vinegar**
- **½ teaspoon freshly ground black pepper, plus more for serving**
- **1 tablespoon fresh thyme leaves**
- **Finely chopped carrot tops (optional)**

Farrotto combines the classic technique of rice-based risotto with farro, a chewy, delicious type of whole-grain wheat. In this plant-based rendition, you'll simmer the grains in a carrot-infused stock and top them with spears of roasted carrot. Just like making classic risotto, this one likes you to hover and stir.

Buying farro can be confusing because it goes by many names. Semi-pearled farro is my top choice for this recipe, but other types will also work (see Tips).

1. Set an oven rack in the center position and preheat the oven to 375°F (190°C). Line a rimmed baking sheet with parchment paper or a silicone mat.

2. Place the carrots on the prepared baking sheet and toss with 1 tablespoon of the oil and ½ teaspoon of the salt. Spread them in a single layer and bake for 30 to 35 minutes, tossing once, until the carrots are golden brown and starting to get crispy.

3. Meanwhile, make the farrotto. Warm the carrot juice and stock in a small saucepan over medium-high heat. Reduce the heat to low and keep warm on the stove.

4. Heat the remaining 1 tablespoon oil in a large skillet over medium-high heat. Add the shallots, sprinkle with the remaining ½ teaspoon salt, and cook, stirring often, until golden brown, 4 to 6 minutes. Add the garlic and cook until fragrant, about 1 minute. Add the farro, stirring well to coat the grains.

5. Using a ladle or a measuring cup, transfer ½ cup (120 ml) of the stock mixture to the pan. Adjust the heat so the sauce

continued

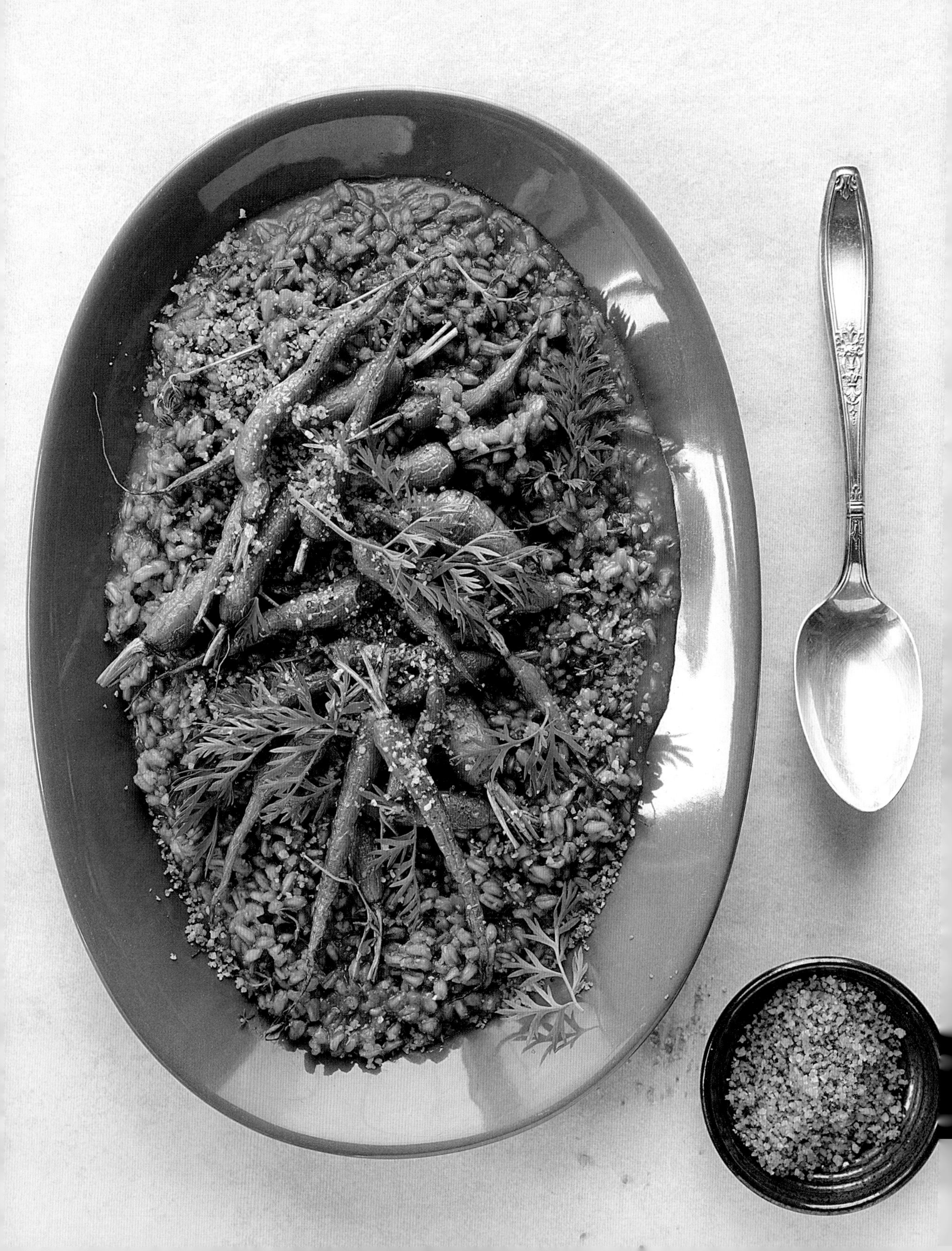

gently simmers, and cook, stirring often, until almost all the liquid has been absorbed, 3 to 5 minutes. Add the remaining stock ½ cup (120 ml) at a time and continue to add the liquid in stages until the farro is tender but still chewy, 30 to 40 minutes total.

6. Stir in ¼ cup (30 g) of the "Parm," the vinegar, and the pepper. Divide the farrotto between shallow bowls, then top with the roasted carrots and the remaining ¼ cup (30 g) "Parm." Sprinkle with the thyme and carrot tops, if using. Finish with more pepper, if you like.

TIPS: *Carrot tops are rich in folate and vitamin K, but they are so often thrown out. Look for slender, rainbow-colored carrots with the greens still attached.*

Different types of farro vary in cooking times, a reflection of how processed the grain is. Pearled farro cooks up the quickest but has had all of its bran removed as well as most of its fiber. Semi-pearled farro retains more bran and is my farro of choice—it gives you more fiber and takes just a few more minutes to cook than pearled. Whole-grain farro is not processed at all and so retains the greatest amount of fiber, balanced by a cooking time of up to 1½ hours. (An overnight soak speeds that up.) The freshness of the grain matters, too, so if your farro is old, it will take longer to cook.

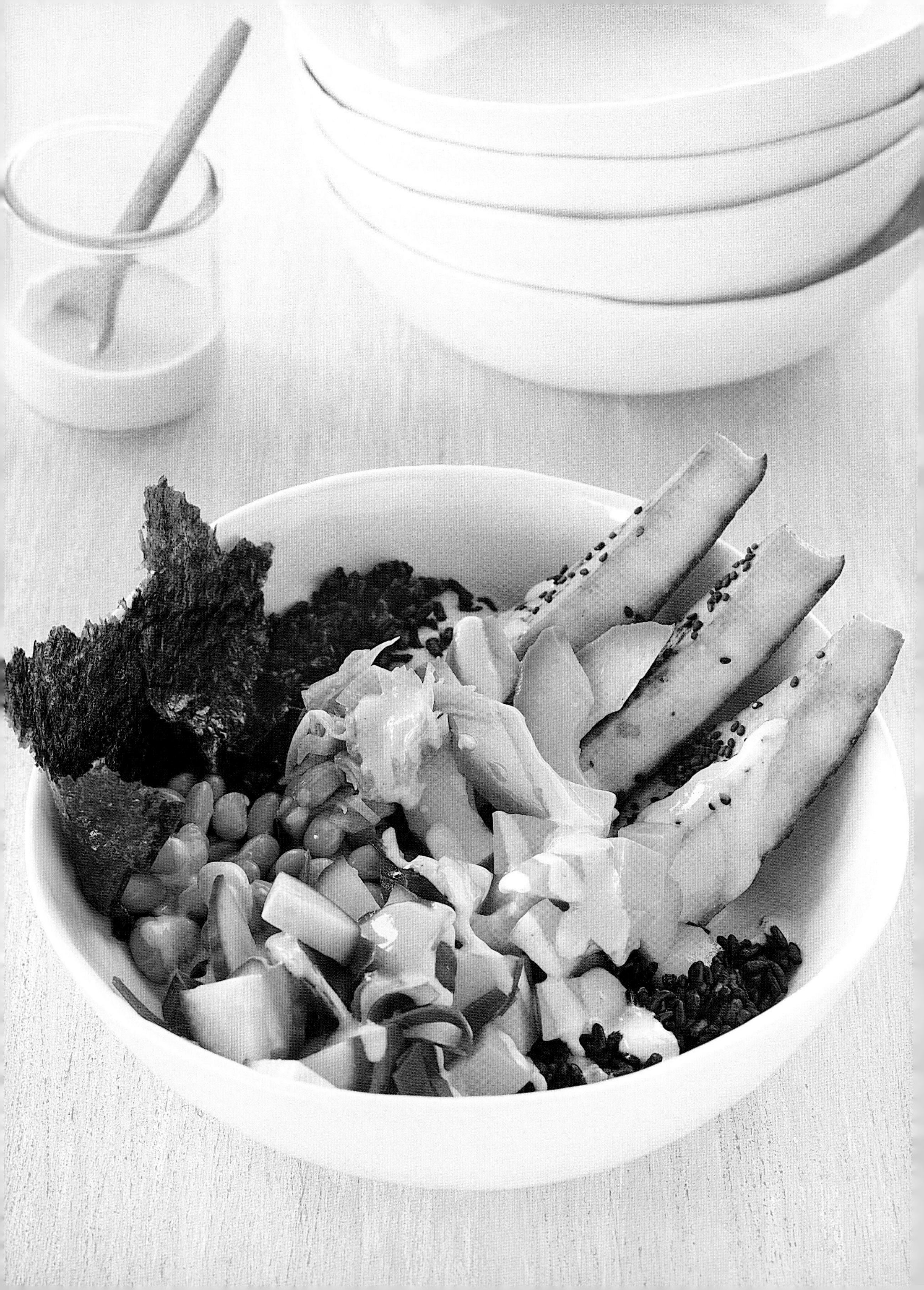

SUSHI ROLL GRAIN BOWLS

SERVES 4

One 14-ounce (400 g) block extra-firm tofu, halved horizontally through the center and cut into triangles

2 cups (500 ml) water

1 cup (210 g) Forbidden Rice (black rice)

½ teaspoon kosher salt

1 tablespoon plus 1 teaspoon tamari or low-sodium soy sauce

1 tablespoon unhulled white or black sesame seeds

½ ounce (15 g) wakame, precut or cut into 1-inch (2.5 cm) strips

1 medium Persian cucumber (8 ounces/225 g), sliced ½ inch (1.25 cm) thick, each slice quartered

¼ cup (40 g) pickled ginger, thinly sliced, plus 3 tablespoons of the pickling liquid (see Tip)

2 cups (290 g) shelled edamame beans

1 teaspoon dried wasabi powder

½ cup (120 ml) Almost Instant Cashew Cream (page 370) or vegan mayo

½ teaspoon sriracha or other hot sauce

1 mango, peeled and cut into ½-inch-thick (1.25 cm) cubes

1 avocado, sliced ½ inch (1.25 cm) thick

1 sheet nori, torn or cut into bite-size pieces

This vibrant recipe reimagines a veggie-packed sushi roll as a grain bowl. You'll top a pile of black rice (also called Forbidden Rice) with tamari-infused tofu, a vinegary cucumber salad, and a creamy wasabi sauce. If you are new to sea vegetables, you may be surprised at how easy they are to prepare at home, not to mention how much their sea-forward flavors add to simple foods.

If you can't find Forbidden Rice, swap in long-grain brown rice instead.

1. Line a small rimmed baking sheet with a clean kitchen towel. Place the tofu on top in a single layer and cover with another towel. Top with a second baking sheet and weight it with something heavy, such as a cast-iron pan. Let sit for at least 30 minutes (or refrigerate up to overnight).

2. Set an oven rack in the center position and preheat the oven to 375°F (190°C). Line a rimmed baking sheet with parchment paper.

3. Bring the water, rice, and salt to a boil in a medium saucepan with a tight-fitting lid. Reduce the heat to a low simmer, cover, and cook until the rice is tender, 35 to 40 minutes. Remove from the heat and steam, covered, for 5 minutes.

4. Meanwhile, squeeze as much water as you can from the tofu, then place on the parchment-lined baking sheet. Pour 1 tablespoon of the tamari over top, flipping the slices to evenly coat. Sprinkle with the sesame seeds and bake for 25 to 35 minutes, until golden brown and crispy along the edges.

5. While the tofu bakes, place the wakame in a medium bowl and cover with hot tap water. After 5 minutes, drain then

TIP: When shopping for pickled ginger (sometimes called sushi ginger), look for a jar without added sugar or artificial ingredients, like aspartame or food dye FD&C #40 that makes it bright pink. (See Resources, page 390, for suggested brands.) You'll use the pickling liquid from the jar to make the wasabi mayo; alternatively, you could substitute unseasoned rice vinegar.

squeeze dry with a clean towel. Place back in the bowl along with the cucumber and 2 tablespoons of the ginger pickling liquid. Toss together.

6. Place the edamame in a shallow microwaveable bowl with 1 inch (2.5 cm) water. Cover tightly with a plate and microwave on high for 2 minutes, or until soft.

7. For the dressing, stir together the wasabi powder and the remaining 1 tablespoon ginger pickling liquid to make a smooth paste. Stir in the cashew cream, sriracha, and the remaining 1 teaspoon tamari.

8. To serve, divide the rice between bowls. Top with the cucumber salad, edamame, avocado, mango, nori, and tofu. Add the pickled ginger and drizzle with wasabi dressing.

SCIENCE BITE:

SEA VEGETABLES ARE BRAIN FOOD

Think of sea vegetables as the leafy greens of the sea. These include the edible seaweeds—nori, wakame, dulse, arame, hijiki, and kombu, the dried kelp that helps make beans more digestible (see page 218). Technically types of algae, sea vegetables add briny nuance and umami flavor to foods, along with a bounty of neuroprotective nutrients.

Sea vegetables are one of the few plant-based sources of vitamin B12 and EPA (see page 42), the essential omega-3 fatty acid found in fish and seafood. They provide an impressive array of minerals, like calcium, iron, folate, and potassium. And there's more: sea vegetables are rich in alginic acid, which can bind with harmful heavy metals in the body and assist in their removal.

It's the marine-based carotenoids, however, that make sea vegetables a particularly brain-healthy food. These potent antioxidants—such as fucoxanthin, fucoidan, and astaxanthin (page 155)—quell inflammation in the brain by turning off FOXO3—one of the genes that regulate inflammatory pathways.

A diet rich in sea vegetables is one of the unique characteristics of people living on the Japanese island of Okinawa, a Blue Zone. Other Okinawan dietary staples, such as turmeric, purple yams, and green tea, have also been found to downregulate FOXO3. This is just one piece of the puzzle that may explain why Okinawans who eat a traditional diet are spared from the neurodegenerative diseases.

CHUNKY WHOLE-GRAIN CHOCOLATE CHIP COOKIES

MAKES 16 COOKIES

- ¾ packed cup (180 g) light brown sugar
- ¾ cup (180 ml) tahini, well stirred and at room temperature
- ½ cup (120 ml) extra-virgin olive oil
- 1 teaspoon pure vanilla extract
- 1 spooned-and-leveled cup (140 g) whole-wheat flour
- ½ cup (70 g) buckwheat flour
- ¼ cup (40 g) oat bran cereal or ¼ cup (25 g) rolled oats
- 3 tablespoons cacao powder
- 1 teaspoon baking powder
- 1 teaspoon kosher salt
- 2 eggs
- 6 ounces (170 g) bittersweet chocolate (60% to 80% cacao), chopped into ½-inch (1.25 cm) chunks (or 1 cup dark chocolate chips)
- Flaky salt (optional)

This go-to treat answers the craving for a classic chocolate chip cookie but also keeps brain health in mind. It's got a soft, chewy interior, crisp outsides, and a lot of chocolate.

The three whole-grain flours aren't just a smart swap for white flour, they create a cookie with a distinctive, nutty taste. Whole-wheat flour adds an earthy flavor, buckwheat brings out the fruity qualities in good dark chocolate, and oat bran adds a nubby texture, making the cookies feel more substantial.

Instead of butter, the dough features a blend of tahini and olive oil for a brain-friendly fat profile. Plus, there's half the added sugar of a regular chocolate chip cookie.

1. Set oven racks in the upper- and lower-third positions and preheat the oven to 350°F (180°C). Line two rimmed 18-by-13-inch (46 by 33 cm) baking sheets with parchment paper or silicone mats.

2. Whisk together the sugar, tahini, oil, and vanilla in a large bowl. Let sit for 10 minutes.

3. Meanwhile, whisk together the whole-wheat flour, buckwheat flour, oat cereal, cacao powder, baking powder, and kosher salt in another large bowl.

4. Beat the eggs one at a time into the sugar-tahini mixture, scraping down the sides of the bowl between additions, until smooth and well incorporated. Add the flour mixture to the bowl and stir until you have a thick dough with no streaks of flour remaining. Set aside 2 tablespoons of the larger pieces of chocolate to top the cookies. Add the rest of the chocolate, including any shards on the cutting board, to the cookie dough and mix until evenly combined.

continued

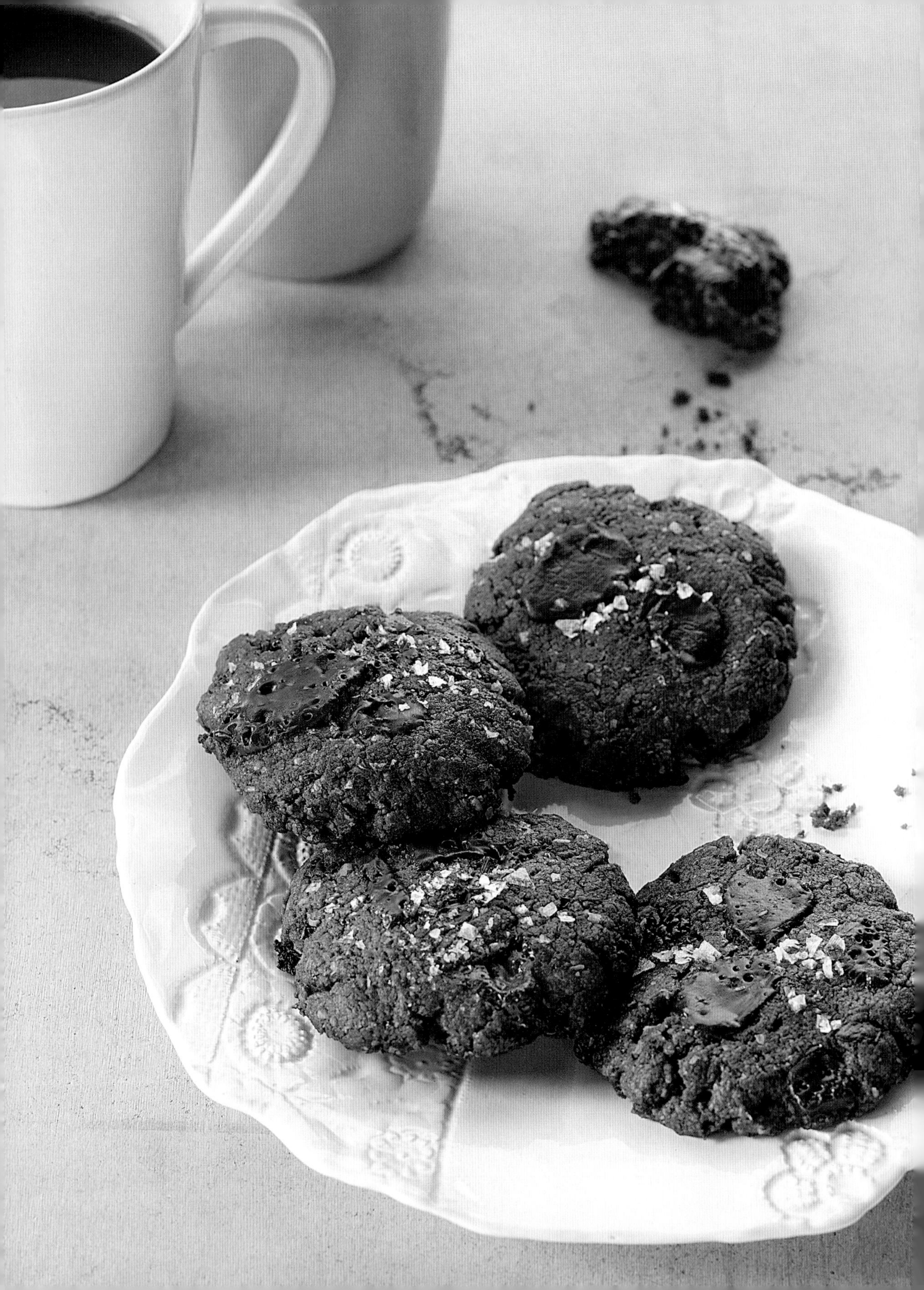

TIPS: *The size here is strategic: rolling the dough into a 1½-inch (3.8 cm) ball and flattening it into a 2-inch (5 cm) puck creates a cookie that's soft and chewy, with a slightly craggy texture. Keep a close eye on them toward the end of baking and pull from the oven when the centers are still soft.*

These cookies are still good if you use chocolate chips instead of chopped chocolate, but they won't have the same texture that comes from the melted shards and chunks.

5. Using a tablespoon measure, scoop out scant 3 tablespoons (55 g) for each cookie and roll into a 1½-inch (3.8 cm) ball, then press down to form a 2-inch-wide (5 cm) puck. Place on the prepared baking sheets leaving 3 inches (7.5 cm) between cookies, or eight to a sheet. Press a few pieces of the reserved chocolate into the tops of each cookie and sprinkle with a pinch of flaky salt (if using).

6. Bake for 8 to 10 minutes, or until set on the edges and still soft in the center. Let sit a few minutes then transfer to a rack to cool.

7. These cookies are best eaten the same day as or the day after baking. Cookie dough freezes well in an airtight container for up to 3 months. Or freeze the baked cookies, tightly wrapped, in the freezer for up to 3 months.

SCIENCE BITE:

OAT BRAN LOWERS LDL

A recent meta-analysis confirms oat bran's reputation as a cholesterol-lowering food. That's because oat bran, a more whole form of oats, contains enough beta-glucan (a type of fiber) to lower harmful LDL cholesterol. This was found to be especially true for those at risk for heart disease and Alzheimer's because they have diabetes and high levels of LDL. Just one serving of oat bran cereal (made from ⅓ cup/40 g dry oat bran) will provide 6 grams of fiber, most of it beta-glucan.

That being said, one cookie doesn't provide enough beta-glucan (the cholesterol-lowering fiber) from the oat bran to impact your blood cholesterol. If you buy a bag of oat bran cereal to make these cookies, use the rest for breakfast porridges.

GRANOLA, TWO WAYS

Eating better-for-you food doesn't have to mean sacrificing flavor or crunch in your granola. In these two recipes, the whole-grain oats bake up pleasingly crisp. Each recipe pairs two brain health superstar ingredients—matcha and sesame, and turmeric and black pepper.

Enjoy this energy-dense granola in small amounts (closer to a small handful than a whole bowl) and with other brain-healthy foods, like berries and unsweetened almond milk.

MATCHA GRANOLA

MAKES ABOUT 6 CUPS (700 G)

5 cups (500 g) rolled oats

¼ cup (30 g) hulled pumpkin seeds (pepitas)

¼ cup (40 g) unhulled sesame seeds, black, white, or a mix

¼ cup (35 g) hemp seeds

3 tablespoons culinary-grade matcha green tea powder

1 teaspoon kosher salt

½ cup (120 ml) pure maple syrup

½ cup (120 ml) extra-virgin olive oil or pecan oil

1 teaspoon pure vanilla extract

1 teaspoon orange oil, flavor, or extract (see Resources, page 390)

If you love a matcha latte, then this is the recipe for you. The powdered green tea adds a sophisticated note to the breakfast staple, which is balanced by maple syrup and vanilla. Thanks to its high catechin content, matcha is a brain-healthy addition to your granola (see page 344).

1. Set an oven rack in the center position and preheat the oven to 350°F (180°C). Line a rimmed 18-by-13-inch (46 by 33 cm) baking sheet with parchment paper or a silicone mat.

2. Combine the oats, pumpkin seeds, sesame seeds, hemp seeds, matcha, and salt in a large bowl.

3. Whisk together the maple syrup, oil, vanilla, and orange oil in a small bowl or 2-cup (480 ml) measuring cup. Pour over the oat mixture and stir until well coated. Scrape onto the prepared baking sheet and spread out in an even layer (see Tip).

4. Bake for 20 minutes, then rotate the baking sheet front to back and bake for 5 to 10 minutes longer, until golden brown throughout and darker on the edges. Let cool completely in the pan, then break into clusters. Use the parchment paper as a funnel to transfer the granola into an airtight container.

5. To store, keep in an airtight container, away from heat and light, for up to 3 weeks.

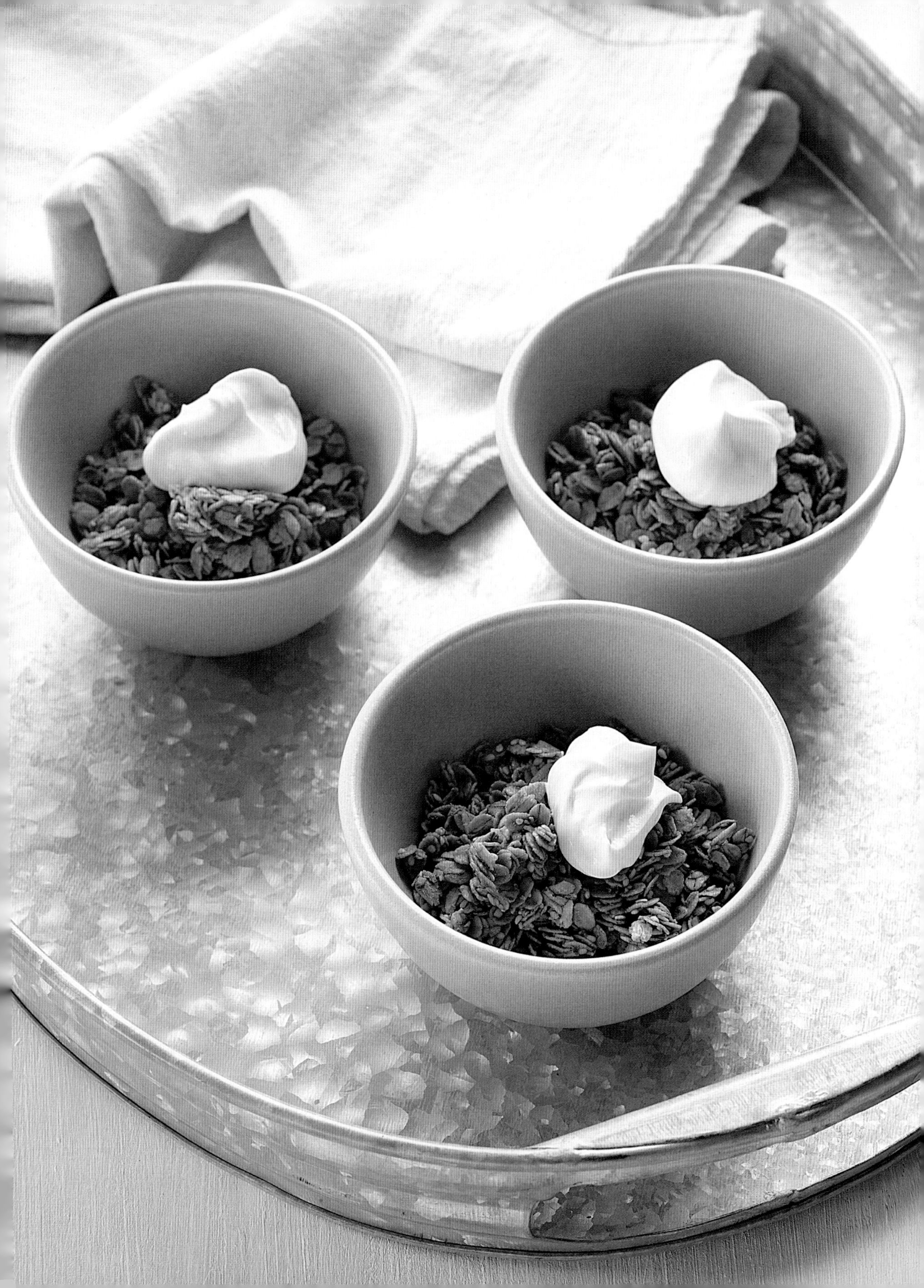

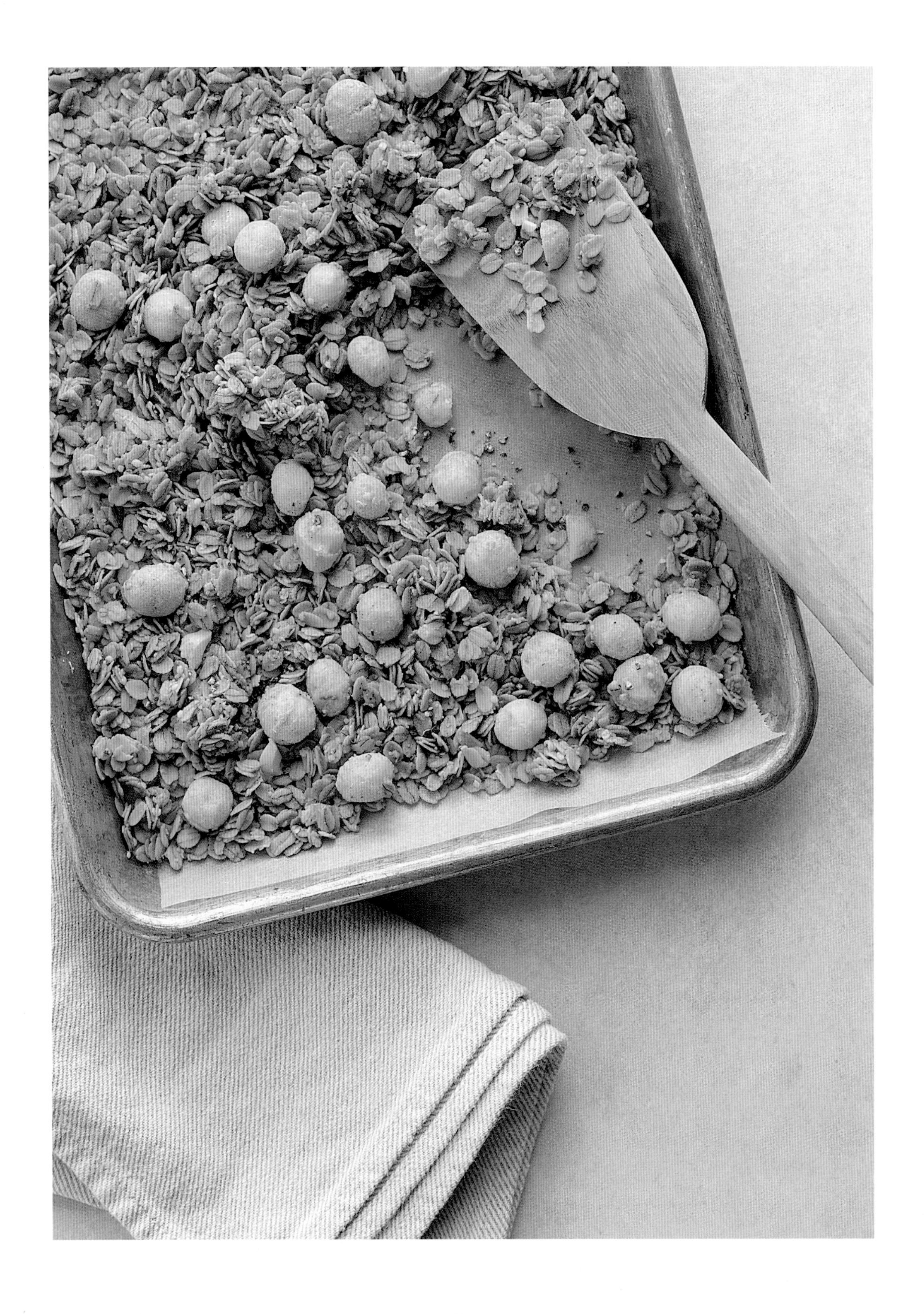

TURMERIC AND BLACK PEPPER GRANOLA

MAKES 6 CUPS (700 G)

5 cups (500 g) rolled oats

1 cup (140 g) raw cashews or macadamia nuts

½ cup (70 g) hemp seeds

2 teaspoons ground turmeric

½ teaspoon finely ground black pepper

1 teaspoon kosher salt

½ cup (120 ml) pure maple syrup

½ cup (120 ml) virgin unrefined coconut oil, melted, or extra-virgin olive oil

Turmeric is rich in curcumin, a phytonutrient with potent antioxidant properties. In this slightly savory granola, it's paired with black pepper, which provides more than a kick. That's because the peppercorns contain piperine, an alkaloid with brain health benefits that enhances the bioavailability of curcumin. The fat in the coconut oil helps you absorb more of turmeric's antioxidant nutrients, but you could also use extra-virgin olive oil if you prefer a more savory, less coconutty, flavor.

1. Set an oven rack in the center position and preheat the oven to 350°F (180°C). Line a rimmed 18-by-13-inch (46 by 33 cm) baking sheet with parchment paper or a silicone mat.

2. Stir together the oats, cashews, hemp seeds, turmeric, pepper, and salt in a large bowl.

3. Whisk together the maple syrup and oil in a small bowl or 2-cup (480 ml) measuring cup. Pour over the oat mixture and stir until well coated. Transfer to the prepared baking sheet and smooth into an even layer (see Tip, page 272).

4. Bake for 20 minutes, then rotate the baking sheet front to back and bake for 10 to 20 minutes longer, until golden brown throughout and darker on the edges. Let cool completely in the pan, then break into clusters. Use the parchment paper as a funnel to transfer the granola into an airtight container.

5. To store, keep in an airtight container, away from heat and light, for up to 3 weeks.

continued

TIPS: *For the best clusters, spread the granola evenly atop the baking sheet and gently press with the back of a spatula. Don't stir during baking, and let cool completely in the pan before breaking into clusters with your hands.*

Buy an oven thermometer, an inexpensive gadget that can help ensure the success of your baking. Many ovens run fast or slow, which can result in a different cooking time than a recipe states and, with it, over- or undercooked food. Place the thermometer in your oven and turn it on. Compare the temperature on the thermometer to the one you set. Even a small difference of 50°F (10°C) could alter your baking time, or even worse, lead to a pan of burnt granola. If your oven is off, get it calibrated so that it's accurate or adjust the baking temperature accordingly.

WHAT ABOUT GLUTEN?

There's a lot of confusion about gluten, a family of proteins found in wheat, barley, and rye. People with celiac disease (about 1 percent of the population) become very ill when they consume gluten. Another group of people (about 4 percent) should avoid eating wheat because they have an allergy or a food sensitivity to it. If you fall into one of these categories, wheat (and barley and rye) is off the plate; going gluten-free is the recommendation.

For the remaining 95 percent of the population, whole grains—whether they contain gluten or not—are anti-inflammatory foods. What's confusing is that as many as one-third of Americans choose to be gluten-free even though they don't suffer from a gluten disorder. That's probably because there's a health halo (see page 50) that surrounds going gluten-free. Or many who suffer from undiagnosed problems stemming from their digestion assume gluten, or grains in general, are the culprit. The problem with going gluten- or grain-free (if you don't need to do so for health reasons) is that unless you are strategic about eating gluten-free whole grains, you could end up eliminating an entire food group with proven benefits for your body and your brain. And if you've cut out all grains, your gut microbiota can suffer without a steady and diverse diet of the prebiotic fiber grains provide.

Even if you have celiac disease or a wheat allergy/sensitivity, you can still enjoy many of the whole-grain recipes in this chapter. Thankfully, some of the lesser-known grains like buckwheat and Forbidden Rice are the most delicious ones and are also naturally gluten-free.

CARAMELIZED APPLE AND QUINOA PANCAKES

SERVES 4

½ cup (100 g) quinoa

¾ cup (100 g) quinoa flour

½ cup (45 g) hazelnut flour or meal

1 teaspoon baking powder

1 teaspoon baking soda

1 teaspoon ground cinnamon

1 teaspoon kosher salt

1½ cups (360 ml) unsweetened plant-based milk, homemade (page 363) or store-bought

1 egg

2 tablespoons fresh lemon juice

1 tablespoon pure maple syrup, plus more for drizzling (optional)

1 teaspoon pure vanilla extract

Extra-virgin olive oil, for the pan

2 large apples, such as Gala or Honeycrisp, thinly sliced

4 teaspoons hemp seeds

Plain, unsweetened yogurt (coconut, whole milk, or nut-based)

Stirring cooked quinoa into batter transforms pancakes into something unique and delicious. These are fluffy yet hearty with a delightfully chewy texture. Hazelnut flour enhances quinoa's nutty notes while also boosting vitamin E and adding more fiber. Both ingredients are protein rich, too, meaning they'll sustain you long after breakfast is over.

Even if the surface seems crowded, layer as many apple slices as will fit on each pancake. You can replace the apple slices with 1 cup (190 g) blueberries or 1 cup (170 g) chocolate chips.

Pancakes don't like to wait, so it's ideal to use a large griddle to cook these pancakes if you want to serve a group at once. Or use a small skillet and serve in batches.

1. If you want to serve the pancakes all together, set an oven rack in the center position and preheat the oven to 300°F (150°C).

2. Bring a medium pot of salted water to a boil and add the quinoa. Boil, uncovered, until the quinoa is fluffy and tender, about 12 minutes. Drain well. You should have about 1½ cups (215 g).

3. Meanwhile, whisk together the quinoa flour, hazelnut flour, baking powder, baking soda, cinnamon, and salt in a large bowl until no lumps remain.

4. Whisk the milk, egg, lemon juice, maple syrup, and vanilla in a medium bowl until combined. Pour over the flour mixture and fold until no streaks of flour remain. Fold in the cooked quinoa. Let the batter sit for 10 minutes.

5. Heat a griddle or large nonstick skillet over medium heat and coat with a few drops of oil. Pour in ⅓ cup (80 ml) of

the batter and arrange as many apple slices as will fit on the surface. Cook until the underside is crispy and brown and the center is set, 4 to 5 minutes. Using a rigid spatula, carefully flip the pancake and cook until golden brown on the other side and the center is dry, another 3 to 4 minutes. Serve right away or transfer to a plate and place in the oven to keep warm. Repeat with the remaining batter.

6. Serve hot, sprinkled with 1 teaspoon hemp seeds per serving, topped with a dollop of yogurt, and drizzled with maple syrup, if you like.

TIPS: *Though boiling quinoa like pasta takes only about 12 minutes, these pancakes come together in a snap with leftover cooked quinoa.*

Quinoa flour adds even more toasty quinoa flavor and is a nice addition to your whole-grain pantry. If you don't have any, though, use white whole-wheat or oat flour instead. *(See the DIY oat flour on page 132.)*

SCIENCE BITE:

QUINOA: THE TINY SEED WITH NUMEROUS BRAIN HEALTH NUTRIENTS

Quinoa has been a traditional food of people living in the high country of South America for thousands of years. Harvesting the tiny seeds is a labor-intensive process that pays off big in its unique flavor and nutrient density. Quinoa earned "superfood" status by health-conscious Westerners because it provides all nine of the essential amino acids—the building blocks of protein that must come from our diets since the human body cannot produce them.

With more fiber than other whole grains, quinoa is a boon for metabolic health. It's one of the richest food sources of flavonoids like quercetin, catechin, epigallocatechin (EGCG). Quinoa also provides brain-healthy isoflavones like daidzein and genistein (see page 230) and twenty-nine different phenol compounds that exert powerful antioxidant, antidiabetes, and anti-inflammatory actions.

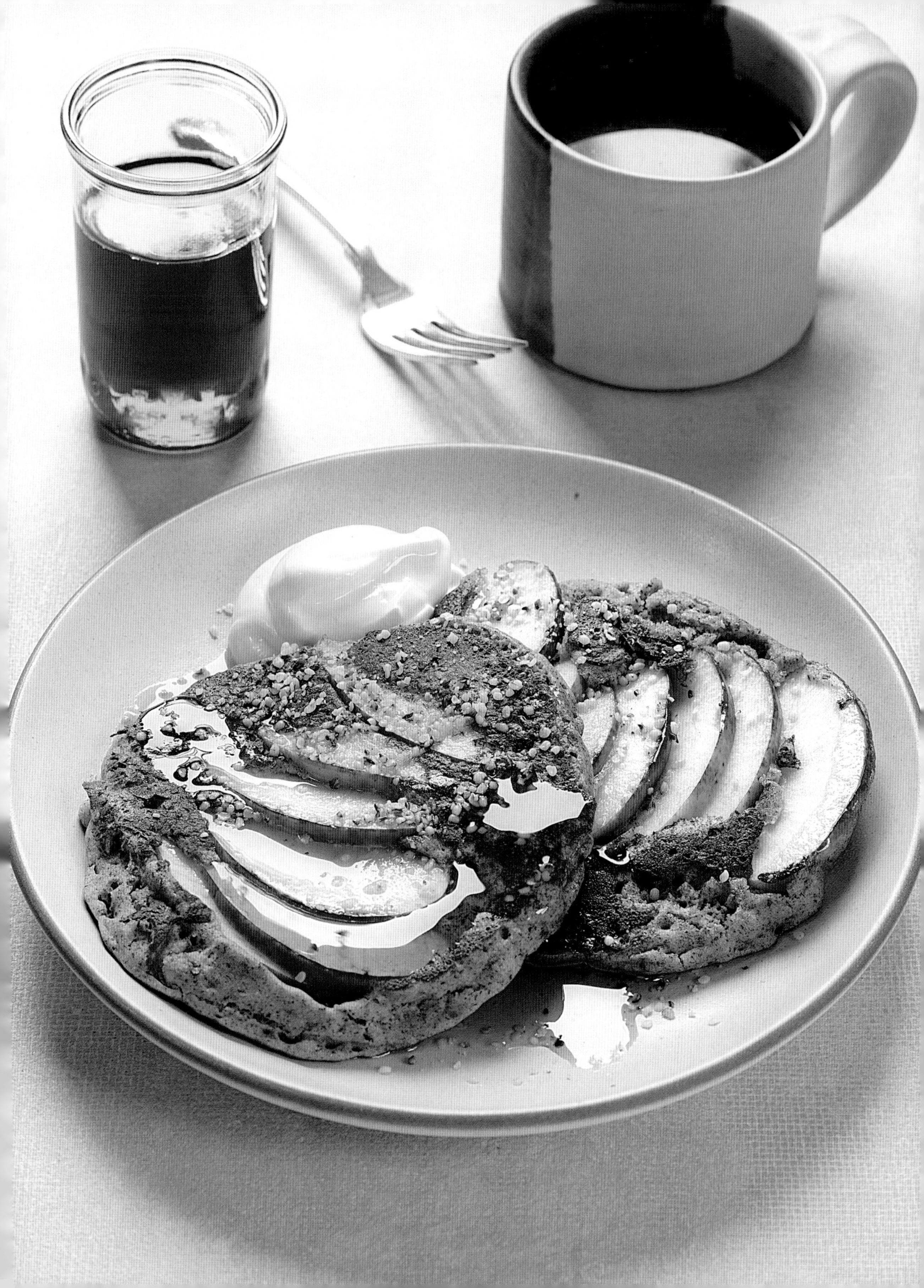

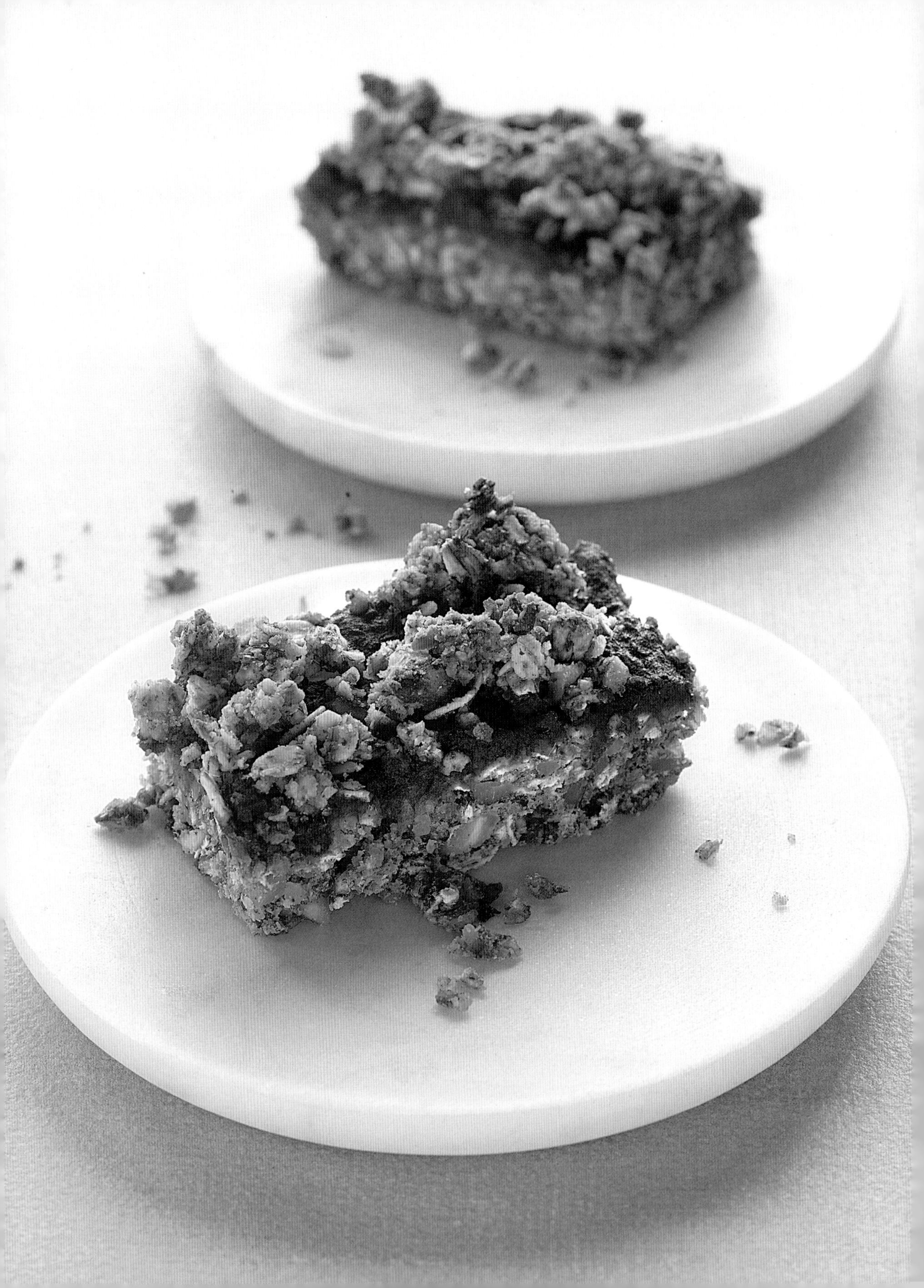

COFFEE, DATE, AND OAT BARS

MAKES 12 BARS

Extra-virgin olive oil or olive oil cooking spray, for the pan

1½ loosely packed cups (170 g) pitted dates (10 to 12 large Medjool dates), roughly chopped

1 cup (250 ml) freshly brewed coffee

1 teaspoon orange oil, flavor, or extract (see Resources, page 390)

1 cup (140 g) toasted almonds (see page 190 for toasting instructions)

2 cups (200 g) rolled oats

½ cup (60 g) almond flour or meal

1 egg

1 teaspoon kosher salt

1 cup (200 g) dried figs, stems removed and coarsely chopped

These fig-packed chewy bars are packed with brain-healthy ingredients like almonds, oats, dates, and flavonoid-rich dried figs. Thanks to this roster of fiber-rich ingredients—and a cup of fresh coffee—these decidedly grown-up bars keep you feeling satisfied all morning.

1. Set an oven rack in the center position and preheat the oven to 350°F (180°C). Line an 8-inch (20 cm) square baking pan with parchment paper so that the edges overhang, and coat with olive oil or cooking spray.

2. Place the dates, hot coffee, and orange oil in the bowl of a food processor. Let sit for 5 minutes to soften. Process on low speed until you have a mostly smooth paste, about 30 seconds. Scrape into a bowl.

3. Place the almonds in the food processor and process on low speed until coarsely chopped, about 30 seconds. Add the oats, almond flour, egg, salt, and ½ cup (150 g) of the date puree and process until the ingredients start to come together, about 30 seconds. Scrape down the sides of the bowl and process for another 30 seconds. Set aside 1 cup (215 g) of the oat mixture to use as a topping and transfer the rest to the prepared pan. Press firmly using your hands to make an even crust with an edge that comes 1 inch (2.5 cm) up the sides of the pan.

4. Spread the remaining date puree over top and smooth into an even layer. Sprinkle with the figs and the remaining oat mixture. Press the toppings firmly into the base so they adhere. Bake for 30 to 40 minutes, until the bars are golden brown on the edges and set in the center. Let cool completely before cutting into bars.

5. To store, wrap tightly and keep in the refrigerator for up to 5 days or in the freezer for up to 3 months.

TIPS: *Use large kitchen shears to snip off the stems of the figs.*

Use decaffeinated coffee if you prefer.

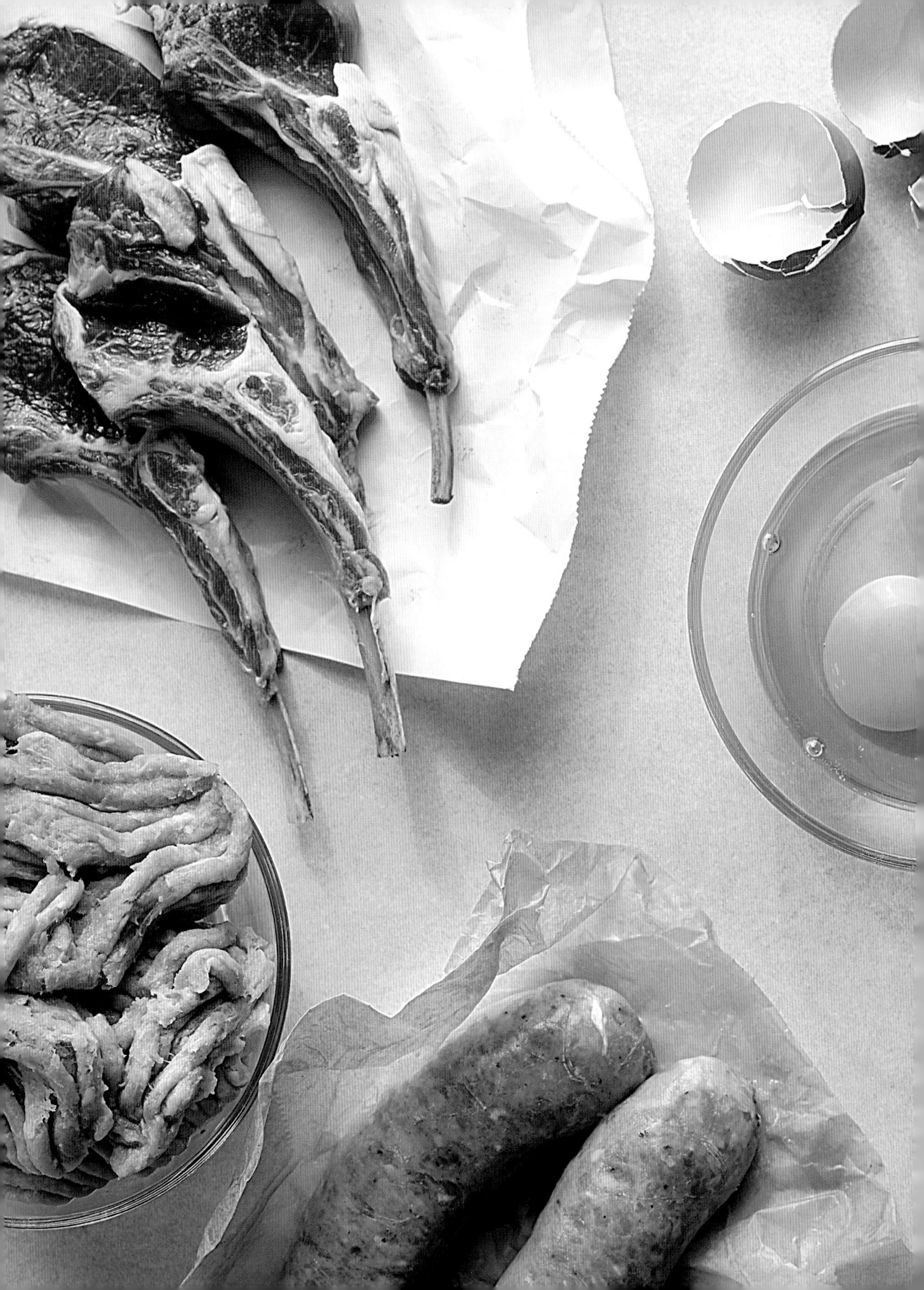

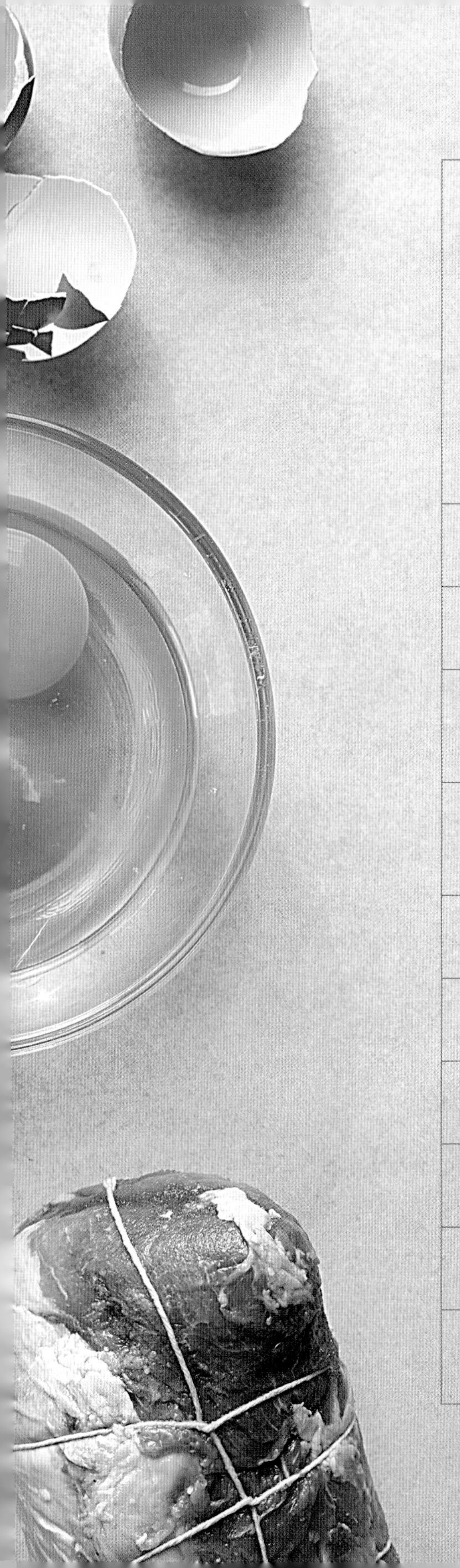

MEAT, POULTRY, AND EGGS

Brain-protective diets all have one thing in common: they are mostly plants. If you choose to eat animal products, the emphasis in this chapter and throughout the book is on quality and quantity—smaller amounts than traditionally consumed in the standard American diet. In fact, a plant-rich dietary pattern that also includes animal products turns the American way of eating upside down. Instead of making meat or chicken or eggs the focus of each meal, treat them more like a side dish, or even a condiment—adding a flourish of richness and a comforting familiarity to your meals while keeping your overall dietary pattern plant based.

Your Brain Health Mindset (page 43) will help guide you if you want to include small quantities of animal products in your cooking. First, seek out the highest-quality products that are raised sustainably and ethically. This means skipping all factory-farmed meat, poultry, and eggs. Instead, your animal products should come from grass-fed meats, ethically raised chicken and turkey, and pastured eggs from reliable sources like small, family-owned farms and farmers' markets.

Next, rethink standard portion sizes. In the traditional Mediterranean lifestyle, eating meat was viewed as a luxury item reserved for Sundays and holidays, seasonal feasting, and other special occasions. The MIND diet recommends limiting red meat to three 3-ounce (85 g) servings or less each week and eating poultry about twice a week. I recommend striving for an even more plant-based diet, keeping meat and poultry under four 3-ounce (85 g) servings each week.

Third, brain-healthy cooking methods are especially crucial when it comes to animal products. Adopting the most gentle techniques, like braising and slow cooking, will reduce saturated fat and minimize advanced glycation end products (AGEs), the brain-harmful substances created during cooking. (More on how to do that is on page 284.)

Finally, always pair meat, poultry, and eggs with an abundance of plant foods. Not only does this keep your overall dietary pattern plant based, but the plants also act as a buffer to prevent the absorption of AGEs. That's why I recommend that whenever you eat meat and poultry, especially, make sure your plate is at least three-quarters full of plant foods like leafy greens and vegetables.

EGGS

A few decades ago, eggs were vilified for their cholesterol content. For years, physicians recommended eating eggs sparingly, if at all, to reduce the risk of heart disease. That's because it was thought that the type of cholesterol in eggs led to higher harmful blood cholesterol, especially LDL. Then nutrition scientists determined that eggs contain less dietary cholesterol than previously thought. The understanding of how dietary cholesterol impacts blood cholesterol evolved as well. Now we know that the cholesterol in the foods you eat has very little effect on your blood cholesterol numbers. It's the saturated fat in your diet that contributes to a rise in harmful LDL, an important risk factor for Alzheimer's. In other words, it's not the eggs, it's the bacon that is usually served with them.

Eggs are an excellent source of protein, omega-3 fatty acids, and key brain health nutrients like B vitamins, folate, choline, and lutein. While the dietary cholesterol in eggs is not thought to be problematic for most people,

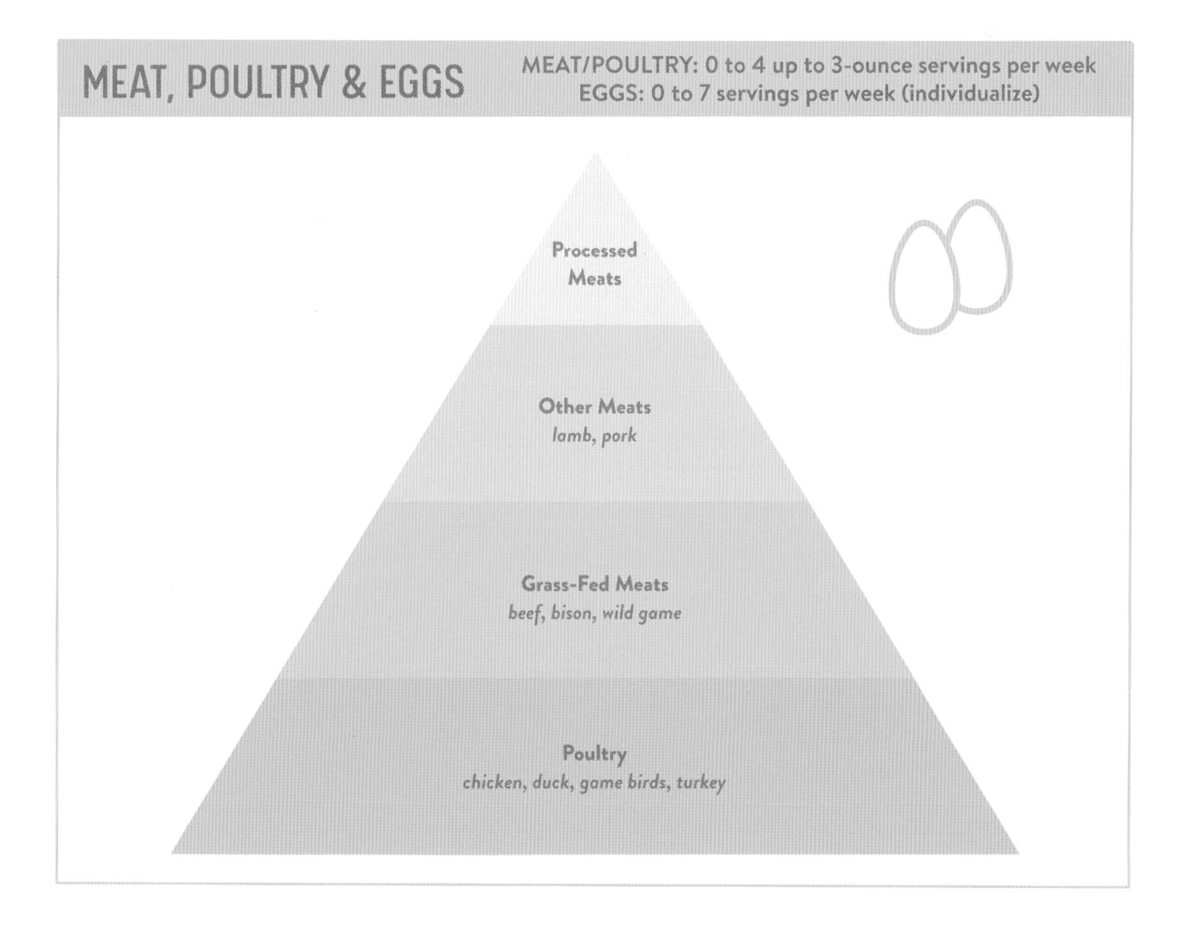

and the majority of their fat is the brain-friendly kind (monounsaturated), they do contain saturated fat (just under 2 grams per large egg).

The current American Heart Association recommendation for eating eggs is based on an analysis of more than fifty studies that have examined the relationship between dietary cholesterol, blood cholesterol, and the risk of heart disease. The consensus: healthy people can eat up to seven eggs per week without increasing the risk of heart disease. A few groups of people, however, should eat less than this: those with dyslipidemia (too much harmful and/or not enough beneficial lipids in the blood), those with diabetes, and those at risk for heart failure. Others can eat more—up to two eggs per day: vegetarians who do not consume meat-based cholesterol-containing foods, and older adults with normal cholesterol levels where the convenience and nutrition eggs provide outweigh the risks.

It may make sense for you to include eggs in your brain-protective dietary pattern within these guidelines. Pair your eggs with carotenoid-rich foods, like tomatoes, leafy greens, and vegetables. The fats from the yolk will help your body absorb more of these brain-healthy nutrients from the plants—lycopene, lutein, zeaxanthin, and beta-carotene.

Gentle cooking methods are the brain-friendliest way to cook eggs. Poaching or braising in a sauce (the method for all the Skillet Egg recipes in this chapter) is ideal. Hard-cooked eggs are fine as long as the yolk isn't overcooked. When scrambling eggs, stir constantly over low heat. Better yet, place them in a bowl over boiling water so not in direct contact with the heat. Avoid any direct and high-heat method, such as sunny-side-down fried eggs; this oxidizes the healthy fats and creates inflammatory substances. (Instead of flipping a fried egg, add a few teaspoons of water to the pan and cover to finish cooking.) The yolks should be cooked until no longer runny, or to a temperature above 160°F (70°C), to reduce the risk of contracting the intestinal pathogen salmonella. The jammy eggs in the breakfast salad (page 106) and the tuna Niçoise (page 331) achieve the sweet spot of an adequately cooked but perfectly molten yolk.

POULTRY

The Mediterranean lifestyle includes small portions of chicken and other types of poultry. Chicken is one of the ten brain-healthy food groups in the MIND diet guidelines. MIND diet researchers chose to include chicken because of promising reports that dietary sources of niacin were associated with reduced Alzheimer's risk. All types of poultry are rich sources of niacin and other B vitamins, choline, lutein, and the amino acid tryptophan—a building block of the neurotransmitter serotonin. How you cook your chicken is key here. This food can be a lean source of protein and nutrients or it can be a saturated fat disaster depending on how you prepare it. (More about this on page 284.)

RED MEAT

Assuming you're following the guidelines outlined above, there may be some advantages to eating meat—beef, lamb, pork, and game—in your brain-protective dietary pattern. Meat can be an excellent source of lean protein, for one. And it provides a good dose of B vitamins, especially vitamin B12, which is crucial for protecting nerve cells. Meat also provides iron in its most

RED MEAT AND ALZHEIMER'S RISK

When researchers try to narrow in on the relationship between eating red meat and Alzheimer's risk, studies are mixed. In a recent review of twenty-nine scientific studies, twenty-one showed no correlation between eating meat and an increased risk of Alzheimer's. Five of twenty-nine studies showed that eating meat about once a week was associated with a reduced risk of Alzheimer's, and a few showed that eating meat increased risk. When a randomized, controlled study looked at adding small servings of lean beef to a Mediterranean dietary pattern, participants had better blood lipid tests than those following a standard American diet. In other words, adding in small amounts of high-quality meat did not alter the benefits of the Mediterranean diet.

In one of the largest studies to date of more than 490,000 people in the United Kingdom, the consumption of processed meat was associated with an increased risk of dementia. Participants who ate unprocessed meat, however, such as high-quality poultry and red meat, had fewer cases of dementia, including Alzheimer's.

The takeaway from these studies is that whether or not you eat small amounts of high-quality, lean red meat may not greatly increase, or decrease, your risk of getting Alzheimer's. But consuming saturated fat, especially the most harmful kinds found in processed meats, is strongly correlated with increased risk.

bioavailable form—heme iron. A deficiency in heme iron has been associated with an increased risk of Alzheimer's. Get too much heme iron in the diet, though, and it can create harmful substances in the body.

DAIRY

Just like other animal products, you may opt to include strategic amounts of high-quality dairy in your brain-protective diet. This could be a dollop of full-fat yogurt with your granola, gut-friendly kefir in your smoothie, small cubes of feta on a salad, or a sprinkle of Parmesan cheese.

The MIND diet guidelines recommend limiting cheese intake to 1 ounce (30 g) per week and butter intake to less than 1 ounce (30 g) per day (about a pat). This may seem austere, but it's a smart strategy for long-term brain health to limit dairy products in your diet. That's because they are a major source of saturated fat in the standard American diet. In addition, processed dairy products harbor some of the highest levels of AGEs of all foods. The Mediterranean diet includes more servings of cheese each week, but traditionally these have been high-quality, unprocessed foods. In the Blue Zone of Sardinia, for example, local goat- and sheep-milk cheeses are a dietary staple and a source of gut-friendly probiotics. Throughout the Mediterranean, cheese may be served as a dessert course in small portions and rich cheeses (like a triple-creme brie) are reserved for special occasions, such as a holiday meal.

Throughout the book, dairy is used minimally to achieve a favorable balance between brain-friendly fats and saturated fats. Fortunately, there are many plant-based dairy products available at the supermarket now, as well as some easy ones you can make at home (page 363).

THE BEST WAY TO COOK MEAT AND POULTRY FOR BRAIN HEALTH

Reducing AGEs (see page 280) in your food starts before you cook. Using an acidic marinade, such as one with lemon juice, vinegar, or yogurt, for at least an hour before cooking reduces AGE formation by about half. The marinades in this chapter are triple duty: they marinate, provide a barrier to direct heat while cooking, and serve as a finishing sauce. (See the recipes for Marinated

Steak on page 299 and Sheet-Pan Lamb Chops on page 305.)

The best way to cook meat and poultry is "low and slow": braising, stewing, slow roasting, slow cooking, or over the indirect heat of a grill. Sous vide is the ultimate low-and-slow method; the food is placed in a vacuum-sealed bag and immersed in a bath of circulating warm water. Microwaving does not raise AGEs to the same extent as other high-heat cooking methods, as long as the cooking time is brief (about 6 minutes or less). In the Wild Rice, White Bean, and Turkey Soup recipe (page 289), you'll employ a gentle braising technique to enhance the flavor and texture of these lean ground meats while draining off most of the fat. You'll use this same technique to lock in flavor while reducing fat in the chicken sausage skillet eggs (page 308) and the bison chili (page 302).

All foods, especially meat and poultry, rack up AGEs if cooked with high and dry methods, such as frying, high-heat grilling, searing, broiling, and high-heat roasting. If the food is also slathered with a sugary sauce, such as barbecue sauce, honey, or marmalade, AGE levels skyrocket.

AVOID PROCESSED MEATS FOR MAXIMUM BRAIN HEALTH

Processed meat is a large category of meat best avoided in your neuroprotective diet. The World Health Organization's definition of processed meat is: "meat that has been transformed through salting, curing, fermentation, smoking, or other processes to enhance flavor or improve preservation." This includes bacon, cured ham, smoked and canned meat, hot dogs, sausages, salami, lunch meats, and beef jerky. These meats are high in saturated and trans fats as well as sodium, and they rack up AGEs during processing. Does this mean never enjoying a piece of bacon ever again? The occasional piece of bacon is not likely to change the outcome of how your brain ages. However, if you eat bacon many days of the week, it becomes a part of your dietary pattern, working against all the other brain-healthy efforts you may make.

SHEET-PAN CHICKEN COBB WITH KEFIR-AVOCADO DRESSING

SERVES 4 TO 6

- **¾ pound (340 g) fingerling potatoes, sliced lengthwise**
- **4 plum tomatoes (12 ounces/340 g total), cut in half lengthwise**
- **2 tablespoons extra-virgin olive oil**
- **1 teaspoon kosher salt**
- **¼ teaspoon freshly ground black pepper, plus more for serving**
- **1 pound (455 g) boneless, skinless chicken thighs**
- **¾ cup (180 ml) plain, unsweetened kefir**
- **1 loosely packed cup (20 g) fresh flat-leaf parsley leaves**
- **1 small avocado (4 ounces/115 g)**
- **1 tablespoon fresh lemon juice**
- **1 small garlic clove**
- **Up to ¼ cup (60 ml) water (optional)**
- **10 cups (355 g) romaine lettuce, hearts cut into 2-inch (5 cm) pieces, leaves torn**
- **2 ounces (60 g) feta cheese, cut into 1-inch (2.5 cm) cubes (about ½ cup)**
- **4 hard-cooked eggs (page 282), sliced lengthwise**
- **Flaky salt (optional)**

Most Cobb salads include sliced avocados, but for this one you'll blend ripe avocado with kefir for a buttermilk-like herbaceous dressing packed with gut-friendly probiotics. For the optimal Cobb experience, get a mix of the contrasting textures and flavors in each bite—crispy, creamy, salty, and tangy on top of crunchy chilled romaine.

1. Set an oven rack in the center position and preheat the oven to 400°F (200°C). Line a rimmed baking sheet with parchment paper.

2. Toss the potatoes and tomatoes on the prepared baking sheet with the oil, ¼ teaspoon of the kosher salt, and the pepper. Separate the two veggies so the potatoes sit on one half of the sheet, cut side down, and the tomatoes are on the other, cut side up. Nestle the chicken pieces between the vegetables, drizzle with the remaining 1 tablespoon oil, and sprinkle with ¼ teaspoon of the kosher salt. Roast for 25 to 30 minutes, until the tomatoes collapse, you can easily insert a fork in the potatoes, and the chicken is cooked through (an instant-read thermometer should register 165°F/75°C when inserted in the thickest part of the chicken).

3. Meanwhile, place the kefir, parsley, avocado, lemon juice, garlic, and the remaining ½ teaspoon kosher salt in a blender. Blend on high speed until completely smooth, adding more water, if needed, to loosen.

4. When the chicken has cooled, slice ½ inch (1.25 cm) thick.

5. Toss the lettuce and half the dressing in a shallow bowl. Top with the chicken, tomatoes, feta, eggs, and potatoes. Drizzle with more dressing and finish with flaky salt, if using.

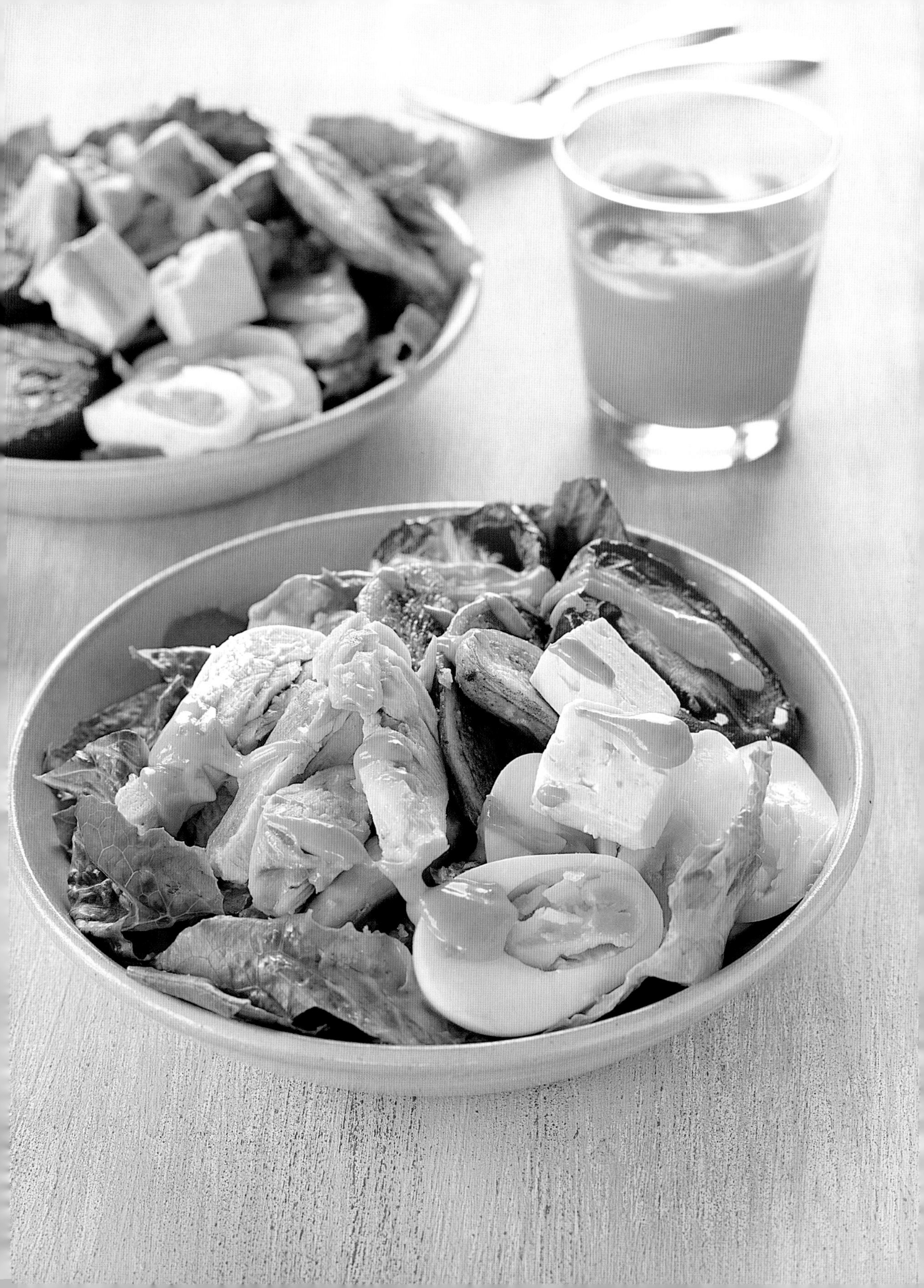

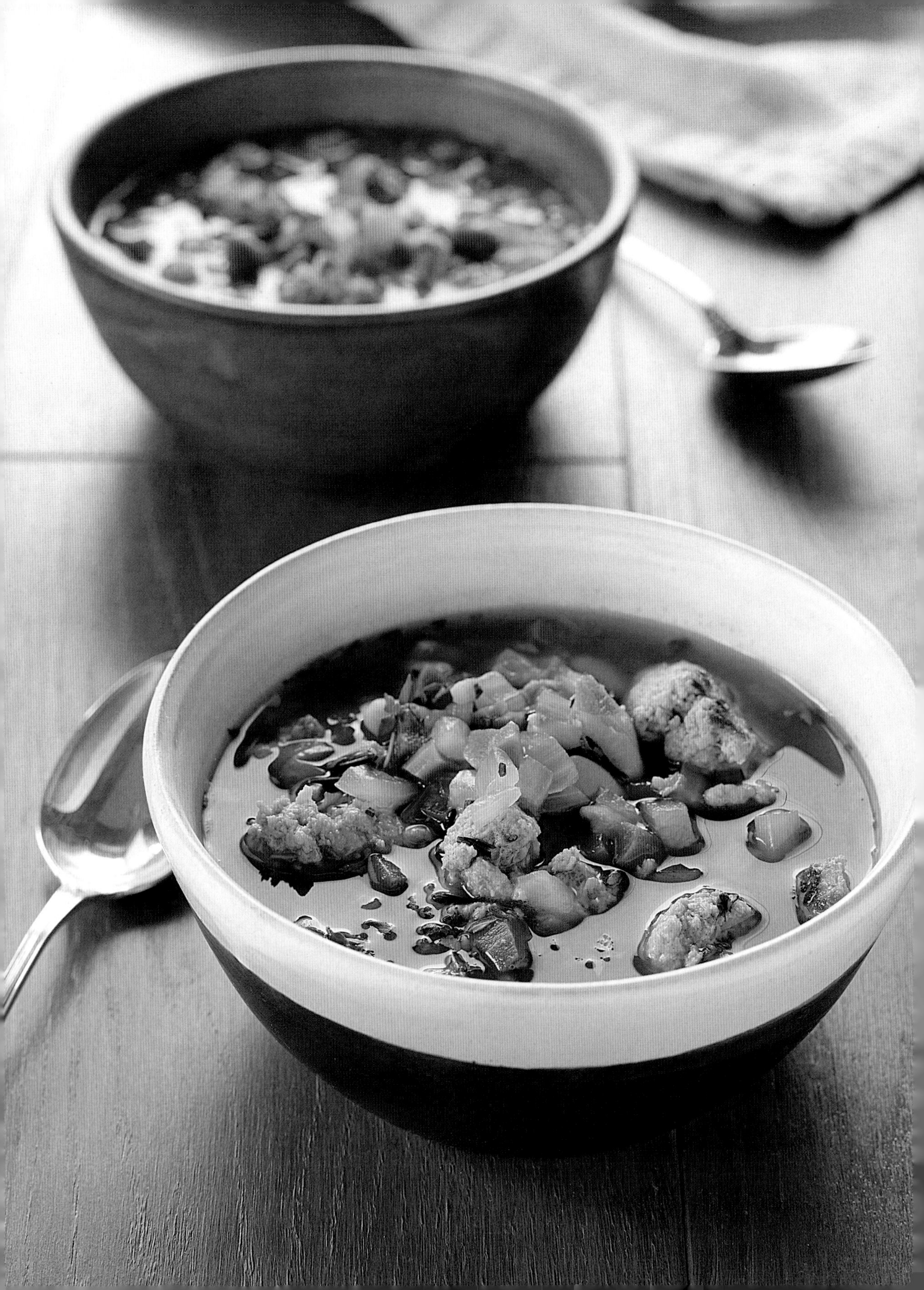

WILD RICE, WHITE BEAN, AND TURKEY SOUP

SERVES 6 TO 8

- **1 pound (455 g) 98 percent lean ground turkey**
- **½ cup (120 ml) water**
- **¾ teaspoon kosher salt**
- **¾ teaspoon freshly ground black pepper, plus more for serving**
- **2 tablespoons extra-virgin olive oil**
- **1 large yellow onion (12 ounces/340 g), finely chopped (about 2 cups)**
- **3 medium carrots (12 ounces/340g total), scrubbed and finely chopped (about 1½ cups)**
- **4 celery stalks (7 ounces/ 200 g total), finely chopped (about 1 cup)**
- **¾ cup (180 ml) dry white wine**
- **8 cups (2 L) chicken or vegetable stock, homemade (page 374) or low-sodium store-bought**
- **½ cup (100 g) uncooked wild rice**
- **1 tablespoon finely chopped fresh rosemary leaves**
- **1 tablespoon finely chopped fresh sage leaves**
- **1 tablespoon finely chopped fresh thyme leaves, plus more for serving**
- **1 to 2 tablespoons low-sodium soy sauce or tamari**
- **1½ cups (265 g) cooked white beans (page 215) or one 15-ounce (425 g) can, drained**

Brothy, substantial, and delicious—this is the soup for cold nights and cozy evenings. Gently braising the ground turkey in water and salt not only keeps the lean meat tender and flavorful, it's also best for brain health.

As with any soup, the flavor will depend on the stock you use. Homemade stock (page 374) is richer and more flavorful than store-bought, but in a pinch, a carton of low-sodium stock works, too. Season to taste with the soy sauce and don't skimp on the fresh herbs.

1. Combine the turkey, water, ¼ teaspoon of the salt, and ¼ teaspoon of the pepper in a large heavy-bottomed pot over medium heat. Cook, stirring often, until the meat is broken into clusters and no longer pink, 3 to 5 minutes. Using a slotted spoon, transfer the turkey to a bowl.

2. Into the same pot add the oil, onion, carrots, celery, and remaining ½ teaspoon salt and cook until soft, 5 to 7 minutes. Add the wine and cook until the liquid has evaporated, 3 to 5 minutes. Stir in the stock, rice, rosemary, sage, and thyme. Bring to a boil over high heat and reduce to a gentle simmer. Stir in 1 tablespoon of the soy sauce and cook, stirring occasionally, until the rice is tender, 45 to 55 minutes.

3. Stir in the beans and turkey and continue cooking over a gentle simmer until the beans are hot, about 10 minutes longer. Taste; add another tablespoon of soy sauce, if you like.

4. To serve, ladle the soup into shallow bowls and finish with more pepper and thyme.

TIP: *When shopping for herbs, look for a package that includes a mix of "poultry" herbs including rosemary, sage, thyme, and parsley, then sprinkle chopped parsley on the finished dish.*

GRILLED CHICKEN WITH ANCHOVY BUTTER, BROCCOLINI, AND TOMATO BREAD

SERVES 4

4 tablespoons (60 g) unsalted butter, preferably grass-fed, at room temperature

4 anchovy fillets, preferably packed in olive oil, finely chopped (about 1 heaping teaspoon)

1 large garlic clove, minced (about 1 teaspoon)

1 tablespoon fresh lemon juice

½ loosely packed cup (10 g) fresh flat-leaf parsley leaves, finely chopped, plus more for serving

2 large boneless, skinless chicken breasts (1¼ pounds/570 g total), cut horizontally, leaving a 1-inch (2.5 cm) edge attached as a hinge

2 tablespoons extra-virgin olive oil

½ teaspoon kosher salt

¼ teaspoon freshly ground black pepper

1 bunch broccolini (6 ounces/170 g)

Crusty whole-grain bread, cut into 1-inch (2.5 cm) slices

1 large tomato (7 ounces/200 g), chopped

Flaky salt (optional)

All too often, healthy eating advice boils down to "eat a chicken breast with some veggies." This recipe reinvents that combination. You'll stuff the chicken with an omega-3-rich anchovy butter and pair with Broccolini and a quick pan con tomate to soak up the juices. The result is a dinner that stays within the brain-healthy range of about 4 ounces (115 g) of chicken per portion.

1. Preheat a grill to medium-high with a rack 4 to 6 inches (10 to 15 cm) from the heat source. Alternatively, use a grill pan.

2. Mash together the butter, anchovies, garlic, and lemon juice in a small bowl until smooth. Fold in the parsley until evenly distributed.

3. Open the chicken breasts like a book and smear one side of each piece with 1 tablespoon of the anchovy butter. (You should have about half the anchovy butter remaining; chill in the fridge until you are ready to serve.) Close the chicken back up, brush both sides with 1 teaspoon of the oil, and sprinkle with ¼ teaspoon of the kosher salt and the pepper.

4. Toss the broccolini with 2 teaspoons of the oil and sprinkle with the remaining ¼ teaspoon kosher salt. Place the broccolini on one side of the grill and the chicken on the other. Grill the broccolini until it is crisp-tender and charred in some spots, 5 to 7 minutes. Grill the chicken until golden on one side, 5 to 7 minutes. Flip the chicken over and grill on the other side, about 5 minutes, or until an instant-read thermometer registers 165°F (75°C) in the thickest portion. Let the chicken rest for 5 minutes, then divide each breast into two pieces.

continued

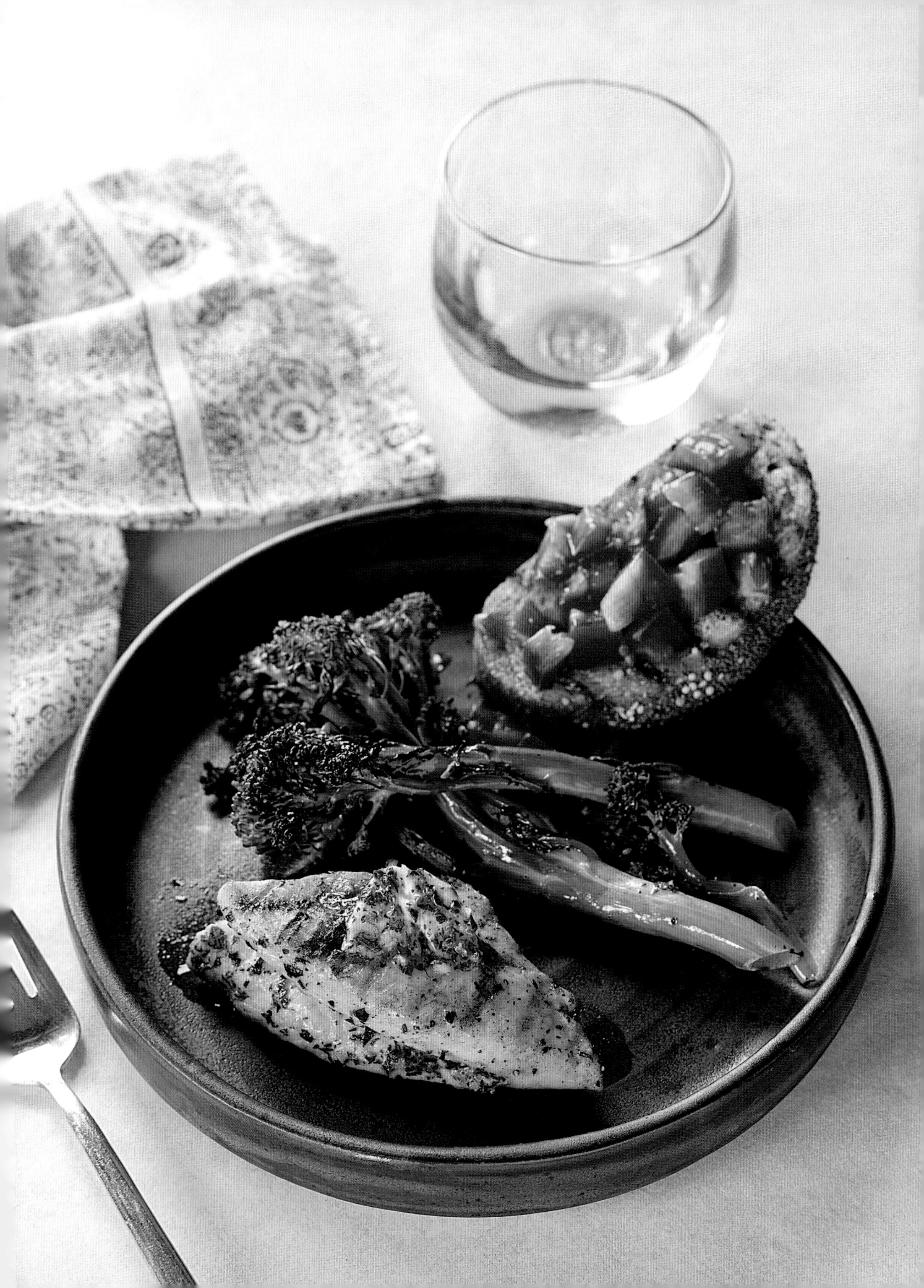

5. Place the bread on the least hot part of the grill and watch closely to toast it without burning, turning halfway through, 3 to 4 minutes total. Drizzle with the remaining 1 tablespoon oil.

6. To serve, divide the chicken between plates with the broccolini. Top each piece of chicken with some of the remaining anchovy butter and spoon the chopped tomato onto the bread. Finish with flaky salt, if you like.

TIPS: *If using a grill pan to cook the chicken on the stove, steam the broccolini instead. Place a steamer basket inside a large pot that has a lid and fill with 2 inches (5 cm) of water. Bring to a boil and add the broccolini; steam until crisp-tender, 4 to 5 minutes. Let sit in the steamer basket with the lid off to cool slightly.*

Double the anchovy butter and store the rest in the fridge for up to 2 weeks or the freezer for up to 3 months. Dab it on fish and seafood (like grilled scallops or cod), fold into warm grain bowls, and stir into pasta with vegetables.

BRAIN-HEALTHY GRILLING TIPS

Cooking meat and poultry on the grill doesn't have to be a recipe for AGEs (see page 280). This process may look a little different from the way you are used to grilling, but the results will be both delicious and better for you.

- Keep your grill sparkling clean (no char clinging to the grates) and oil before each use.
- Avoid grilling too close to the heat source. Grill baskets and wood planks can protect meat from the heat.
- Grilling with hardwood chips will make it easier to cook meat at a lower temperature.
- Create a high-heat zone and a low-heat zone on your grill. Place the meat in the low zone so it cooks by indirect heat.
- Avoid grill marks; those black char lines harbor high concentrations of AGEs. Grill marks also contain heterocyclic amines (HCAs), substances long considered carcinogenic.
- Don't slather your meat with sugary sauces; use a dry rub instead to infuse flavor with spices while providing a barrier between the surface of the meat and the heat source.
- Serve grilled meats with an abundance of plants—a green salad, plenty of fresh herbs, and cruciferous vegetables.

SUMAC-SPICED CHICKEN WITH APPLES AND CURRANT-PISTACHIO RICE PILAF

SERVES 4 TO 6

One 3½- to 4-pound (1.6 to 1.8 kg) roasting chicken, patted dry with paper towels

2 teaspoons kosher salt

½ teaspoon freshly ground black pepper

2 tablespoons ghee, at room temperature, or extra-virgin olive oil

2 tablespoons sumac

4 large baking apples (1½ pounds/680 g total), such as Honeycrisp, Jonagold, or Fuji, cored and cut into ½-inch (1.25 cm) wedges

1 large yellow onion (12 ounces/340 g), cut into ¼-inch (6 mm) rounds, 2 tablespoons finely chopped and set aside

1 cup (240 ml) water

1 tablespoon lemon zest (from 1 large lemon)

¼ cup (60 ml) fresh lemon juice

1 teaspoon ground cardamom

1 tablespoon extra-virgin olive oil

1½ cups (300 g) long-grain brown rice, rinsed

1 quart (1 L) chicken stock, homemade (page 376) or store-bought

continued

Slow roasting is a brain-friendly cooking technique that is mostly hands-off, not to mention it creates the tenderest meat. After a quick dry rub to draw moisture from the meat, you'll brush the skin with ghee—aka clarified butter—and sprinkle it with tart sumac—a flavonoid-packed spice (page 57)—for an elegant take on classic roast chicken. Using a low temperature means the chicken creates fewer AGEs (see page 280) as it roasts and allows all the juices to drip onto the bed of apples and onions. You'll pair these with a Persian-inspired rice pilaf, studded with pistachios, pomegranate seeds, and herbs. Though rice is called for here, you can doctor up already cooked grains, like farro or quinoa, for quicker prep.

1. Rub the chicken all over with 1 teaspoon of the salt and the pepper. Place on a wire rack set over a plate or baking dish. Refrigerate, uncovered, for at least 4 hours and up to overnight.

2. When ready to cook, set an oven rack in the lower position and preheat the oven to 300°F (150°C). Using paper towels, pat the chicken dry, rubbing off any excess salt. Brush the surface of the chicken with the ghee and rub in 1 tablespoon of the sumac.

3. In the bottom of a 9-by-13-inch (23 by 33 cm) baking dish, combine the apples, onion slices, water, 2 teaspoons of the lemon zest, the lemon juice, cardamom, remaining 1 tablespoon sumac, and ½ teaspoon of the salt. Nestle the chicken, breast side down, into the apple mixture. Bake on the lower rack for 2½ to 3 hours, basting the chicken every

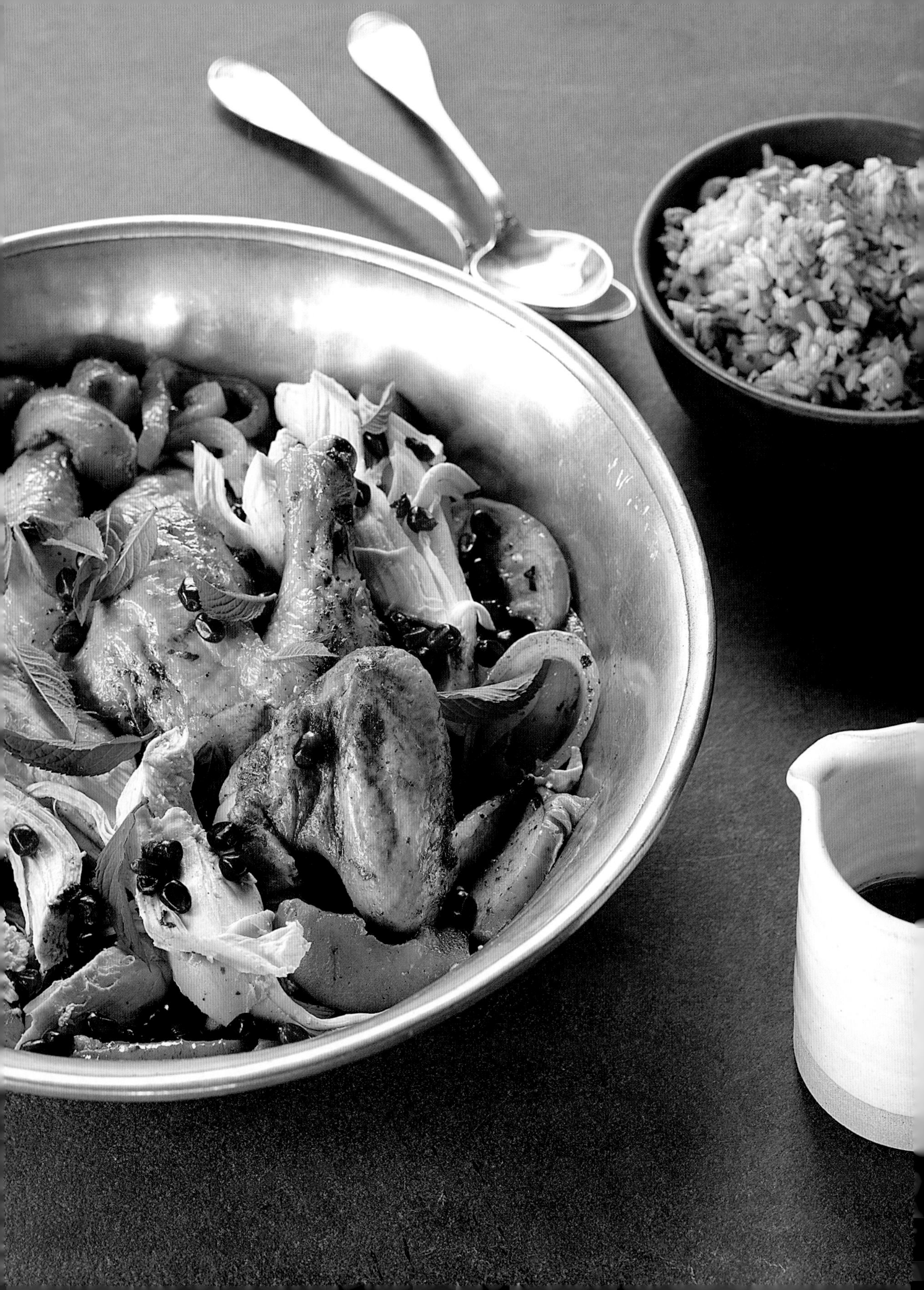

- ½ cup (80 g) dried currants, golden raisins, or raisins
- Pomegranate seeds
- Fresh mint leaves
- 1 cup (100 g) toasted pistachios (see page 190 for toasting instructions)
- 1 loosely packed cup (20 g) fresh flat-leaf parsley leaves, finely chopped

hour with the pan juices, until the skin is a deep reddish brown and the meat is starting to fall off the bones (an instant-read thermometer should register 165°F/75°C in the thickest part of the thigh).

4. An hour before you plan to eat, make the pilaf. Warm the oil in a large saucepan or Dutch oven with a tight-fitting lid over medium heat. Add the 2 tablespoons chopped onions and cook, stirring often, until soft, about 5 minutes. Add the rice and stir to coat the grains. Stir in the stock, currants, and the remaining ½ teaspoon salt. Bring to a gentle simmer, then reduce the heat to low. Cover and cook, undisturbed, until the grains are tender and most of the liquid has been absorbed, 35 to 45 minutes. Cover and set aside.

5. When the chicken is done, transfer it to a cutting board, cover with foil, and let sit for 10 minutes to rest. Meanwhile, use a slotted spoon to transfer the apples and onions to a large shallow serving bowl, then pour off any pan juices into a small pitcher. Carve the chicken (or just pull the meat apart, saving the bones to make stock) and pile the meat in the center of the bowl atop the apples. Sprinkle with pomegranate seeds and mint leaves.

6. Fluff the rice with a fork and stir in the pistachios and parsley. Divide the chicken, apples, onions, and rice pilaf between plates, drizzle with pan juices, and finish with the remaining 2 teaspoons lemon zest and more pepper, if you like.

TIP: *Use the leftover chicken bones to make stock (page 376).*

WHOLE-WHEAT SPAGHETTI WITH TURKEY-ZUCCHINI MEATBALLS

SERVES 4 TO 6

2 medium zucchini (7 ounces/200 g each), one spiralized, the other grated (about 1¼ cups) and squeezed dry

1 teaspoon kosher salt

1 pound (455 g) ground turkey, 93% to 98% lean

½ cup (45 g) whole-grain breadcrumbs

¼ cup (30 g) Walnut "Parm" (page 184) or freshly grated Parmesan cheese, plus more for serving

1 egg

¼ teaspoon crushed red pepper flakes

1 tablespoon extra-virgin olive oil or olive oil cooking spray

½ pound (225 g) whole-wheat spaghetti (see Resources, page 390)

1 quart (1 L) marinara sauce, homemade (page 379) or from a jar (see Resources, page 390)

½ cup (10 g) fresh basil leaves, larger leaves torn, smaller ones left whole

The nostalgic elements of spaghetti and meatballs are all here in this brain-healthy twist on the comfort-food staple, from the tangle of pasta in garlicky tomato sauce to the tender meatballs. Folding in grated zucchini to stretch the meat further and using Walnut "Parm" rather than cheese make for a wonderfully light meatball that's lower in saturated fat. Tossing spirals of zucchini with the spaghetti is a delicious and colorful way to add an extra dose of vegetables to your plate.

1. Set an oven rack in the center position and preheat the oven to 375°F (190°C). Line a rimmed baking sheet with parchment paper.

2. Place the spiralized zucchini in a colander and sprinkle evenly with ¼ teaspoon of the salt. Toss and set aside in the sink to drain.

3. Combine the grated zucchini, turkey, breadcrumbs, "Parm," egg, red pepper flakes, and ½ teaspoon of the salt in a large bowl. Using wet hands, gently toss together until all the ingredients are uniformly distributed. Shape into 2-inch (5 cm) meatballs (about 2 ounces/60 g each), pressing firmly so they hold together. You should have about fifteen meatballs. Place the meatballs on the baking sheet and brush or spray with the oil. Bake for 20 to 25 minutes, until golden.

4. Meanwhile, bring a large pot of salted water to a boil over high heat. Add the pasta, stirring as the water comes back to a boil, and cook until almost cooked through, about 1 to 2 minutes less than the package directions. Drain the pasta in the colander with the zucchini. Toss gently; set aside.

TIP: *If you don't have a spiralizer, use store-bought zucchini noodles (about 2 cups/200 g) and pat dry before using, or increase the pasta to ¾ pound (340 g) total. If using Parmesan cheese instead of Walnut "Parm," add 1 teaspoon minced garlic to the meatball mix.*

5. Return the pot to the stove and add the marinara sauce. Warm over medium heat until bubbling. Reduce the heat to a low simmer and gently slide the meatballs into the sauce, stirring until all are evenly coated. Cook with the lid ajar, stirring occasionally to make sure nothing sticks to the bottom of the pot, until the meatballs are hot and an instant-read thermometer registers 165°F (75°C) when inserted into the center, 2 to 3 minutes.

6. Using tongs, add the pasta and zucchini noodles to the sauce and toss gently to coat. Cook over medium-low heat until the sauce coats the pasta and the pasta is tender and slightly chewy, 1 to 2 minutes.

7. Divide the pasta and meatballs between shallow bowls and sprinkle with the basil leaves and more "Parm," if you like.

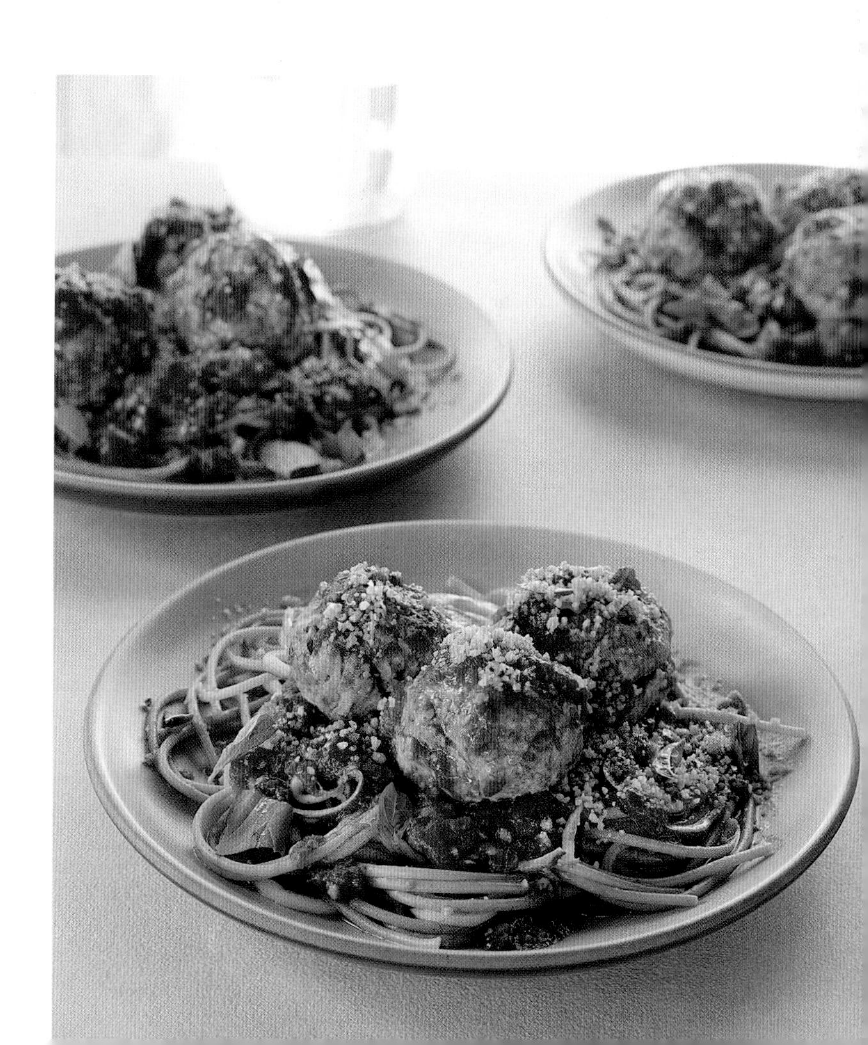

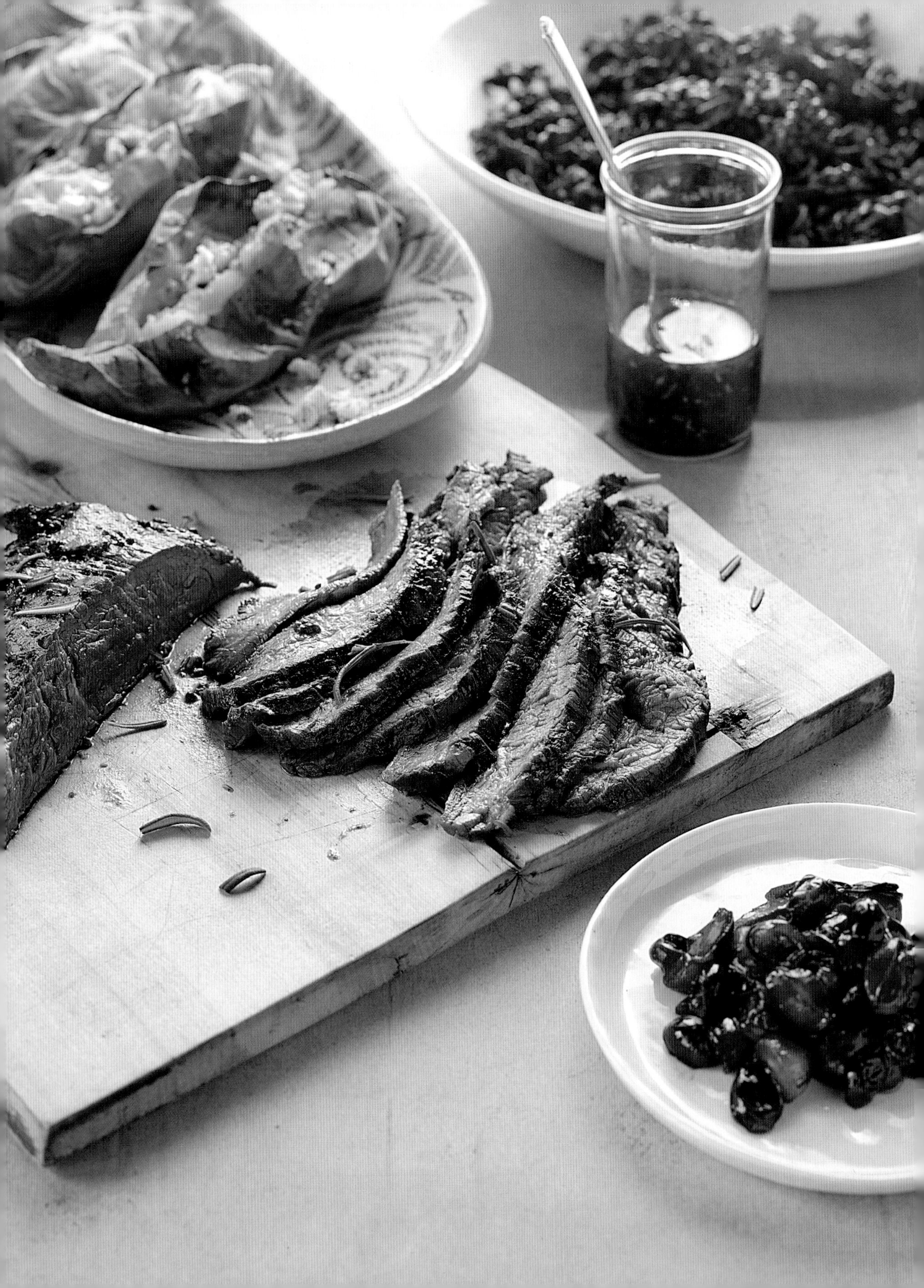

MARINATED STEAK WITH WARM KALE SALAD AND SWEET POTATOES

SERVES 4

⅓ cup (80 ml) balsamic vinegar

1 tablespoon whole-grain mustard

2 large garlic cloves, minced (about 2 teaspoons)

1 tablespoon fresh rosemary, finely chopped

1½ teaspoons kosher salt

½ teaspoon freshly ground black pepper

¼ cup plus 1 tablespoon (65 ml) extra-virgin olive oil

¾ pound (340 g) skirt or flank steak, trimmed of visible fat, preferably grass-fed

4 long and skinny sweet potatoes (1¾ pounds/790 g total), scrubbed and patted dry

1 bunch lacinato kale (aka Tuscan or dinosaur kale) (6 ounces/170 g), leaves thinly sliced (about 4 cups)

6 ounces (170 g) seedless black or red grapes, halved lengthwise (about 1 cup)

2 ounces (60 g) blue cheese, crumbled

Flaky salt (optional)

Yes, you can eat steak and prioritize brain health. Step 1: Start with high-quality meat (preferably 100 percent grass-fed). Step 2: Marinate before you cook, a technique that reduces formation of advanced glycation end products (AGEs; see page 280). Step 3: Grill it over indirect heat. Step 4: Serve with an abundance of vegetables. A good rule of thumb is to fill your plate three-quarters full of fiber-rich plants, like the kale salad and sweet potatoes here. Not only is this a delicious pairing, but vegetables blunt the absorption of AGEs and saturated fat from the meat.

1. Whisk together the vinegar, mustard, garlic, rosemary, ½ teaspoon of the kosher salt, and ¼ teaspoon of the pepper in a small bowl. Keep whisking while you slowly add ¼ cup (60 ml) of the oil until fully incorporated. Measure out ¼ cup (60 ml) to use as a dressing; set aside. Place the steak in a glass or ceramic dish and pour the remaining marinade over top. Flip the steak to coat, cover tightly, and refrigerate for at least 4 hours and up to overnight.

2. An hour before you plan to eat, set an oven rack in the center position and preheat the oven to 400°F (200°C). Line a rimmed baking sheet with parchment paper.

3. Use a fork to poke holes on all sides of each sweet potato and place on the prepared baking sheet. Rub each potato all over with 1 teaspoon of the oil and sprinkle them all with ¼ teaspoon of the kosher salt. Bake for 45 to 50 minutes, then turn the potatoes over and push them to one side of the pan. Put the kale and grapes on the other side, drizzle with the remaining 2 teaspoons oil, and sprinkle with ¼ teaspoon

of the kosher salt. Toss well and spread in an even layer on the pan. Bake for 5 to 10 minutes longer, until the grapes have collapsed, the kale is wilted, and you can easily insert a knife into the center of the potatoes.

4. Meanwhile, heat a grill to medium-high (375°F/190°C) with a rack 4 to 6 inches (10 to 15 cm) from the heat source; alternatively, get out a grill pan. Remove the steak from the marinade and let the excess drip off. Discard the marinade. Sprinkle the steak with the remaining ½ teaspoon salt and ¼ teaspoon pepper. Grill the steak until browned, 5 to 7 minutes. Flip and cook on the other side for another 2 minutes for rare or 3 minutes for medium-rare. Transfer the steak to a cutting board, tent with foil, and let rest for 5 minutes.

5. Split each sweet potato down the middle and sprinkle each one with 1 teaspoon blue cheese crumbles; divide between the plates. Thinly slice the steak and divide between the plates with the kale and grapes. Drizzle the reserved ¼ cup (60 ml) dressing over the steak and kale, dividing evenly, and sprinkle with flaky salt (if using) and more pepper, if you like.

SHOPPING SMART: ANIMAL PRODUCTS

EGGS. At the supermarket, you'll be bombarded with meaningless marketing buzzwords on the carton: *natural*, *hormone-free*, *antibiotic-free*, *cage-free*, *vegetarian-fed*, *farm-fresh*, and *free-range*, to name a few. Ignore all of those terms. Instead, look for organic eggs from chickens that are pastured (allowed to forage), often indicated by a Certified Humane Raised & Handled logo or an Animal Welfare Approved seal. Expect to pay a bit more (an additional few dollars per carton) for these eggs to ensure the farms you support treat their animals with the highest ethical standards. If you have access to eggs from a local farm or neighbor with a small flock, these are almost always the best choice.

CHICKEN AND OTHER POULTRY. Seek out the highest-quality product available. Just as with eggs, ignore meaningless marketing terms like *free-range* and instead look for organic birds that are pastured and display the Certified Humane or Animal Welfare Approved seal. Expect to pay more for birds from farms with high ethical standards. If purchasing poultry at the farmers' market, be sure to ask the farmer what the birds eat; a diverse diet of natural forage, kitchen scraps, and non-GMO feed (sometimes boosted with omega-3 fatty acids) is ideal.

BEEF, PORK, AND LAMB. Shopping for beef, pork, and lamb requires your most stealth supermarket skills. Most of the meat at the grocery store comes from factory farms where animals are kept in close quarters, given antibiotics to hasten growth, and fed what's akin to a junk-food diet. Skip all industrially produced meats and seek out reliable indicators of high standards: USDA Organic, Animal Welfare Approved, American Grassfed, and Certified Humane stamps or seals. Natural beef, pork, and lamb are raised without antibiotics or hormones. *Organic* is a good indicator of antibiotic- and hormone-free meat from animals who have good living standards. If you buy from local ranchers, be aware that they may be raising animals organically, even though they can't afford the official USDA stamp.

If you can, choose 100 percent grass-fed beef: When cows are fed only grass, without corn or other types of feed, the meat retains a higher concentration of alpha-linolenic acid (ALA), a type of omega-3 fatty acid from the grass. This gives the meat a higher ratio of anti-inflammatory omega-3s to pro-inflammatory omega-6s. Grass-fed cows also have a superior quality of life compared to those clustered in the concentrated animal feeding operations (CAFOs) of factory farms. Seek out small, family-owned ranchers as close as possible to where you live who raise their animals in traditional, more planet-friendly methods.

BISON AND BLACK BEAN-CACAO CHILI

SERVES 4 TO 6

1 pound (455 g) ground bison or grass-fed beef

1½ cups (360 ml) water

2 teaspoons kosher salt

1 tablespoon extra-virgin olive oil

1 large yellow onion (12 ounces/340 g), chopped (about 2 cups)

2 large poblano peppers (10 ounces/285 g total), seeded and chopped (about 2 cups)

3 large garlic cloves, minced (about 1 tablespoon)

1 tablespoon chipotle chiles in adobo, finely chopped, plus 1 tablespoon adobo sauce

1½ teaspoons ground coriander

1½ teaspoons ground cumin

Two 28-ounce (800 g) cans crushed tomatoes

1½ cups (250 g) cooked black beans, homemade (page 215) or one 15-ounce (425 g) can, drained

2 tablespoons natural cacao powder

Almost Instant Cashew Cream (page 370) or plain, unsweetened yogurt

Fresh cilantro leaves, torn, and tender stems, finely chopped

Quick-Pickled Pomegranate Red Onions (page 383) or store-bought (optional)

Ground bison is low in fat and big on flavor, making it a good choice for this brain-healthy chili packed with fresh poblanos, roasted chipotles, and your favorite beans. Adding cacao powder to a savory dish has been a part of Mexican cooking traditions since ancient times. The cacao accentuates its savory flavors while providing flavonoid compounds with antioxidant properties. The result is a deeply flavorful bowl of chili that's ready in about an hour.

Braising the meat in water and salt is a brain-friendly cooking method that gently cooks it without browning, minimizing the production of advanced glycation end products (AGEs, page 280). The fat dissolves into the water, making it easy to pour off, while keeping the lean meat from drying out.

Load up this chili with toppings, keeping them in the brain-healthy camp. Serving the chili with whole grains, such as quinoa or brown rice, makes this a hearty meal.

1. Combine the meat and ½ cup (120 ml) of the water in a large pot or Dutch oven over medium heat. Sprinkle with ½ teaspoon of the salt and cook, breaking the meat up with a wooden spoon until it is in small crumbles and no longer pink, 6 to 8 minutes. Use a slotted spoon to transfer the meat to a bowl. Carefully pour off the liquid into a heatproof container; set aside to discard when cool.

2. Using the same pan, warm the oil over medium heat, then add the onion, poblanos, and remaining 1½ teaspoons salt. Cook over medium-high heat until the onions are soft, 5 to 7 minutes. Add the garlic, chipotles and sauce, coriander, and cumin and cook until fragrant, about 1 minute.

3. Stir in the cooked meat and tomatoes and bring to a lively simmer over high heat. Reduce the heat to a gentle simmer, cover with the lid ajar, and cook, stirring occasionally to

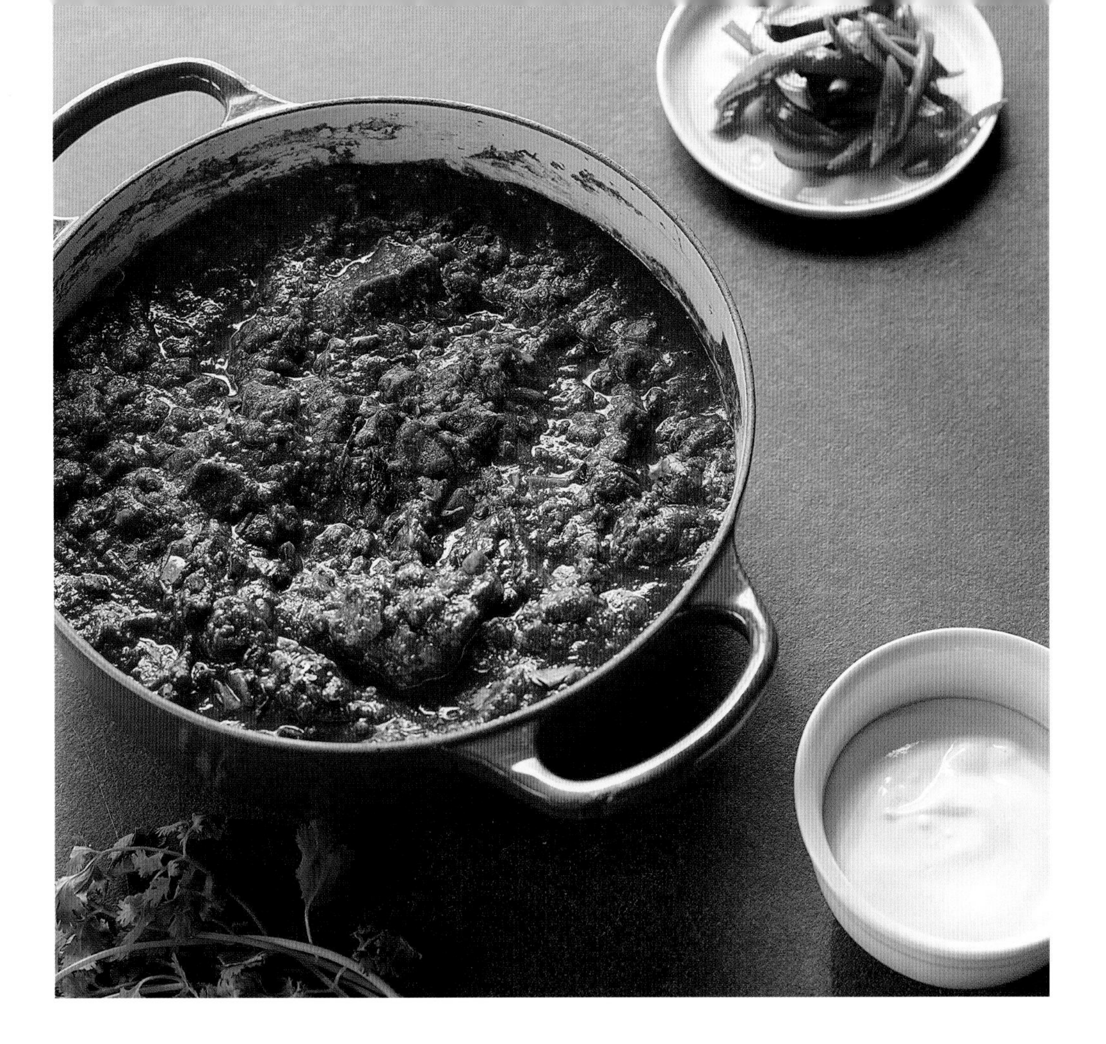

make sure nothing sticks to the bottom of the pot, for 45 to 50 minutes. Stir in the beans, cacao powder, and, if the chili seems too thick, up to 1 cup (240 ml) of the remaining water or some bean stock. Cook for 15 to 20 minutes longer, until the chili is warmed through.

4. Serve topped with cashew cream, cilantro, and pickled onions (if using).

INSTANT POT METHOD

1. Combine the bison, ½ cup (120 ml) of the water, and ½ teaspoon of the salt in the multicooker and push the Sauté button. Use a wooden spoon to break up the meat into smaller

TIP: *Try this with freshly cooked beans using the method on page 215. An heirloom variety of black or red beans, such as Pinquitos, Rio Zapes, or Vaqueros, works well.*

pieces and cook, stirring occasionally until the meat is no longer pink. Use a slotted spoon to transfer the meat to a bowl. Carefully pour off the liquid into a heatproof container; set aside to discard when cool.

2. Combine the bison, oil, onion, poblanos, garlic, chipotles and sauce, coriander, cumin, tomatoes, beans, and 1 teaspoon of the salt in the multicooker. Push the Chili/Bean button or use the High Pressure button, and set the time manually for 22 minutes. Let the pressure release naturally before removing the lid.

3. Push the Sauté button, stir in the cacao powder, and, if the chili seems too thick, up to 1 cup (240 ml) of water or some bean stock. Cook, stirring occasionally, for 15 to 20 minutes longer, until the chili is bubbling gently.

WHY BRAIN-HEALTHY EATING IS ALSO PLANET FRIENDLY

Each time you make a brain-healthy food choice, chances are you are helping to protect the health of the planet, too. That's because eating for brain health means choosing an abundance of resource-savvy foods, like whole grains, legumes and beans, and vegetables. As you bulk up on these plant foods, you weed out many of the inflammatory foods that are not only bad for your brain but contribute greatly to the destruction of the ecosystem, which drives climate change. The more plant-based your diet becomes, the less likely your food choices will take a toll on the health of the planet.

If you do eat animal products, opt out of the industrially produced meat system. Not only are factory farms flooding our food supply with unhealthful meat while raising animals in horrific conditions, they've also become breeding grounds for a new generation of virulent bacteria. Emerging from the guts of animals given subtherapeutic doses of antibiotics, these bugs make it difficult for physicians to treat foodborne illnesses. Consuming only animal products from small producers who practice regenerative agriculture—farming and grazing practices that restore biodiversity and give back to the soil and the land—will help align your health goals with that of the planet's.

SHEET-PAN LAMB CHOPS WITH ASPARAGUS, LEMON, AND PEAS

SERVES 4 TO 6

2 cups (480 ml) plain, unsweetened yogurt (coconut, whole milk, or nut-based)

¼ cup (60 ml) fresh lemon juice

1 large garlic clove, minced (about 1 teaspoon)

2 tablespoons extra-virgin olive oil

1½ teaspoons kosher salt

¾ teaspoon freshly ground black pepper

Six 3-ounce (85 g) lamb loin chops, each about 1½ inches (4 cm) thick

1 pound (455 g) thin asparagus, trimmed

1 small bunch radishes (6 ounces/170 g), quartered

1 small, thin-skinned lemon, thinly sliced and seeds removed, if needed (see Tip)

2 cups (290 g) peas, fresh or frozen

1 cup (15 g) fresh mint leaves, roughly chopped, plus a few leaves for serving

Flaky salt (optional)

This colorful one-pan supper is the essence of spring—yogurt-marinated lamb chops are nestled into asparagus, radishes, peas, and rounds of lemon for a quick roast. The radishes lose their peppery bite and the lemon shifts from tart to caramelized. Roasting asparagus is best for brain health because the spears retain their powerful array of phytonutrients, which can seep out into the water when boiling or steaming.

The garlicky yogurt does double duty in this recipe. Half is for finishing the dish, while the rest acts as a marinade for the lamb chops. Note that regular (not Greek-style) yogurt is the key here so that the marinade easily comes off the chops before roasting.

Because the marinade takes time to work its magic on the chops, it's best to plan to get the prep going at least an hour before you want to eat.

1. Stir together the yogurt, lemon juice, garlic, 1 tablespoon of the oil, ½ teaspoon of the kosher salt, and ¼ teaspoon of the pepper in a large bowl. Set aside half the sauce (in an airtight container in the fridge) to top the finished dish.

2. Pat the lamb dry with paper towels and place in the bowl with the yogurt sauce, flipping them over with tongs to coat. Cover the bowl and marinate in the fridge for at least 1 hour and up to 4 hours.

3. When you are ready to cook, set an oven rack in the center position and preheat the oven to 400°F (200°C). Line a rimmed baking sheet with parchment paper.

4. Place the asparagus, radishes, and lemon together on the prepared pan. Drizzle with the remaining 1 tablespoon oil and

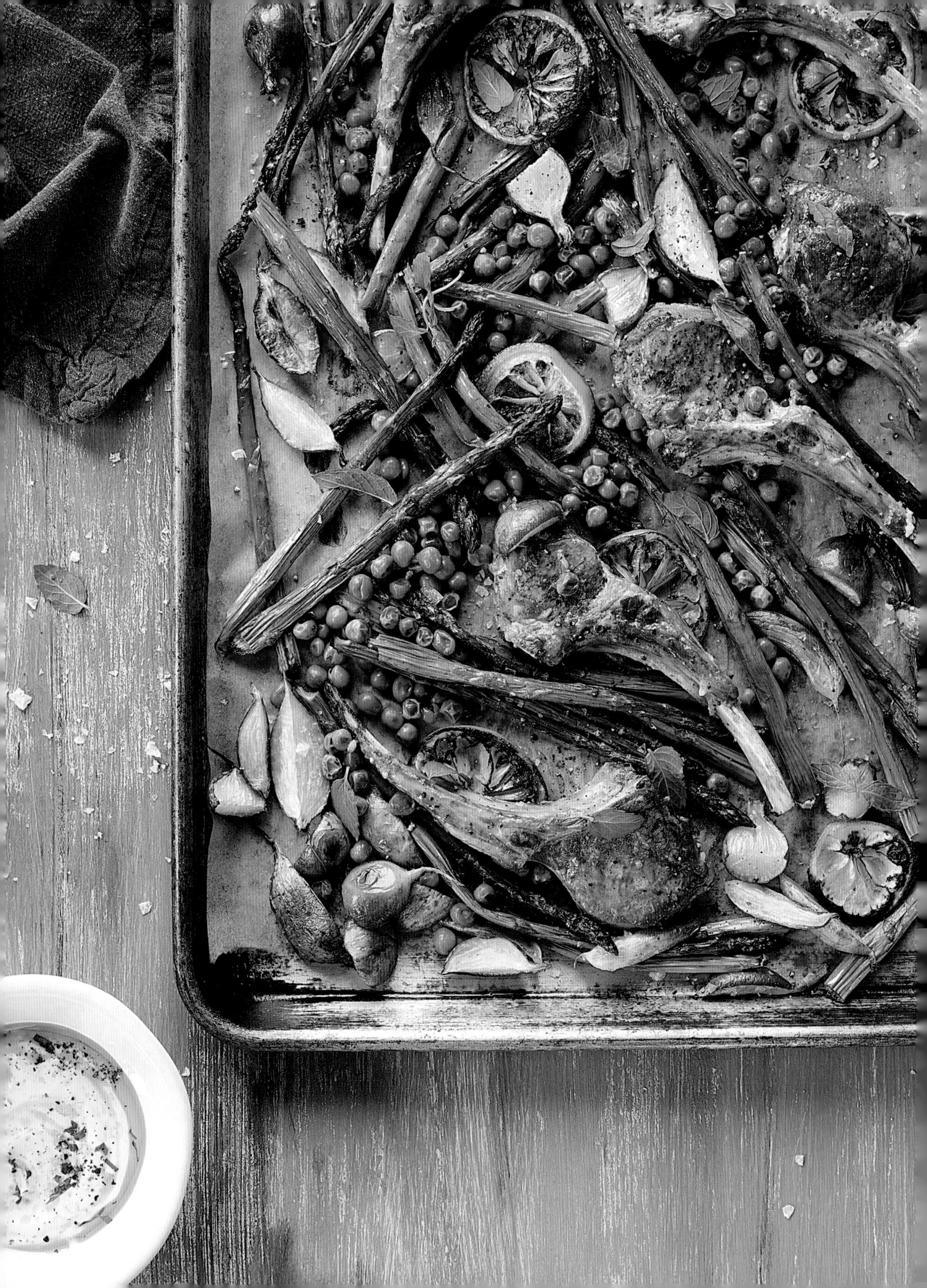

TIPS: *Since you'll eat the lemon rind in this dish, it's worth buying organic. Seedless Eureka and Meyer lemons are good choices because there won't be any seeds to pick out.*

Lamb loin chops are a leaner cut than lamb rib chops and require less cooking time. An added bonus: most loin chops are just the right size (3 ounces/85 g) to keep your serving size within Brain Health Kitchen guidelines. Lamb rib chops will also work in this recipe, but you may need to adjust the cooking time up or down depending on their size.

sprinkle with ½ teaspoon of the kosher salt. Toss to coat and spread evenly over the pan.

5. Using tongs, lift the lamb chops from their marinade and let any excess drip off. Blot dry with paper towels and season on both sides with the remaining ½ teaspoon kosher salt and pepper. Evenly space the chops on the sheet pan, wedging them between the vegetables and lemons. Discard the marinade.

6. Roast for 8 to 10 minutes, then flip the chops and scatter the peas over the pan. Cook for 3 minutes longer for rare or 5 minutes for medium-rare. (If using an instant-read thermometer, the lamb chops are done when the internal temperature reaches 120°F/50°C for rare and 125°F/52°C for medium-rare.)

7. Meanwhile, stir the chopped mint into the reserved yogurt sauce. Serve the lamb and vegetables topped with a dollop of sauce. Sprinkle with mint leaves and flaky salt (if using), and more pepper, if you like.

SCIENCE BITE:

ASPARAGUS IS A BRAIN-PROTECTIVE FOOD

The pairing of asparagus and lamb chops in this recipe is more than a classic spring combo—the folate in asparagus and the vitamin B12 found in high-quality meat are both essential for healthy brain aging. In a study from Tufts University, older adults with robust levels of both folate and B12 performed better on a test of response speed and mental flexibility.

Asparagus is also an excellent source of glutathione, a potent antioxidant that combats oxidative stress in the brain. Thanks to the amino acid asparagine, asparagus acts like a natural diuretic, which serves to lower blood pressure and enhance cardiovascular health.

Asparagus may even have specific anti-Alzheimer's activity. When asparagus is metabolized by the body, it breaks down into sarsasapogenin, a nutrient of interest to Alzheimer's researchers due to its neuroprotective actions, like blocking amyloid formation and the enzyme acetylcholinesterase.

ITALIAN PEPPERS AND CHICKEN SAUSAGE SKILLET EGGS

SERVES 4

½ pound (225 g) bulk mild Italian chicken or turkey sausage

½ cup (120 ml) water

1 small yellow onion (8 ounces/230 g), thinly sliced

2 large orange, red, or yellow bell peppers (12 ounces/340 g total), thinly sliced

½ teaspoon dried oregano

¼ teaspoon crushed red pepper flakes

¼ teaspoon kosher salt

½ cup (120 ml) chicken stock, vegetable stock, or water

4 to 8 eggs

¼ loosely packed cup (5 g) fresh flat-leaf parsley leaves, finely chopped

Freshly ground black pepper (optional)

Look for Italian sausage made from chicken or turkey, which is lower in saturated fat than pork sausage. Avoid precooked sausage. Use any combination of brightly colored sweet peppers you like.

1. Combine the sausage and ¼ cup (60 ml) of the water in a large skillet over medium-high heat. Cook, stirring often, until the sausage is no longer pink and starting to brown, 5 to 7 minutes. Transfer the meat with a slotted spoon to a bowl. Carefully pour off all but 1 teaspoon of the fat in the pan into a heatproof container to discard once cool.

2. Using the same skillet, add the onion, bell peppers, oregano, red pepper flakes, salt, and remaining ¼ cup (60 ml) water. Cook, stirring often, until the vegetables are soft, 5 to 7 minutes. Stir in the stock and sausage and cook until the liquid bubbles gently, about 2 minutes.

3. Use a spoon to make a well in the sauce and crack an egg into it. Repeat with as many eggs as you want to cook and that your skillet allows. Cover and cook over low heat for 7 to 10 minutes, depending on how you like your eggs: about 7 minutes for runny, 8 for jammy, or up to 10 minutes for a fully cooked yolk.

4. When the eggs are done, sprinkle with the parsley. Scoop out some of the sauce and an egg or two into each bowl and finish with black pepper, if you like.

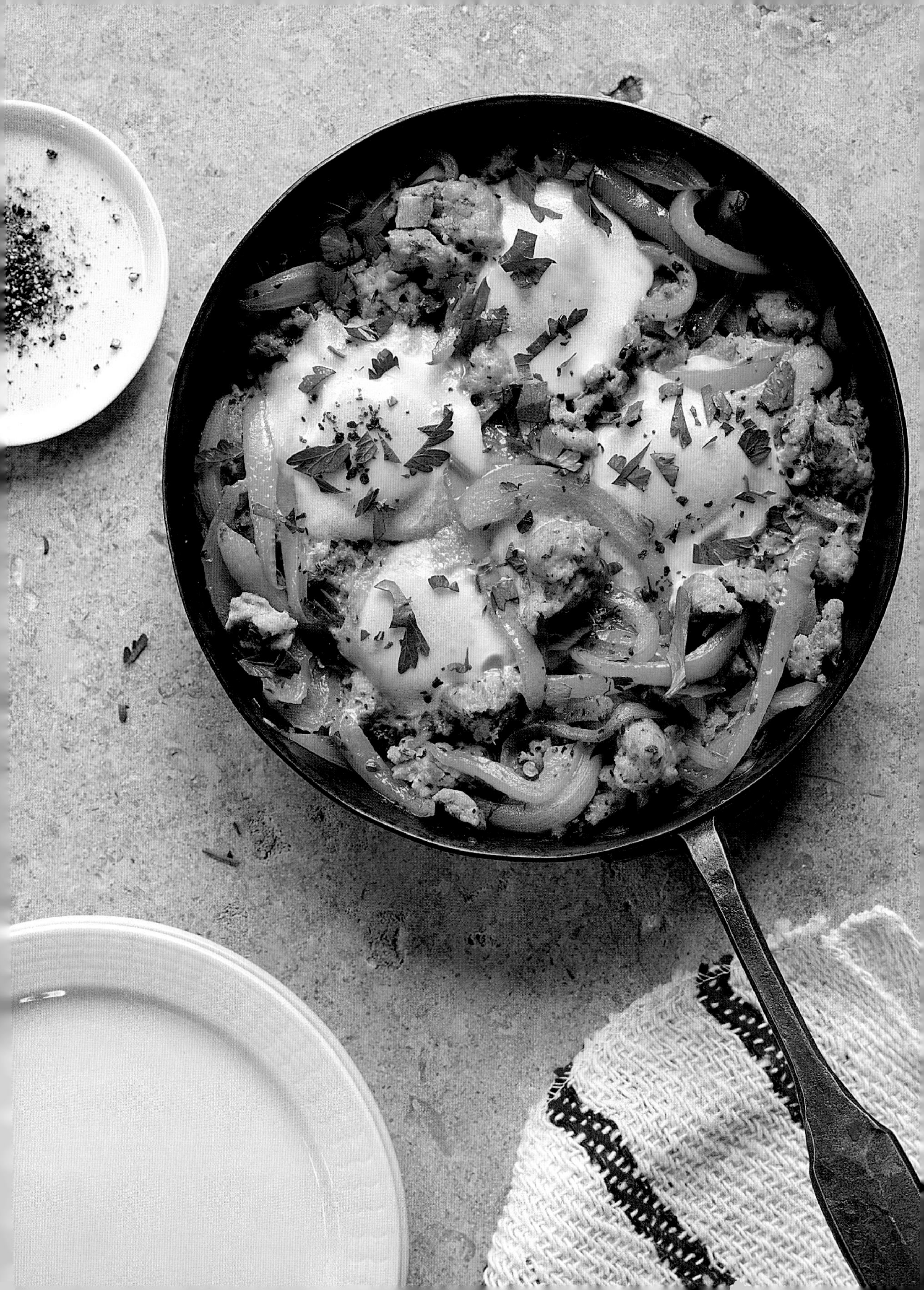

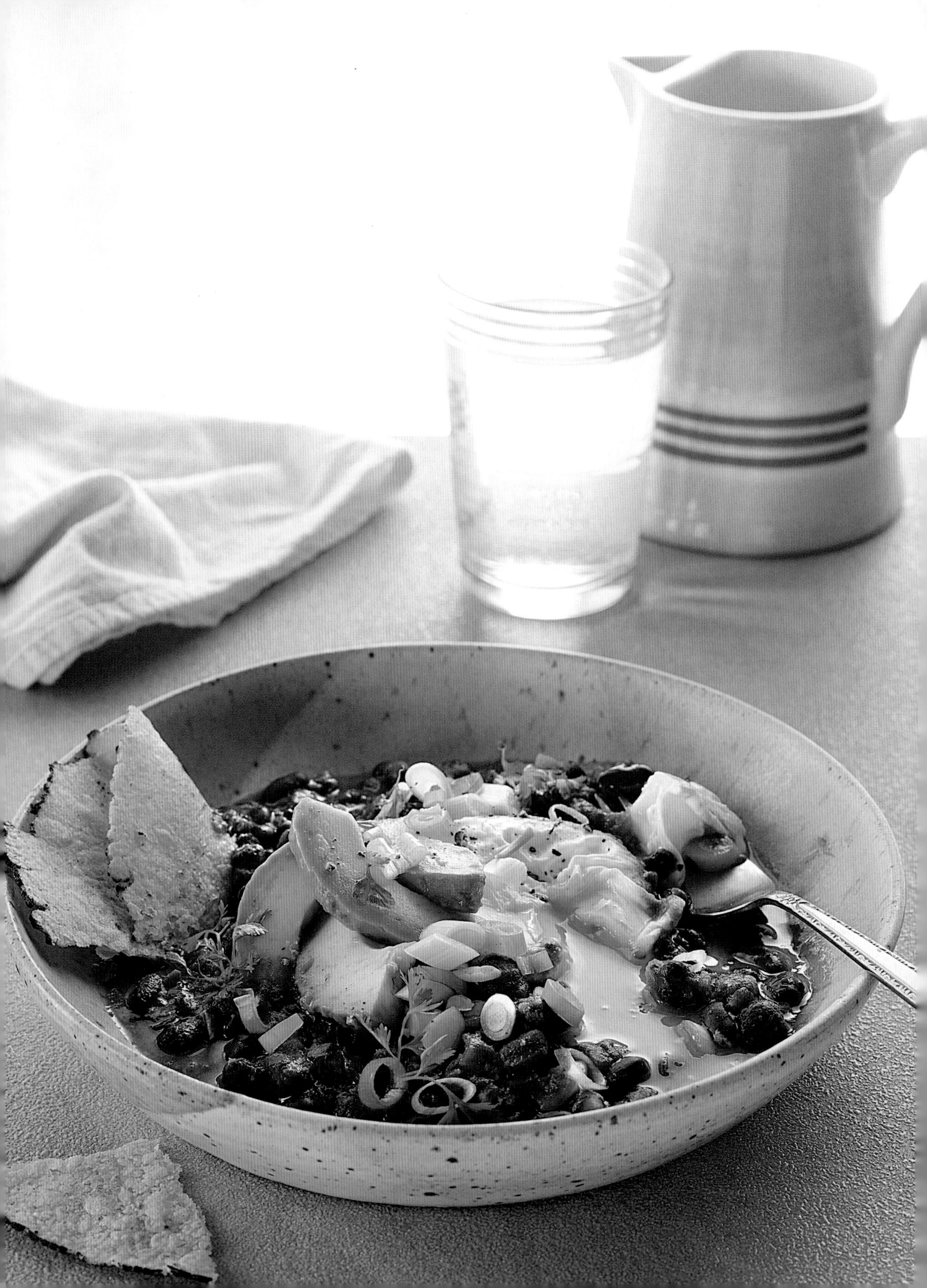

SALSA-POACHED EGGS WITH BLACK BEANS

SERVES 2 TO 4

3 cups (480 g) cooked black beans (page 215) or two 15-ounce (425 g) cans, rinsed

1½ cups (360 ml) jarred salsa, made from red or green chiles (or a mix), mild, medium, or hot

1 cup (240 ml) unsweetened, unflavored nut milk (such as almond, cashew, macadamia, pecan, or other) or water or stock

½ teaspoon kosher salt

4 to 8 eggs

1 avocado, sliced

1 scallion, white and green parts finely chopped (optional)

¼ cup (40 g) fresh cilantro leaves and tender stems, coarsely chopped (optional)

Freshly ground black pepper

Corn tortillas, warmed

This skillet egg dish takes inspiration from the classic Mexican-American dish huevos rancheros. Black beans are a brain-healthier swap for most refried beans, which are often cooked in saturated fat–laden lard. The combination of a good jar of salsa (which provides lycopene, capsaicin, and carotenoids) and a nut milk creates a creamy, nicely spiced sauce that comes together in minutes.

The great thing about skillet eggs is their flexibility. Use this recipe as a jumping-off point for the brain-healthy ingredients you have on hand—leftover roasted vegetables, a pot of your favorite beans, or handfuls of darky leafy greens. This recipe allows you to choose one or two eggs per serving to emphasize the plant-rich accompaniments rather than the eggs.

1. Combine the beans, salsa, nut milk, and salt in a large skillet over medium heat. Bring to a gentle simmer and cook, stirring often, until the mixture starts to thicken slightly, about 10 minutes.

2. Use a spoon to make a well in the sauce and crack an egg into it. Repeat with as many eggs as you want to cook. Cover and cook over low heat for 7 to 10 minutes, depending on how you like your eggs: about 7 minutes for runny, 8 for jammy, or up to 10 minutes for a fully cooked yolk.

3. To serve, scoop out some of the sauce and an egg or two into each bowl. Top with avocado slices and scatter with the scallions and cilantro, if using, then finish with pepper. Serve with warm tortillas on the side.

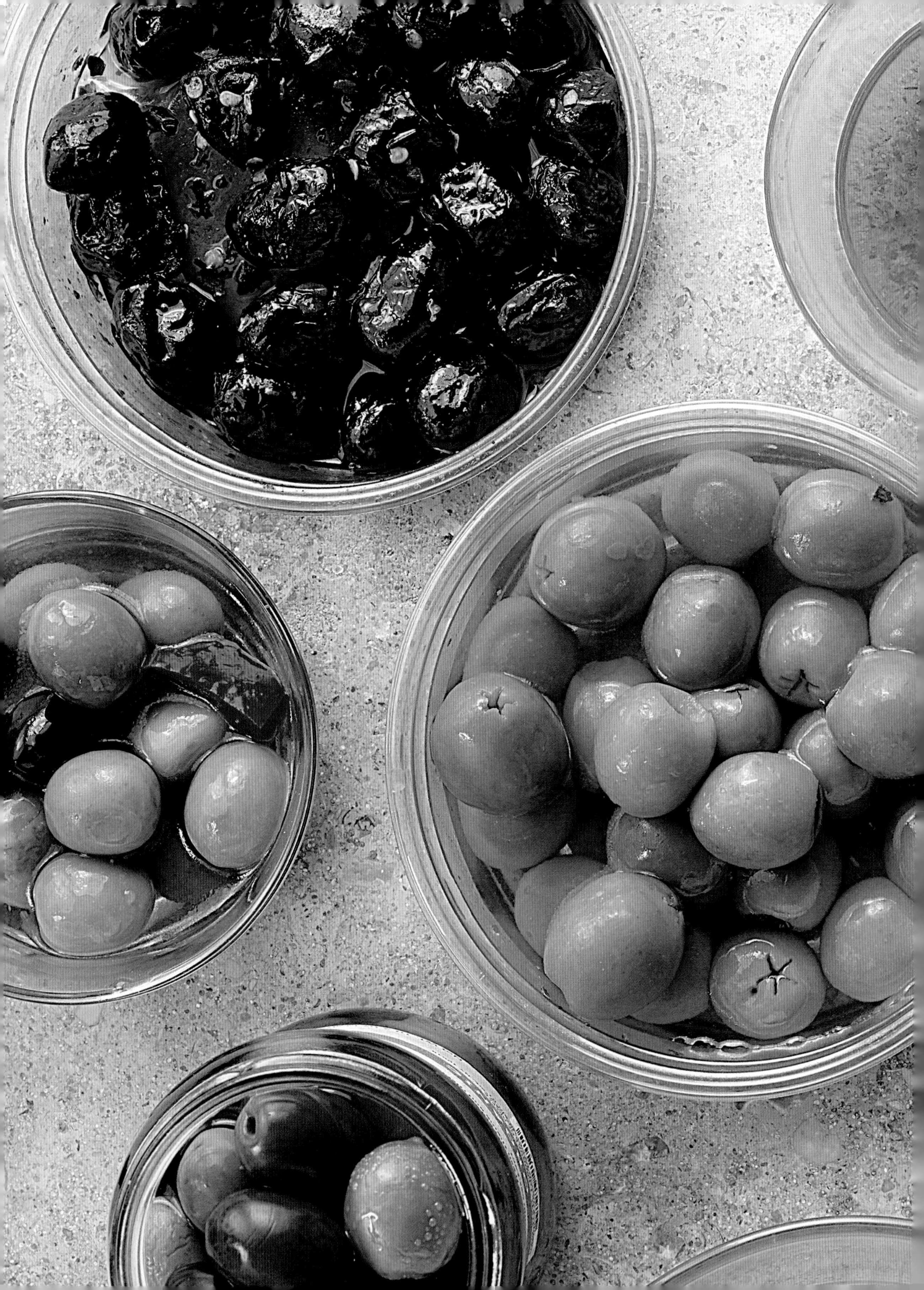

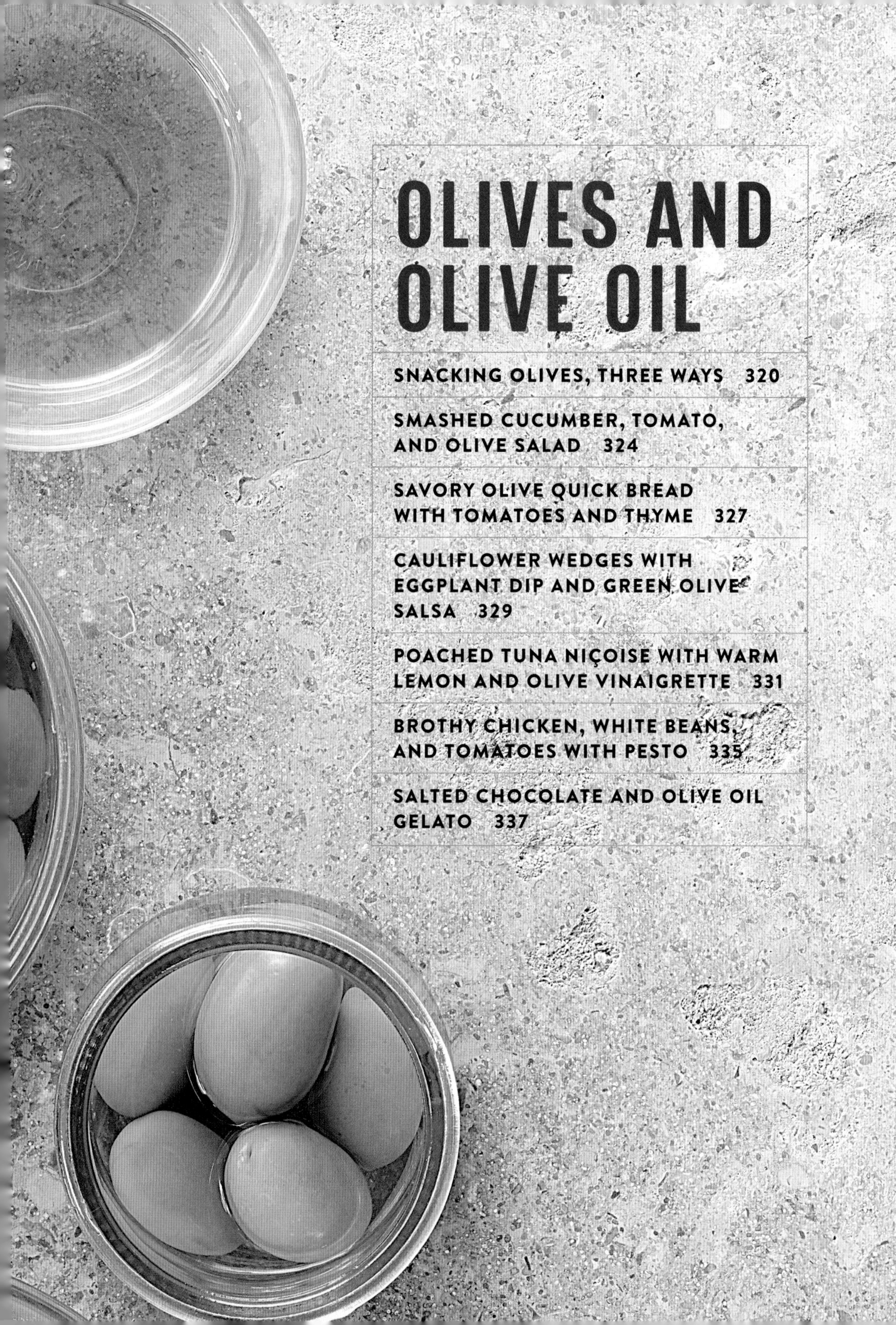

OLIVES AND OLIVE OIL

You may have heard "Let food be thy medicine and medicine be thy food," a saying commonly attributed to Hippocrates. But did you know that Hippocrates was likely talking about olive oil back in 400 BCE? While no one knows if this is exactly what Hippocrates wrote, he called olive oil "the great healer" and prescribed it for hundreds of medical conditions. Other ancient physicians also praised olive oil for its medicinal properties—Galen was a fan, and Homer called it "liquid gold." In those days, olive oil was used not just for cooking but for making medicines and perfumes, to anoint nobility, light lamps, and as currency. Athletes in ancient Greece even rubbed olive oil over their bodies before competitions for good luck!

Thousands of years later, modern science supports what the ancients believed: olive oil provides medicinal substances that enhance longevity. This is an added bonus because olive oil makes everything it touches taste better. I think of olive oil as the "secret sauce" of the Mediterranean diet. It marries and enhances the flavors of all the other brain-healthy food groups, whether it's cooked into dishes or drizzled on top before serving (which allows the beneficial polyphenols to stay intact).

This chapter will help you find delicious new ways to enjoy olive oil as well as snack on olives and work them into everyday meals. Olives take center stage in the smashed cucumber salad on page 324 and the tuna Niçoise on page 331. Or do like the ancients did and offer a plate of warm marinated olives—there are three varieties, including one inspired by pizza (page 323).

Olive oil amplifies the inherent nutrition of many foods. Think of it as a synergy between olive oil and the Mediterranean staple foods: while individual food groups are important on their own, each becomes more potent when drizzled in olive oil. This may be because the healthy fats in the oil act as a conduit to help you absorb the fat-soluble vitamins D, E, A, and K from food. Or the olive oil may blunt the insulin response to a meal, while adding another layer of protection to reduce oxidative stress and inflammation. In addition, the healthy fats in olive oil serve to drive down harmful blood cholesterol, resulting in healthier blood vessels and blood flow to the brain. Whatever the mechanism, most scientists agree: olive oil is probably the most significant reason the Mediterranean diet specifically has been proven, over and over again, as a way of eating that protects the brain and the heart.

USE OLIVE OIL AS YOUR PRIMARY COOKING OIL

Olive oil is the primary cooking oil in the Mediterranean diet and the MIND diet (page 17), both of which are proven to reduce Alzheimer's risk. Though most of the recipes in this book include olive oil, this chapter features it—along with the fruit it comes from—in unique ways.

You'll use olive oil as the poaching liquid for tuna (page 331). When blended with fresh basil, olive oil becomes a verdant finishing drizzle for a brothy, one-pan dish of chicken, olives, and white beans (page 335). You'll even churn the oil into a rich, chocolatey gelato (page 337) and gild it with a drizzle of your best extra-virgin. Baking with olive oil instead of butter is a brain-healthy swap that also gives baked goods an added dimension of flavor: in a savory quick bread (page 327) and a citrusy almond cake (page 203).

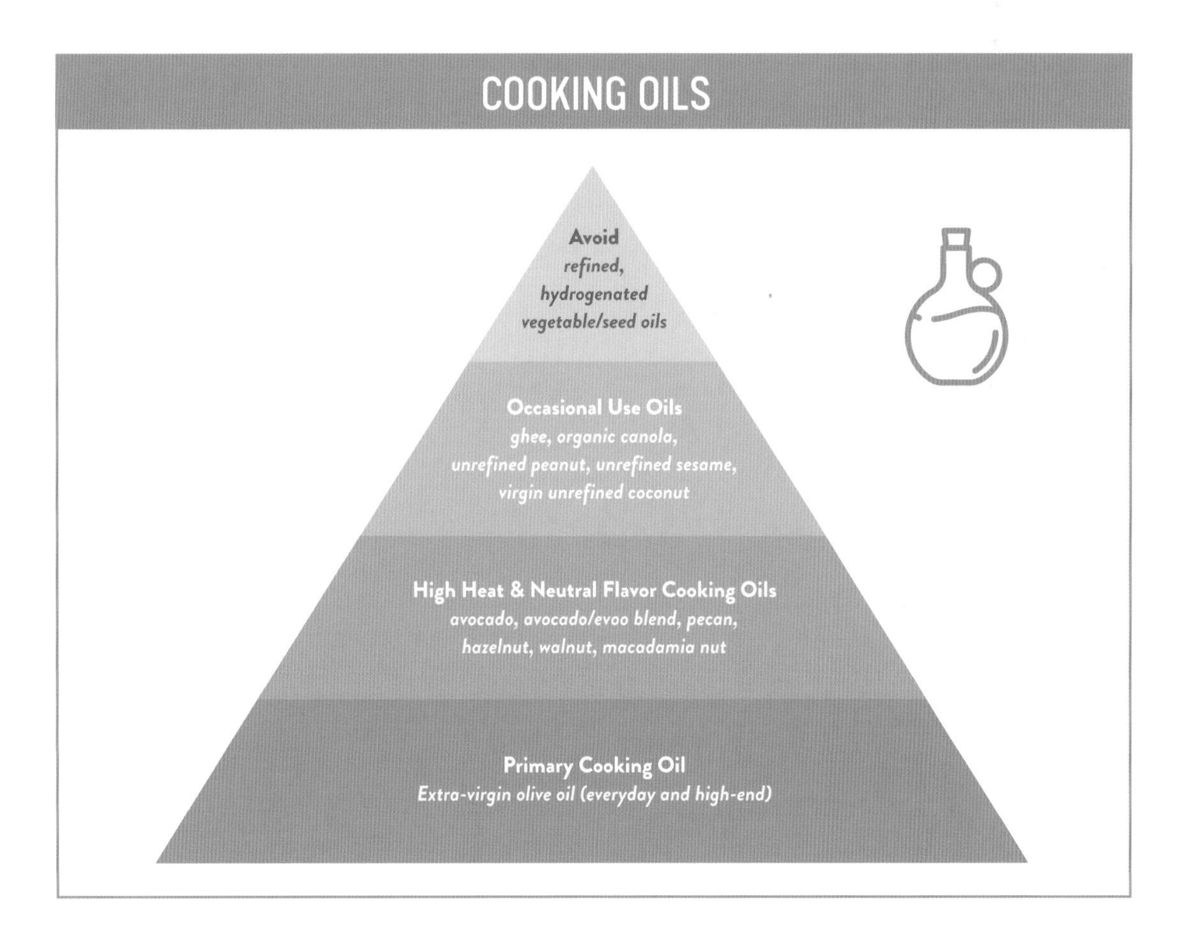

HOW TO PICK AN OLIVE OIL

Stock your pantry with two types of extra-virgin olive oil: an everyday bottle for cooking and baking and a high-end one for raw preparations or drizzling. As long as you choose an oil that is extra-virgin grade, these types both contain healthy fats and are up to 80 percent oleic acid, the monounsaturated fat that provides many health benefits.

You can find everyday extra-virgin olive oils at the supermarket. They may be less expensive than high-end oils, but they should still meet guidelines for quality. Everyday extra-virgin should be the workhorse in your kitchen—use it for baking, sautéing, roasting (below 400°F/200°C), braising, brushing on foods for indirect grilling, making salad dressings, and more. Look for domestic brands from California (which has the most rigorous olive oil standards) or a single country of origin, packed in dark bottles or tins with a harvest date on the label. Certification from the North American Olive Oil Association is a plus.

High-end extra-virgin and fresh, unfiltered olive oils are more expensive because they are pressed in small batches from only the highest-quality olives. And they must adhere to purity standards in concert with the International Olive Council and its country or state's olive oil council. Look for oil packed in dark bottles or tins with a harvest date and country of origin on the label.

CHOOSING THE BEST OLIVES

Olives themselves could be the world's most ancient snack. There is evidence that cave dwellers in Sicily feasted on olives some 10,000 years ago. However, according to Greek food expert Diane Kochilas, the ancient Greeks almost never cooked with olives. Instead, they offered them as a special course called prosfagio, meaning a food to be eaten before the meal.

Olives are an important brain food in their own right. Eating the whole olive provides the same healthy fats and polyphenols as in olive oil, all in a fiber-rich package that stabilizes blood sugar.

It's possible that you haven't already embraced olives, ready for you as a healthy snack or salty little flavor bomb in your cooking. Or maybe your olives have always come from a can and so you've never appreciated a truly flavorful olive? If so, there's a wide world of olives to explore beyond the can and the jar, all with unique fruity, savory, and pleasantly bitter flavors.

SHOPPING SMART: OLIVES

It helps to think of olives as the fruits that they are—grown on trees and usually picked while still unripe and green. When left to ripen on the tree, olives turn from bright green to tawny brown to a purplish black—indicative of an accumulation of anthocyanin, the same brain-healthy polyphenol in berries. Green olives straight from the tree are too bitter to eat (in part because of the brain-healthy compound oleuropein), so they are treated somehow: dry-brined in salt, cured in a saltwater solution, or processed using lye. To make sure you are getting all the health benefits olives provide, shop wisely and pay attention to a few caveats.

The good news is that the olive bars popping up in most grocery stores are an excellent place to get your olives. Like a salad bar for olives, you'll find a dozen or more different types of olives, from the wrinkly, black, salt-cured ones to single varietals stored in buckets of brine. When shopping for olives in brine, make sure they are fully submerged in their brine—this keeps them from being exposed to the air and becoming oxidized, thus losing flavor and polyphenols. Include plenty of that brine as you spoon them into the container to take home. Store your olives in the refrigerator, always under brine, and enjoy them within three weeks.

Other high-quality olives will be found in jars near the condiments. Just like when shopping for olive oil, read the label. Look for a country of origin—Spain, Greece, France, Italy, and Morocco are good bets. And make sure there aren't any artificial-sounding ingredients (like monosodium glutamate) or unhealthy oils (like sunflower oil). Good jarred olives have a short ingredient list: just olives, water, salt, and (sometimes) citric or lactic acid. (See Resources, page 390, for recommended brands.)

Avoid most canned olives, as almost all have been processed with lye to remove their bitter flavors then treated with ferrous gluconate, an iron compound, to turn them black. Unfortunately, this also removes their pleasing flavors and probably all of their polyphenols, resulting in a flavorless olive devoid of nutritional value. While California produces excellent extra-virgin olive oils, avoid California "ripe" olives; these are usually green olives that have been processed with lye.

Buying already pitted olives is undeniably convenient when a recipe calls for a lot of them, like the full cup of chopped olives used to make the vinaigrette for poached tuna (page 331). But there's a price: you may gain time when you don't have to pit yourself, but you lose flavor. Again, think of olives as the fruit that they are, a type of drupe like cherries, apricots, and peaches. A whole olive is juicier, more flavorful, and less likely to soak up the preservative qualities of its brine. This is key if you are watching your sodium intake (because your physician recommends this as a strategy to keep your blood pressure in a healthy range). Whole olives retain less sodium overall.

When you really want to appreciate the nuances of a good olive, as in the Snacking Olives (page 320), go for whole, unpitted olives and pit them yourself. (To quickly and easily pit an olive, see the tip on page 336.)

SHOPPING FOR OLIVE OIL

There are four grades of olive oil: extra-virgin, virgin, pure, and light. For both your high-end and everyday olive oil, buy only extra-virgin olive oil, the highest-quality grade. The others are refined olive oils that have undergone chemical and physical processing to increase shelf life, but that also renders the oil devoid of nutrition. For an oil to be labeled "extra-virgin," it must pass established standards by expert panels. It must be proven authentic, contain a certain concentration of beneficial fatty acids, and be free of known flaws—a list of sixteen official off-flavors and odors described as fusty, rancid, grubby, and metallic, to name a few.

Fresh is best. Unlike wine, olive oil does not improve with age but rather becomes less flavorful and less potent. Good extra-virgin olive oil has two dates on its label: the harvest date and the "best by" date.

The harvest date tells you when the olives were actually picked. Use this date to guide how long your oil will last: consume within eighteen months of harvest, or within six months of opening the bottle, whichever comes first.

The "best by" date is the manufacturer's estimate of how long the olive oil will last on the shelf, usually two years from bottling. If there's no harvest date, use the best by date and subtract six months to determine how long you can use the oil. Beware of bargains on good olive oil (they rarely go on sale), which probably mean they are past their prime.

Good extra-virgin olive oil is sensitive to light and heat, which hasten its lifespan and oxidize its healthy fats and polyphenols. Look for oil sold in tins or dark bottles and leave the clear glass and plastic bottles on the shelf.

Know the place of origin and cultivar. Legitimate extra-virgin olive oil comes from a specific farm where the olives are grown and pressed into oil. Steer clear of olive oils that are pooled from numerous countries. A good sign is that the oil has the stamp of approval from the country or state's olive oil council, such as Italy's DOP (in English, PDO, for Protected Designation of Origin), the California Olive Oil Council, the Australian Olive Association, or the International Olive Council.

Look also for the type of olive—names like Frantoio, Galega, Picholine, Arbequina, and Hojiblanca—from which it is pressed. There are seven hundred types of olives—called cultivars or varietals—that are made into oil. The best olive oils will have both place and cultivar proudly displayed on the label.

It's a good sign when an extra-virgin olive oil is labeled "organic" or "organically grown"—depending on the country, "biologico," "biologique," or "BIO"—because you know it is as free of pesticides as possible. Note that organic designation is a good indicator that the oil is truly "extra-virgin" but does not tell you about the quality of that particular oil.

Ignore marketing terms. You already know that certain descriptors sound good but are actually clues to a poorer grade of olive oil (like pure, light, and virgin). Other red flags are the phrases "bottled in Italy" and "packed in Italy." While Italy does produce some of the world's finest extra-virgin olive oils, it also processes inferior oils grown elsewhere, packs them into bottles on Italian soil, slaps an Italian flag on the label (or a bucolic Tuscan farm scene), and can say it's from Italy. Other marketing terms include "cold-pressed," "first-pressed," and "first cold pressed." In the past, these descriptors of how the oil is pressed were important, but now all extra-virgin olive oil is by definition pressed below 80°F (27°C), and legitimate producers don't declare this on the label.

When shopping for high-end oils, find a store that lets you taste before you buy. It should have an obvious fruity aroma (after all, olive oil is a type of fruit juice). The spectrum of flavors ranges from buttery to herbaceous to peppery to pungent, but good oil is not bland, flavorless, or unpleasantly bitter. Become acquainted with the flavor profiles you like and the ones you don't. Tasting oil also helps you discern when an oil has gone bad or may be fraudulent, meaning you should not consume it.

An extra-virgin olive oil's polyphenol content is an indicator of its antioxidant potency and therefore its usefulness as a cardio- and neuroprotective food. (Read more about polyphenols on page 339.) So why don't olive oil producers put this on the label? Now that the International Olive Council has approved a method of measuring polyphenol content, this is becoming more common. The higher the rating, the better, ranging from 200 mg/kg for good quality up to 800 mg/kg for highest quality.

Store in a cool, dark place. It's fine to keep the oil in its original container; however, if you buy olive oil in large quantities, such as gallon (3.8 L) boxes or tins, it's helpful to pour small amounts of oil into a ceramic or stainless-steel dispenser to have at the ready while you cook. Keep this away from the heat of the stove, oven, and direct sunlight.

SNACKING OLIVES, THREE WAYS

Olives right from the jar are a satiating snack on their own, but warming them in a pan with complementary flavors—citrus peel, spicy touches, and herbs, to name a few—pays off in big ways. Gentle heat coaxes a wide range of flavor from the olives, from light to buttery to fruity to pleasantly bitter. Waiting to add the extra-virgin olive oil at the end of cooking not only preserves the oil's health-promoting polyphenols, it means the warm olives come to the table in a bath of well-seasoned oil, perfect for dunking with a whole-grain cracker or toasted pita, or to save for later to drizzle on pizza, roasted vegetables, or hummus.

Riff on these recipes to suit your taste. While you can enjoy these right away, marinated olives become even more deeply flavored with an overnight rest in the fridge. (Serve at room temperature or warm gently.) Both pitted and whole, unpitted olives work well here. If you have the time, and especially if you are watching your salt intake, buy unpitted olives and remove the pits yourself. Unpitted olives absorb less of the salt from the brine and retain their fresh, fruity flavor longer.

MOROCCAN-SPICED SNACKING OLIVES

MAKES 2 CUPS (340 G)

2 teaspoons coriander seeds

2 cups (370 g) assorted unpitted green olives, such as Castelvetrano and Gaeta, drained

½ tablespoon preserved lemon rind, thinly sliced, or strips of lemon zest from 1 lemon

2 teaspoons harissa (Moroccan red pepper paste)

½ cup (120 ml) extra-virgin olive oil

Use a mix of Castelvetrano, Gaeta, Cerignola, Manzanilla, and Sevillana olives (sometimes called gorditas) in this recipe. Harissa paste (see Resources, page 390) and preserved lemons are traditional ingredients in Moroccan cuisine. If you are lucky enough to have access to a Moroccan food store, look for olive cultivars named Beldi and Meslalla. Serve these Moroccan-spiced olives alongside flavorful small plates, such as grilled eggplant and zucchini, warm whole-grain pita bread, simply grilled chicken or fish, and lemony couscous.

1. Toast the coriander seeds in a medium skillet over low heat until they are fragrant and start to pop, about 1 minute. Transfer to a cutting board and crush using the flat side of a knife.

2. Using the same skillet, reduce the heat to medium-low and add the olives, lemon, and harissa. Stir to combine, then cook, stirring often, until the olives are warm, 3 to 5 minutes. Reduce the heat to low and add the oil. Stir to coat and cook until warmed through, about 1 minute longer. Pour into a bowl, sprinkle with the toasted coriander seeds, and serve warm.

ORANGE AND FETA SNACKING OLIVES

MAKES 2½ CUPS (480 G)

- **2 cups (375 g) small, unpitted black and green olives, such as Niçoise or Nyon, drained**
- **¼ cup (60 ml) fresh orange juice**
- **Five 3-inch (7.5 cm) strips orange zest**
- **1 teaspoon fresh rosemary leaves, finely chopped, plus a few sprigs for serving**
- **¼ cup (60 ml) extra-virgin olive oil**
- **4 ounces (115 g) feta, cut into ½-inch (1.25 cm) cubes (about ½ cup)**
- **1 teaspoon fennel seeds, crushed**

A dish of these fragrant olives is second only to a trip to Greece. Okay, maybe that's going too far, but the woodsy rosemary, sweet orange juice, and earthy fennel seeds do impart the flavors of a Mediterranean island. Look for a firm variety of feta cheese (such as Mt. Vikos, imported from Greece) so that it holds its shape when cut into cubes instead of crumbling, making it easier to spear with a toothpick along with the olives. Serve these on their own as an appetizer, or as part of a meal with small plates that include a fresh fennel salad or a vibrant rice pilaf (page 293).

1. Combine the olives, orange juice, orange zest, and chopped rosemary in a medium skillet and warm over medium-low heat. Cook, stirring often, until the olives are warm, 3 to 5 minutes. Reduce the heat to low, stir in the oil, and cook until warmed through, about 1 minute longer.

2. Place the feta in a shallow bowl and pour the olive mixture over top. Sprinkle with fennel seeds, and finish with rosemary sprigs; serve warm.

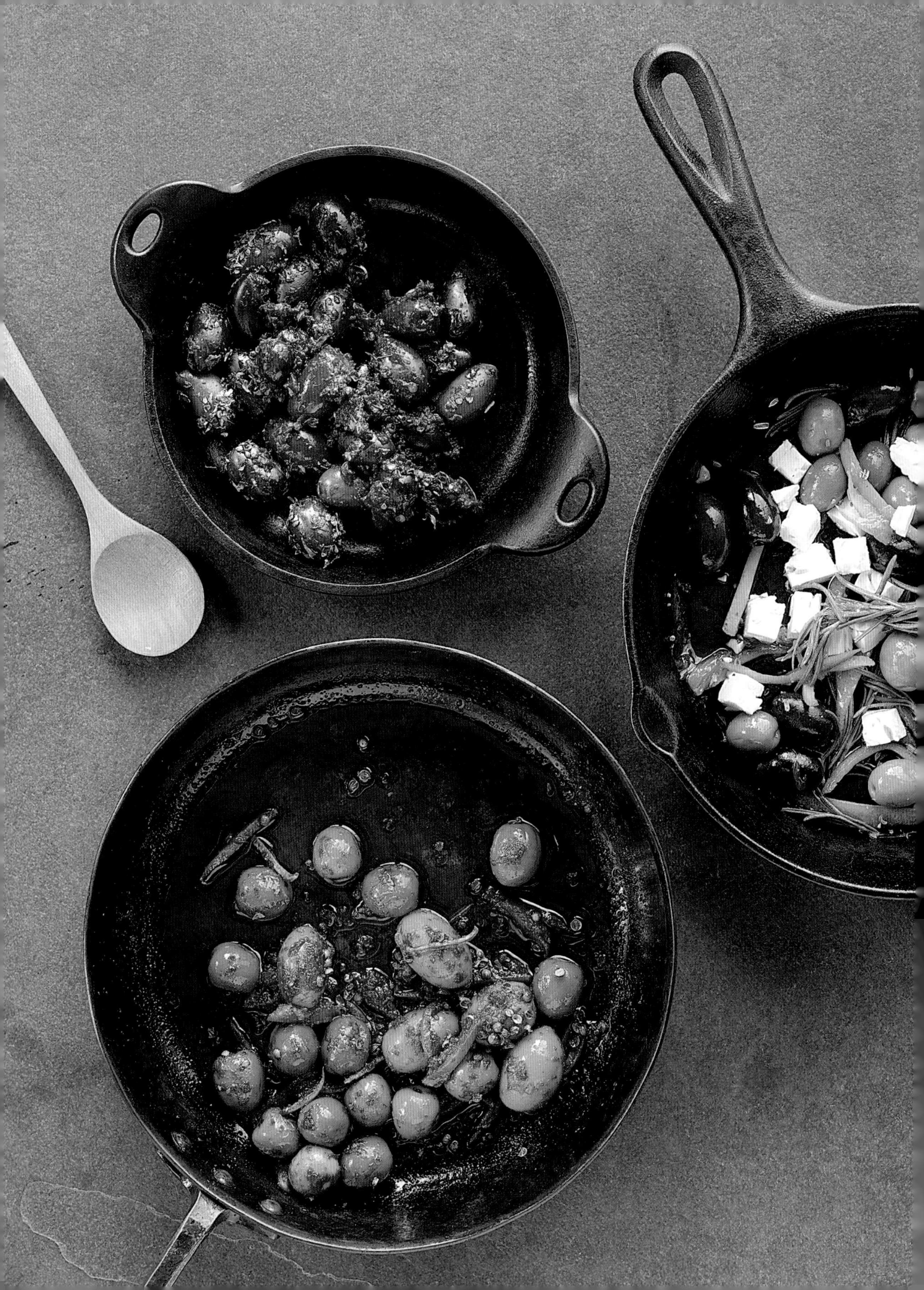

PIZZA-SPICED SNACKING OLIVES

MAKES 2 CUPS (340 G)

- **1 tablespoon tomato paste (from a tube)**
- **1 tablespoon water**
- **2 cups (375 g) unpitted Kalamata olives, drained**
- **1 teaspoon dried oregano, plus more for serving**
- **¼ teaspoon crushed red pepper flakes, plus more for serving**
- **¼ teaspoon garlic powder**
- **¼ cup (60 ml) extra-virgin olive oil**

If you love olives on pizza, then this is the dish for you. Use juicy Kalamata olives from the bulk section of the grocery store or a good, jarred brand in brine. Serve with olive oil breadsticks for snacking, or as an appetizer before an Italian-style meal. You could put these on your pizza, too, for a huge upgrade (in both flavor and brain health nutrition) to canned sliced black olives. Just remember to pit them before proceeding with the recipe below.

1. Combine the tomato paste and water in a medium skillet and cook over medium heat, stirring continuously, until the paste begins to brown slightly and thicken, about 30 seconds. Reduce the heat to medium-low and stir in the olives, oregano, red pepper flakes, and garlic powder. Cook, stirring often, until the olives are warm, 3 to 5 minutes. Reduce the heat to low and pour the oil over top. Stir to coat and cook until warmed through, about 1 minute longer.

2. Transfer to a serving bowl and sprinkle with additional oregano and red pepper flakes, if you like; serve warm.

SMASHED CUCUMBER, TOMATO, AND OLIVE SALAD

SERVES 4

- **1 pound (455 g) English or Persian cucumbers (see Tip)**
- **½ teaspoon kosher salt**
- **1 cup (155 g) Castelvetrano olives, pitted**
- **Half of a 4-inch (10 cm) ball fresh mozzarella (4 ounces/115 g)**
- **1 cup (170 g) cherry tomatoes, halved**
- **⅓ cup (80 ml) extra-virgin olive oil**
- **2 tablespoons white wine vinegar**
- **Fresh basil leaves, larger ones torn**
- **Flaky salt (optional)**
- **Freshly ground black pepper**

Chopped salad gets an upgrade thanks to a clever technique that improves the flavor and texture of cucumbers. You'll use the flat side of a chef's knife to crack the skin, which releases the seeds and creates naturally jagged pieces. The crags in the cucumber help the simple dressing—extra-virgin olive oil, vinegar, and salt—get absorbed rather than slide off into a puddle on the bottom of the bowl.

The deep green Castelvetrano olive is the best choice for this salad. It's meaty, buttery, and large enough to easily tear into pieces with your hands, which adds even more irregular edges to catch the dressing. This variety has a milder flavor than many olives—they're called "dolce" in Italy (translation: sweet)—which makes them a good entry-level choice for the new olive lover. Any large, fruity, and buttery olive works well here, too, such as Cerignola, Frescatrano, or Manzanilla.

1. Cut the cucumbers in half lengthwise and place them cut side down on a cutting board. Gently smash the cucumbers using the flat side of a large knife until they start to break apart. Roughly chop them into 1- to 2-inch (2.5 to 5 cm) pieces and transfer along with any juices to a large bowl. Sprinkle with the kosher salt. Set aside while you prepare the remaining ingredients, for at least 5 minutes and up to 1 hour.

2. Tear the olives into two or three pieces each and tear the mozzarella into 1-inch (2.5 cm) pieces. Add to the cucumbers along with the tomatoes, oil, vinegar, and basil. Toss well and finish with flaky salt (if using) and pepper.

TIP: *The thin-skinned English cucumber works best for this dish.*

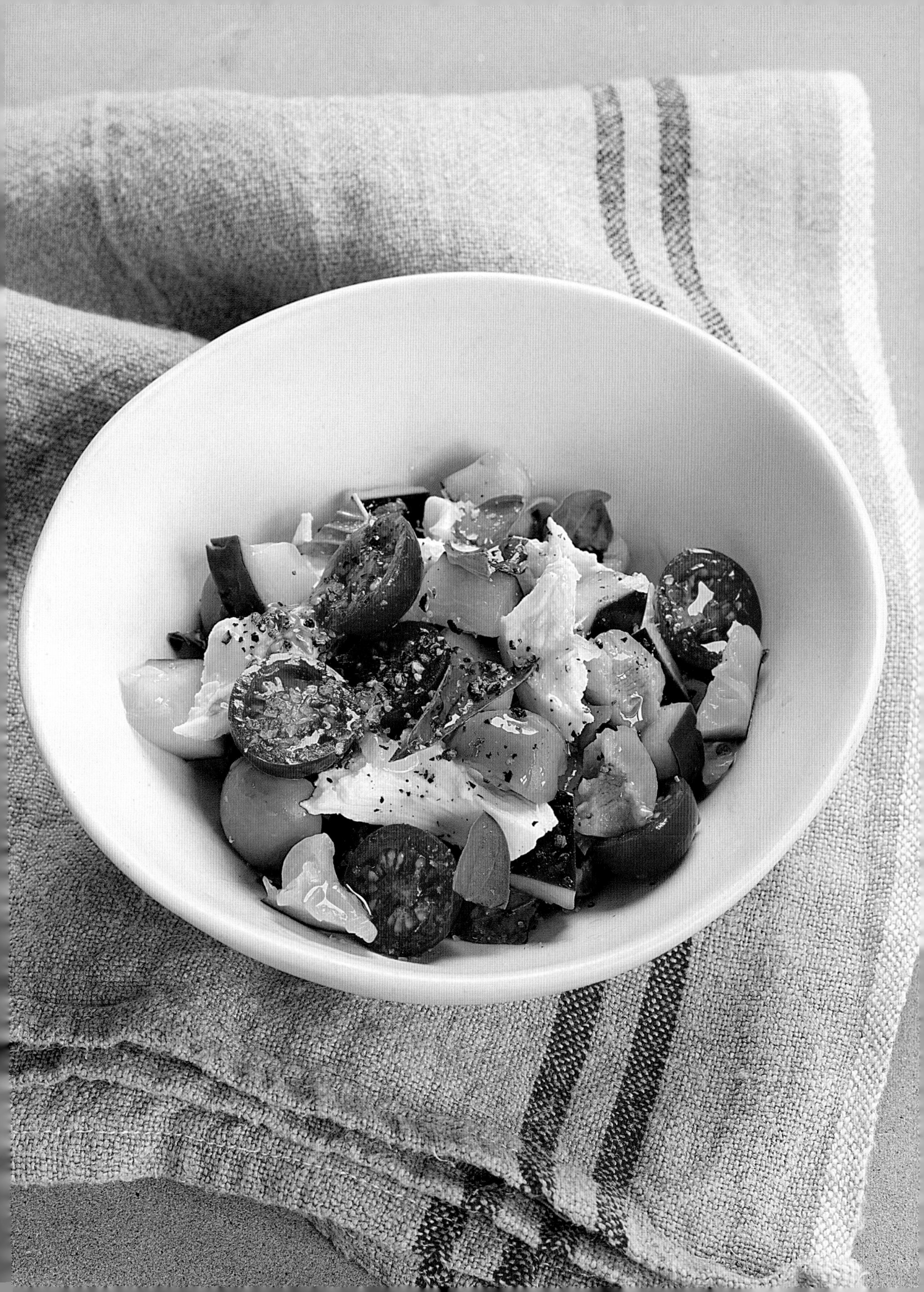

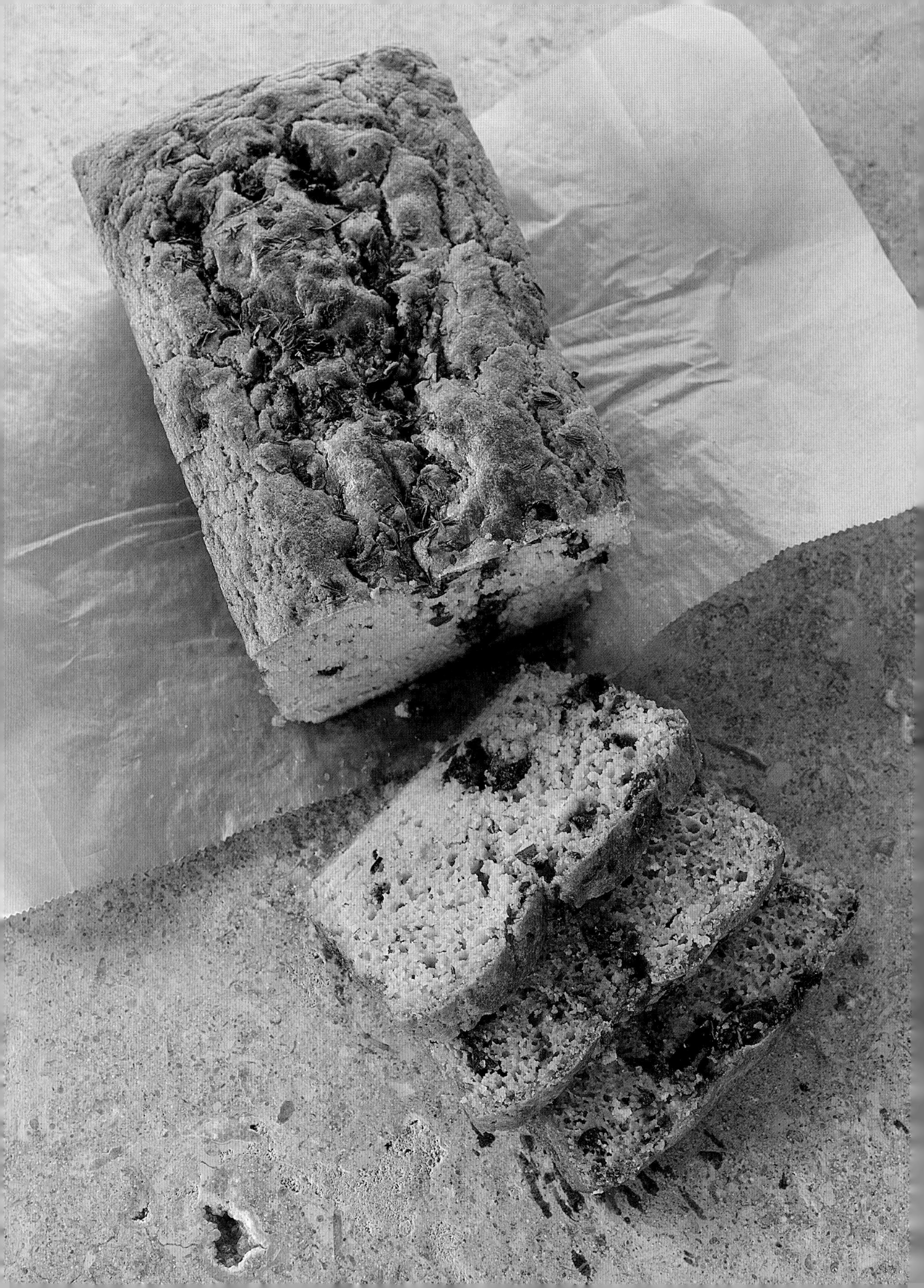

SAVORY OLIVE QUICK BREAD WITH TOMATOES AND THYME

MAKES 1 LOAF; SERVES 8

½ cup (120 ml) extra-virgin olive oil, plus more for the pan

1 cup (240 ml) plain, unsweetened whole-milk yogurt

½ cup (120 ml) plain, unsweetened nut-based or dairy milk (see Tip)

½ cup (115 g) sun-dried tomatoes (packed in olive oil), finely chopped, plus 2 tablespoons of oil from the jar

2 eggs, at room temperature

1 tablespoon lemon zest (from 1 small lemon)

2 tablespoons fresh lemon juice

1 teaspoon fresh thyme leaves, plus more for sprinkling

1 cup (140 g) stone-ground cornmeal (medium or finely ground)

1 spooned-and-leveled cup (140 g) whole-wheat flour

1 teaspoon baking powder

½ teaspoon baking soda

1 teaspoon kosher salt

½ teaspoon freshly ground black pepper

½ cup (115 g) black olives, such as Kalamata or Gaeta, pitted and sliced into ¼-inch (6 mm) rounds

This savory quick bread recipe is a good one to have in your back pocket. Not only does it emerge from the oven smelling like pizza, the bread stays fresh for days, thanks to a combination of olive oil and yogurt in the batter. The olive oil adds flavor, too, accentuating the sun-dried tomatoes, hints of lemon, and juicy black olives, while a combination of whole-grain cornmeal and whole-wheat flour adds both fiber and texture to the loaf.

Even if you haven't eaten a sun-dried tomato since their heyday in the 1990s, this quick bread makes a strong argument for their revival. Ubiquitous across America until a few decades ago, the olive oil–packed sun-dried tomato expanded awareness of Mediterranean foods. Then they mostly disappeared. Here they add a touch of sweetness and a good dose of the antioxidant lycopene. Look for a brand grown in the Mediterranean and packed in extra-virgin olive oil.

1. Preheat the oven to 375°F (190°C). Brush an 8½-by-4½-inch (21 by 11 cm) loaf pan with oil, line it with parchment paper so that the edges overhang, and brush the paper with more oil.

2. Whisk the oil, yogurt, milk, tomatoes and 2 tablespoons oil from the jar, eggs, lemon zest, lemon juice, and thyme in a large bowl until evenly combined.

3. Whisk together the cornmeal, flour, baking powder, baking soda, salt, and pepper in a medium bowl. Add the flour mixture to the wet ingredients and fold with a flexible spatula until only a few streaks of flour remain. Fold in the olives.

continued

4. Scrape into the prepared pan and sprinkle with more thyme leaves. Bake for 50 to 60 minutes, until the edges are brown, the center is set, and a tester inserted into the center comes out clean or with just a few moist crumbs clinging to it.

5. When the bread is completely cool, lift it out of the pan by grasping the parchment overhang on each side. To serve, cut into 1-inch (2.5 cm) slices and enjoy warm or at room temperature.

TIP: *You can use any unsweetened, unflavored milk to make this quick bread, but my preference is to use a nondairy milk that is also rich in monounsaturated fats, such as almond or cashew milk. This shifts the fat profile toward more monounsaturated fats (from the olive oil, olives, and the nut milk) and less saturated ones. For the yogurt, though, go for the full-fat whole-milk kind. It's key here for giving the bread a moist, delicate crumb.*

SCIENCE BITE:

OLIVE OIL IS GOOD FOR THE HEART AND THE BRAIN

It's long been known that small amounts of olive oil in the diet can protect the heart and blood vessels. First, the Spanish PREDIMED study showed that boosting the Mediterranean diet with an extra ¼ cup (60 ml) olive oil daily, when compared to a low fat diet, reduced heart attacks and stroke by 30 percent. Then, in a similar U.S. study, Harvard researchers described what happens when you replace margarine, butter, mayonnaise, and dairy products with olive oil. For every teaspoon of these saturated fat-laden foods replaced with olive oil, participants enjoyed a 5 to 7 percent lower risk of heart disease.

Olive oil's cardioprotective impact translates to less dementia, too. The latest study (of more than 90,000 participants over 28 years) shows that even a few teaspoons of olive oil each day not only reduces the chance of dying from heart disease by 19 percent, but also neurodegenerative diseases (like Alzheimer's) by 29 percent. What's the optimal dose of olive oil? No one knows for sure. But researchers note that consuming just one teaspoon daily can reduce the risk of dying from any cause by 12 percent.

CAULIFLOWER WEDGES WITH EGGPLANT DIP AND GREEN OLIVE SALSA

SERVES 4 AS A LIGHT SUPPER, 6 TO 8 AS A SIDE

2 medium or 3 small globe eggplants (2 pounds/ 910 g total)

1 large or 2 small heads cauliflower (2 pounds/ 910 g total), cut into ¾-inch (2 cm) wedges

3 large garlic cloves

6 tablespoons extra-virgin olive oil

1 teaspoon kosher salt

½ cup (80 g) Castelvetrano olives, or another large green olive, pitted

¼ cup (40 g) pomegranate seeds

¼ cup (35 g) toasted walnuts, roughly chopped (see page 190 for toasting instructions)

1 tablespoon lemon zest (from 1 large lemon)

¼ cup (60 ml) fresh lemon juice

½ cup (120 ml) tahini

½ loosely packed cup (10 g) fresh flat-leaf parsley leaves

½ teaspoon freshly ground black pepper, plus more for serving

Warm pita bread, cut into wedges (optional)

This vegetable-forward recipe combines two brain-healthy principles: putting plants first and eating small "suppers" rather than big dinners. Of course, this dish also works as a side. The green olive salsa served on top is inspired by the tangerine and pecan gremolata (page 195), made instead with walnuts, pomegranate seeds, and meaty green olives. The salsa doubles easily to keep extra green olive salsa on hand to dress up store-bought hummus or sprinkle on grilled fish or chicken.

Cutting the cauliflower into wedges instead of steaks means more of the cauliflower will stay intact. Make wedges by slicing the cauliflower from the crown so that each piece includes some stem to help hold it together. Use two small heads of cauliflower to yield more pieces, if you like.

1. Set an oven rack in the center position and preheat the oven to 400°F (200°C). Line a rimmed baking sheet with parchment paper.

2. Poke holes all over the eggplants with a fork and place on one side of the baking sheet. Place the cauliflower and garlic on the other side of the sheet. Brush all the vegetables with 2 tablespoons of the oil and sprinkle with ½ teaspoon of the salt. Roast for 50 to 55 minutes, until the eggplants collapse, the garlic is toasty brown, and the cauliflower is golden brown on the edges and a fork can be inserted easily into the stem. Keep an eye on the garlic and remove it sooner if turning dark brown.

3. Meanwhile, make the olive salsa. Chop or tear the olives into pebble-size pieces and combine in a medium bowl with the pomegranate seeds, walnuts, lemon zest, and 2 tablespoons of the lemon juice; set aside.

continued

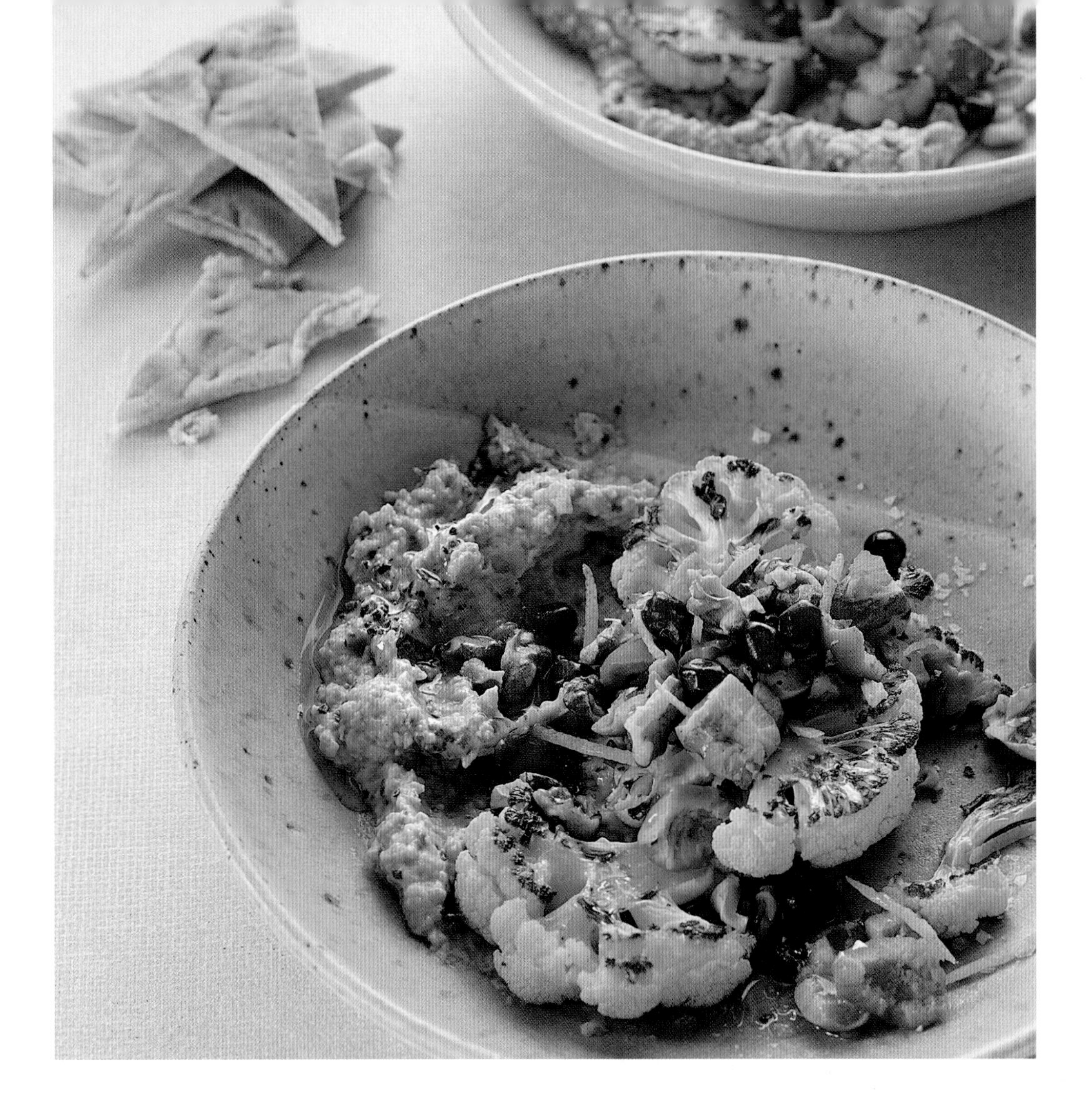

4. Slice the eggplant in half lengthwise on a cutting board and scrape the flesh from the skin using a large spoon. Discard the skin and place the eggplant pulp in the bowl of a food processor with the tahini, parsley, roasted garlic, pepper, and the remaining ¼ cup (60 ml) oil, remaining 2 tablespoons lemon juice, and remaining ½ teaspoon salt. Blend on high speed until smooth, about 1 minute.

5. To serve, use a spoon to smear about ¼ cup (60 ml) of the eggplant puree in shallow bowls. Top each with a wedge or two of cauliflower and a few spoonfuls of olive salsa. Finish with more pepper and a drizzle of oil, if you like. Serve with warm pita bread, if using.

POACHED TUNA NIÇOISE WITH WARM LEMON AND OLIVE VINAIGRETTE

SERVES 4 TO 6

2 or 3 albacore or ahi tuna fillets (1½ pounds/680 g total), cut into 2-by-3-inch (5 by 7.5 cm) pieces

½ teaspoon kosher salt

¼ teaspoon freshly ground black pepper

½ pound (225 g) green beans, stems trimmed

1 pound (455 g) small new potatoes

4 eggs

½ cup (120 ml) extra-virgin olive oil

1 large shallot (5 ounces/140 g), finely chopped (about ½ cup)

1 cup (230 g) black or green olives, such as Niçoise, pitted

1 Meyer lemon, halved, seeds removed, finely chopped (both peel and flesh), or another small, thin-skinned lemon (see Tips)

2 anchovy fillets or 2 teaspoons anchovy paste

1 tablespoon fresh tarragon leaves, coarsely chopped

Flaky salt (optional)

All the quintessential elements of the classic are here—crisp-tender green beans, creamy new potatoes, and boiled eggs—along with a few brain-healthy twists, like a whole lemon and olive dressing spiked with anchovies. To turn this salad into a hearty meal, you'll serve it with olive oil–poached ahi tuna steaks instead of the usual tuna from a can. Rather than searing or grilling the tuna, poaching in olive oil creates tender, flaky fish that is infused with flavor. Plus, it locks in beneficial omega-3 fatty acids that can seep out with higher-heat methods.

You'll use the same pot of boiling water to blanch the green beans and boil the eggs. Bring the pot of water back to a boil to cook the potatoes while you get a saucepan going to poach the fish and make the vinaigrette. For a simplified version, swap in arugula for the green beans.

1. Blot the tuna dry and sprinkle on all sides with ¼ teaspoon of the kosher salt and the pepper. Set aside to come to room temperature.

2. Fill a large bowl with ice water.

3. Bring a large pot of salted water to a boil. Add the green beans and cook until crisp-tender, 5 to 7 minutes. Use a slotted spoon to transfer the beans to the ice water. When completely cool, transfer to a kitchen towel and blot dry; pile on one side of a serving platter. Replenish the ice water with ice.

4. Return the water in the pot to a boil and add the potatoes. Cook until tender when pierced with the tip of a knife, 10 to 15 minutes. Transfer to a bowl and cut in half. Transfer to the serving platter.

continued

TIPS: *Meyer lemons, with their thin skin and sweeter flesh, are perfect for this vinaigrette because you will use the whole lemon, including the peel. If you can't find them, look for a ripe lemon with a thin skin, preferably an organic one.*

Allowing the fish to come to room temperature helps it cook more evenly. Blotting it dry with a paper towel minimizes splatter when it comes in contact with the oil.

5. Use a slotted spoon to gently lower the eggs into the pot of hot water. Reduce the heat to a low simmer. Cook for 10 minutes, then transfer to the ice water. Just before serving, tap gently all over each egg to loosen the shell. Starting at the pointy end, peel the eggs and quarter them lengthwise; place on the platter with the green beans.

6. Meanwhile, place the pieces of tuna in a saucepan just large enough to hold them without touching and pour the oil over top, then flip over to coat evenly in oil. Bring to a low simmer over medium heat; the oil should be barely bubbling. (If you have an instant-read thermometer, the oil should be around 200°F/90°C.)

7. Cook the tuna, lifting the bottoms of the fish occasionally so they don't stick to the bottom, and spooning the oil over them frequently, until the undersides are pearly white, 2 to 3 minutes. Flip over and cook for another 1 to 2 minutes, for a total of up to 3 minutes for rare or 5 minutes for medium-rare. Using tongs, carefully transfer the tuna to the center of the platter.

8. Place a fine-mesh strainer on top of a heatproof measuring cup. When the oil has cooled slightly, strain then return it to the saucepan and heat over medium-low. Add the shallots and sprinkle with the remaining ¼ teaspoon kosher salt. Cook, stirring often, until starting to brown, 4 to 6 minutes. Add the olives, lemon, and anchovies, and cook until the lemons are soft and the anchovies have dissolved, another 4 to 6 minutes. Spoon over the potatoes, tuna, eggs, and green beans and sprinkle with the tarragon. Finish with more pepper and flaky salt (if using).

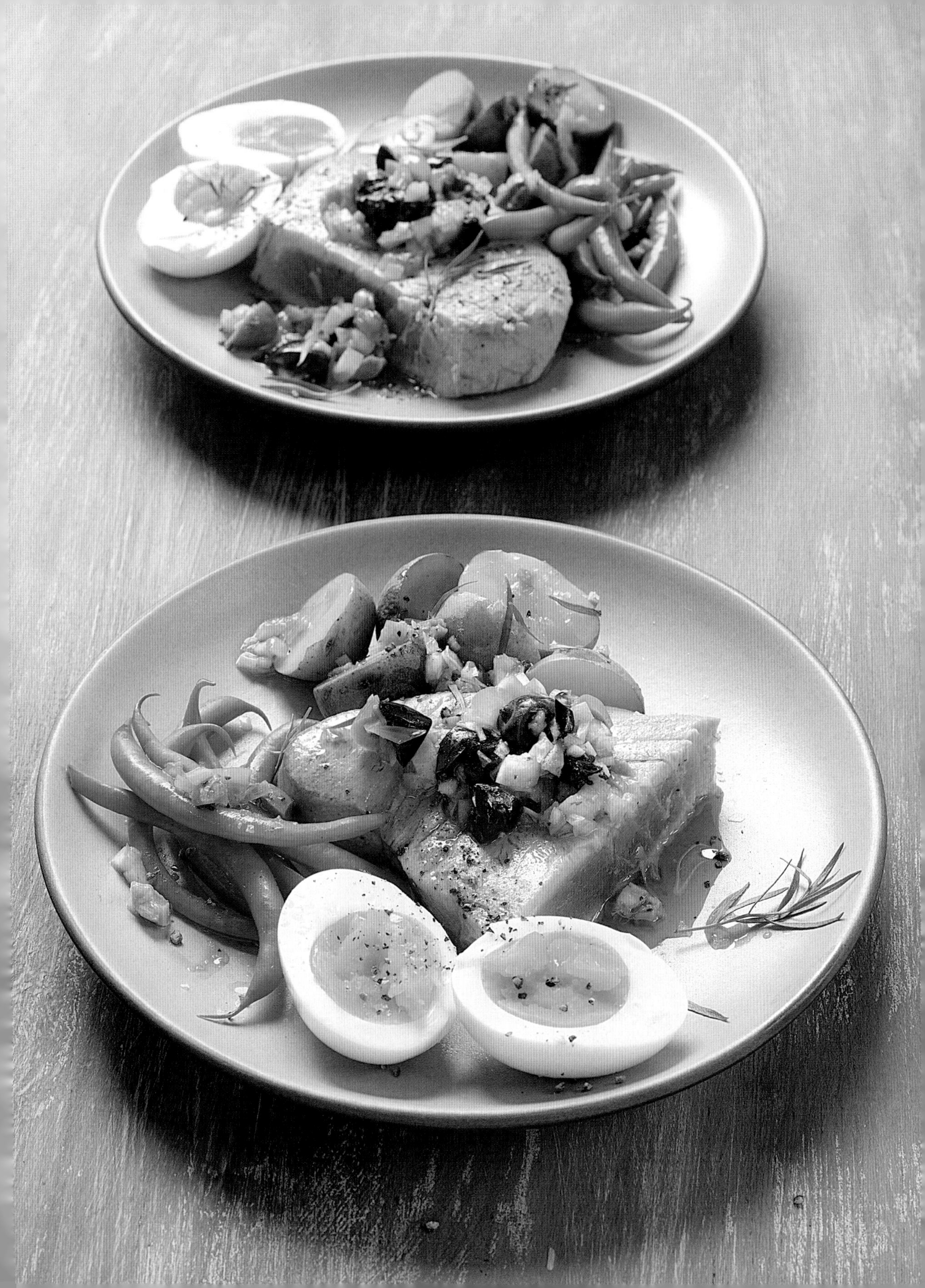

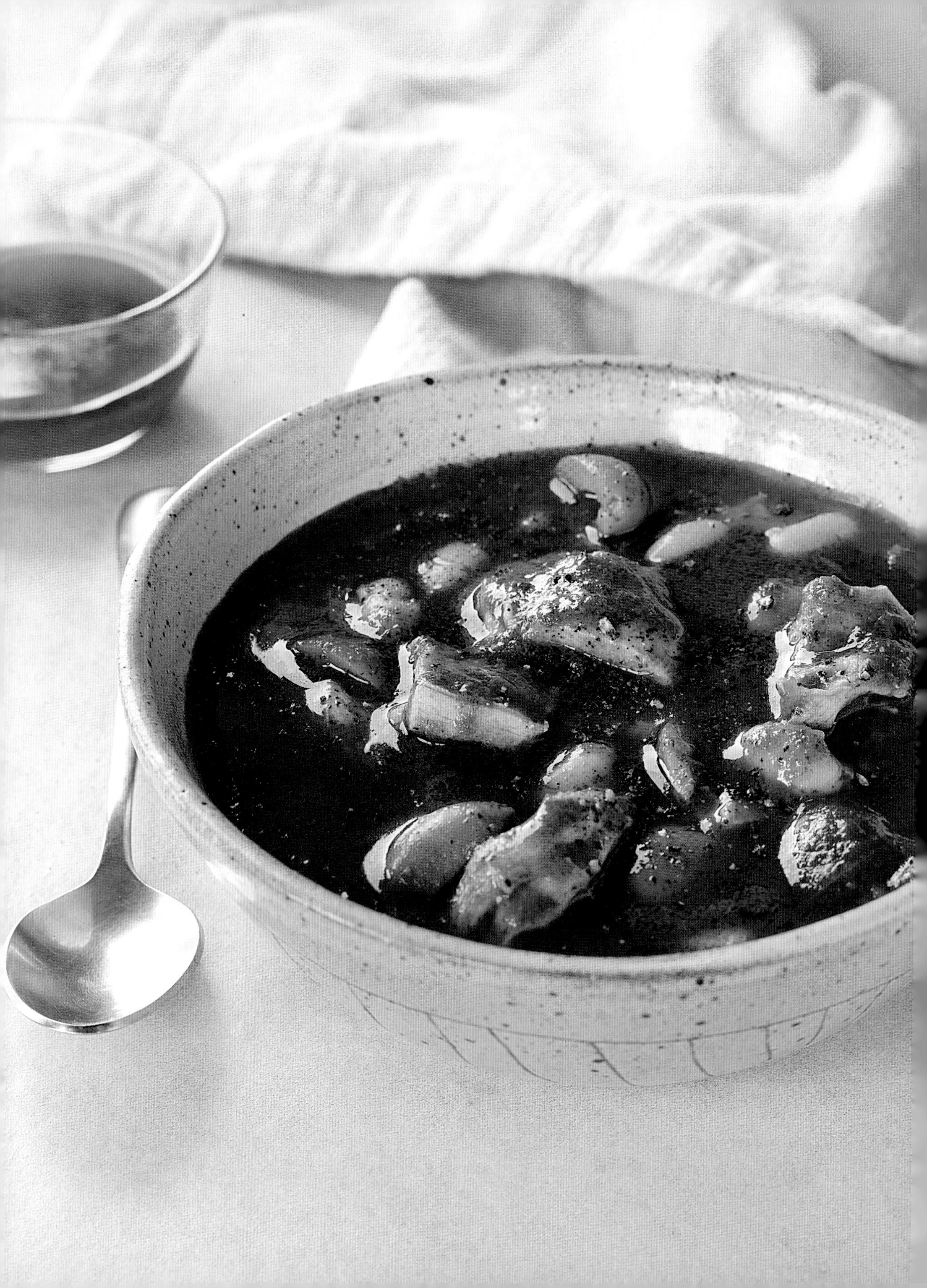

BROTHY CHICKEN, WHITE BEANS, AND TOMATOES WITH PESTO

SERVES 4 TO 6

1 tablespoon extra-virgin olive oil

1 large shallot (5 ounces/ 140 g), finely chopped (about ½ cup)

¼ teaspoon freshly ground black pepper, plus more to finish

1 teaspoon kosher salt

1 cup (230 ml) dry white wine

1½ cups (265 g) cooked cannellini or gigante beans (see page 215) or one 15.5-ounce (440 g) can, rinsed

One 14-ounce (395 g) can whole peeled tomatoes

1 cup (155 g) green olives, such as Frescatrano, pitted and halved lengthwise (see Tip)

1½ cups (360 ml) chicken stock, vegetable stock, or bean stock from freshly cooked beans

Two 6-inch (15 cm) rosemary sprigs

2 pounds (910 g) boneless, skinless chicken thighs, cut into 3-inch (7.5 cm) pieces

¼ cup (60 ml) pesto

Brain-healthy cooking doesn't always have to be about fresh vegetables. Sometimes, it can be a hearty one-pot chicken dinner that uses mostly pantry staples. This one features both olives and olive oil for an abundance of healthy fats and flavor. Braising the chicken in the tomatoes and stock is a health-promoting cooking technique that both concentrates the lycopene content of the tomatoes and keeps this low-fat cut of chicken tender. Though making the basil oil is an extra step, it merits a place in your regular routine. The peppery oil brightens simple meals like grain bowls, avocado toast, or minestrone soup (page 229).

1. Warm the olive oil over low heat in a large saucepan with a tight-fitting lid or a Dutch oven. When the oil starts to shimmer, add the shallots, pepper, and ½ teaspoon of the salt. Cook, stirring often, until the shallots begin to brown, 4 to 6 minutes. Add the wine, bring to a boil, and use a wooden spoon to scrape up any small bits of shallot from the bottom of the pan. Cook until the liquid is slightly reduced, about 2 minutes.

2. Stir in the beans, tomatoes and their juices, olives, stock, and rosemary. Bring to a boil then reduce the heat to a lively simmer. Cook, stirring often, breaking the tomatoes into pieces with your spoon, until the sauce starts to thicken, about 10 minutes. Season the chicken with the remaining ½ teaspoon salt and nestle the pieces in the sauce. Reduce the heat to a gentle simmer, cover, and cook until the sauce thickens slightly and the chicken is cooked through (an instant-read thermometer should register 165°F/75°C when inserted in the thickest part of the chicken), 10 to 15 minutes.

continued

Don't go too far, you want the dish to still be brothy. Discard the rosemary sprigs.

3. Serve in shallow bowls. Sprinkle with more pepper, if you like, and drizzle with the pesto.

TIP: *If you happen to have a cherry pitter—a handheld tool that efficiently punches out the pit like a stapler—you can use it to pit olives, too. If not, the type of olive you are pitting will dictate the best method. For soft, oily olives with tender flesh, just squeeze the olive between your thumb and forefinger and the pit will pop out. For meatier, more hefty olives, like Castelvetranos, lay them on a cutting board and smash them with the flat side of a chef's knife. If the pit doesn't pop out right away, finish by using your fingers.*

OLIVE OIL SMOKE POINTS

It's true that high-heat cooking can blunt the antioxidant activity of the polyphenols in olive oil and break down its healthy fats. But olive oil can withstand more heat than you may think. The fats in extra-virgin olive oils can tolerate temperatures as high as 375°F (190°C), making them a good choice for almost all of the cooking in your kitchen.

There are more reasons to keep temperatures low, too. Low-and-slow methods like braising, poaching, and slow cooking are brain-friendly cooking techniques (see page 145) that preserve the nutrients in all foods, which makes them perfectly suited for cooking with extra-virgin olive oil.

If you want to cook with your high-end extra-virgin oil, it's best to use gentle methods like low-temperature sautéing. Adding it in the last few minutes of cooking at low heat, as in the warm olives (page 320), is a good option, too, since that won't damage the oil's polyphenols and flavor. Ideally, your high-end olive oil is better suited for raw preparations like salad dressings and sauces or for drizzling on foods that have already been cooked because its health-promoting properties are part of the reason high-end olive oil costs more. Don't let me dissuade you from dipping into your best olive oil frequently in your cooking, but use it gently.

For high-heat cooking—roasting above 400°F (200°C), brushing grilled foods, frying, searing, and high-heat sautéing, use a cooking oil with a higher smoke point, such as avocado or pecan oil. (See the Cooking Oils Pyramid on page 315.)

SALTED CHOCOLATE AND OLIVE OIL GELATO

MAKES 6 CUPS (1.4 KG)

2 cups (300 g) raw cashews, soaked in warm water for at least an hour

Two 13.5-ounce (398 ml) cans unsweetened coconut milk

⅔ cup (80 g) natural cacao powder

⅔ cup (160 ml) extra-virgin olive oil, plus more for drizzling

½ cup (120 ml) pure maple syrup

2 tablespoons vodka (optional)

1 teaspoon almond extract

½ teaspoon kosher salt

Flaky salt, to finish

Cacao nibs

While tasting plant-based gelatos as part of my culinary training in Italy (I know, hard work!), I learned to use a bright and fruity olive oil to round out the bitterness that's inherent to high-quality dark cacao. And because this "gelato" forgoes classic ingredients like cow's milk and cream, the olive oil adds a silky texture while providing brain-healthy fats. The magical part, though, comes from the interplay of the oil's grassy and peppery nuances, which magnify the cacao's floral and berry qualities. The resulting gelato is sweet but not cloying and, thanks to natural cacao powder, full of decadent chocolate flavor.

If you don't have an ice cream machine, you can get nearly the same results by stirring the gelato as it sets up in the freezer. The optional addition of vodka keeps the gelato from freezing solid, which makes it easier to scoop. If you omit the alcohol, store any leftover gelato in single-serving portions in the freezer for built-in portion control and ease of softening.

The toppings make this dessert truly spectacular. A drizzle of olive oil accentuates the fruitiness of the cacao, a small sprinkle of salt intensifies the sweetness, while cacao nibs—slightly bitter bits of fermented and roasted cacao beans—add crunch.

1. If using an ice cream machine, freeze the container until solid.

2. Drain the cashews and place them in a blender with the coconut milk. Blend on high speed until completely smooth, about 2 minutes. Add the cacao powder, oil, maple syrup, vodka (if using), almond extract, and kosher salt. Blend on high speed until it is the consistency of melted ice cream, about 1 minute.

continued

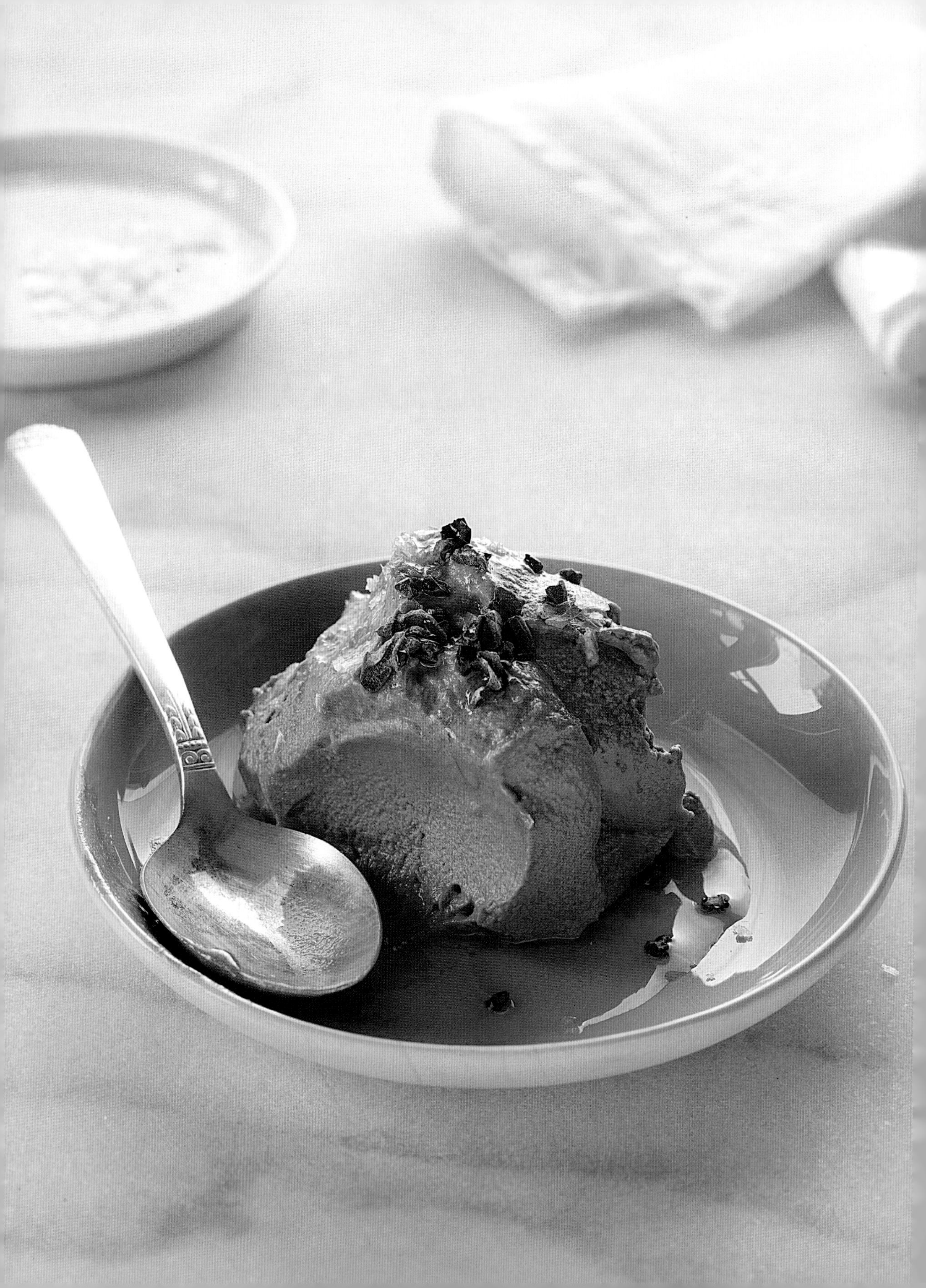

3. Pour the gelato base into your ice cream maker and churn until you have the consistency of soft-serve. Or pour into a container with deep sides—such as a 9-by-13-by-2-inch (33 by 22.8 by 5 cm) glass baking dish—and place in the freezer until it starts to become more solid than liquid, about 1 hour. Stir with a fork to break up the crystals, scraping them from the sides of the pan. Repeat once each hour, and every 30 minutes after that, until you have the consistency of soft-serve ice cream, up to 4 hours. Serve right away or freeze solid for later.

4. To serve, allow the gelato to soften at room temperature until glossy and easy to scoop, at least 10 minutes. Drizzle each serving with oil, then sprinkle with flaky salt and cacao nibs.

5. To store, scrape the gelato into an airtight container, press a piece of parchment or waxed paper against the surface, cover, and freeze for up to 3 weeks.

USING OLIVE OIL TO TREAT MEMORY PROBLEMS

If you swallow a spoonful of good olive oil and feel a pleasantly peppery burn on the back of the throat, that's an oil high in brain-healthy polyphenols. Part of the flavonoid family of plant nutrients, polyphenols contain one or more phenolic hydroxyl groups. Most high-end extra-virgin oils possess more of the polyphenols essential for brain health than lower-grade oils. One polyphenol in particular—oleocanthal—has been found to block inflammatory pathways in the body as effectively as a dose of ibuprofen. This makes extra-virgin olive oil a potent anti-inflammatory food.

A fresh, unfiltered olive oil will have the highest polyphenol content of all. Bottled right from the olive press, these oils (sometimes called "early harvest" or "high phenolic type olive oil") have a deep green color and a bold aroma, and they may even be a little cloudy due to the small pieces of olives. This category of olive oil has been studied for its ability to improve cognitive symptoms in early Alzheimer's. In one randomized, controlled trial from Greece, participants with mild cognitive impairment given 2 tablespoons (50 ml) of unfiltered olive oil daily did better on cognitive testing, such as memory and recall skills, than those given filtered oil with a moderate polyphenol content and those following a Mediterranean diet without supplemental olive oil.

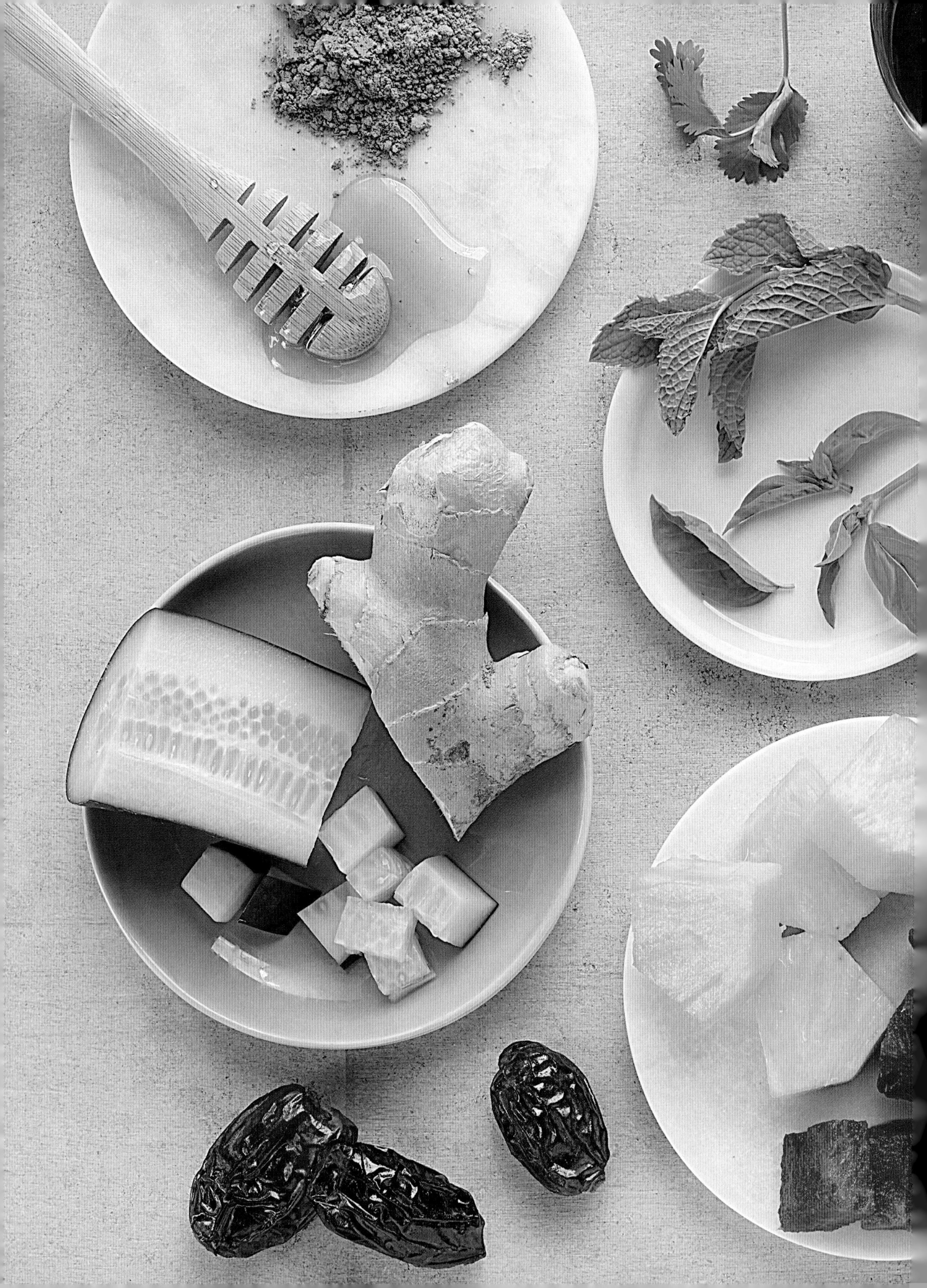

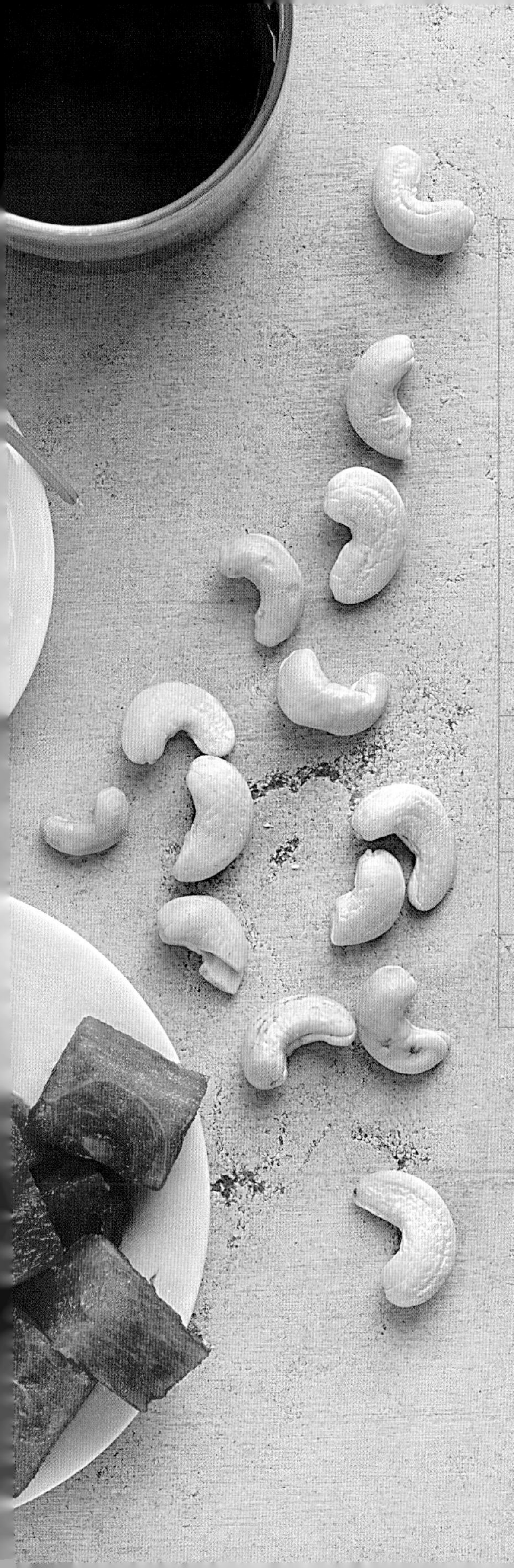

COFFEE, TEA, AND OTHER DRINKS

While knowing what to eat for brain health can be complex, what to drink is refreshingly straightforward. The best way to hydrate your brain is to drink plain water throughout the day. Even a small amount of dehydration (3 to 4 percent) can cause brain fog, fatigue, headaches, and mood swings. Make water your beverage of choice, and your brain will perform better and age more gracefully.

So many products are marketed to be brain-boosting beverages. Coffee, tea, juice, energy drinks, alcoholic beverages, and an infinite list of bubbly and fizzy drinks claim health benefits, but only some of these drinks can complement your neuroprotective diet. Once you know the details about what's brain healthy or brain harming, it's simple to navigate the world of beverages.

The five recipes in this chapter each play a role in helping you stay hydrated while also providing key brain health nutrients. Not only will they add a splash of refreshment and color to your day, they serve as better-for-you alternatives to drinks like fancy coffee shop lattes or alcoholic beverages.

Get into the habit of drinking water consistently throughout the day, starting with a glass first thing in the morning. Most people require 8 to 10 cups (about 2 L) of water each day, more if physically active. As you get older, your brain requires more water, too. Meeting most of your hydration needs during the day (before the evening meal) assures you'll maintain a high level of energy without the need for sleep-interrupting bathroom breaks from guzzling water before bed.

Eating water-rich foods can help hydrate your brain. Watermelon, not surprisingly, has the highest water content (93 percent) and is rich in brain-healthy lycopene, too. Other water-rich foods that provide brain health benefits include cantaloupe, celery, cucumbers, lettuces, peaches, strawberries, and raw zucchini.

The best type of water to drink is the kind that tastes good to you. Ideally, your tap will provide water you can drink straight up. If it has an off taste, as many municipal waters do, filter it yourself with a device that screws into your faucet or by letting it drain through a filtered pitcher. If you have concerns about your tap water, have it tested to rule out harmful chemicals.

If plain water doesn't do it for you, give it a flavor boost with a splash of pomegranate juice or a squeeze of lemon. If you enjoy the fizz of a sparkling beverage, these are a good way to mix up your water intake. There are a plethora of choices: sparkling, seltzer, club soda, and soda water are all carbonated water with or without minerals. Avoid tonic water, though—it is not really water but a mixer that also contains quinine and added sugar.

Skip bottled water, which not only gets expensive but also creates wasteful plastic and glass bottles. If you do need to buy water, for instance when you are traveling, spring water is best. Avoid purified water, which is devoid of minerals, and beware of flavored waters—many have added sugar.

Coconut water is extracted from young green coconuts into an electrolyte-rich drink. It's more like juice than water, though. Even unsweetened coconut water has as much as 9 grams of sugar (about 2 teaspoons) per 8-ounce (240 ml) cup. Coconut water is too sugary to become a fixture in your brain-protective diet; drink sparingly, if at all.

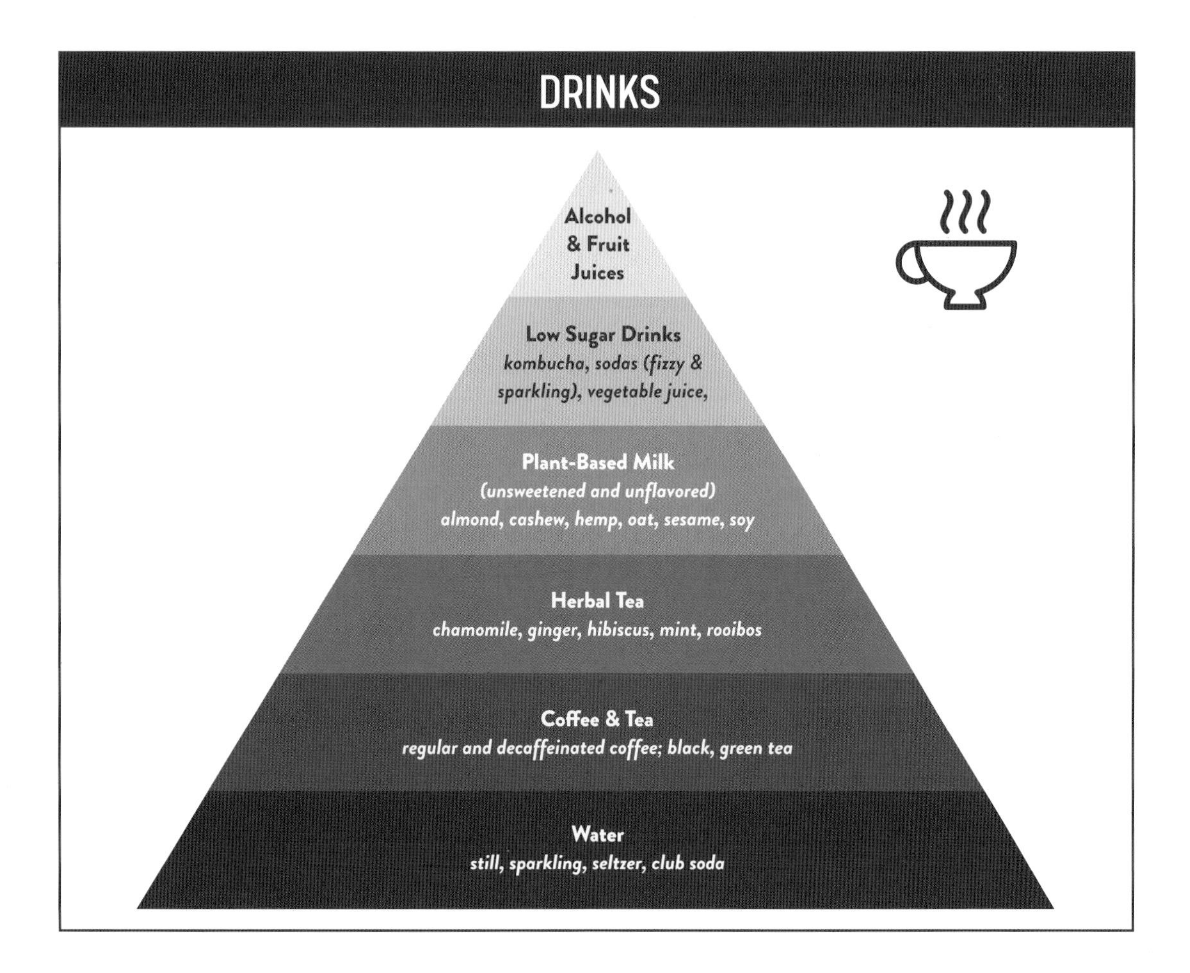

TEA

Black, green, oolong, and white teas are varieties of tea from the same plant—*Camellia sinensis*—that provide an abundance of polyphenols, such as catechins, theaflavins, tannins, and flavonoids. These phytonutrients specifically protect the brain by blocking oxidative stress and combating the accumulation of amyloid protein in the brain.

The tea leaves and buds are left to oxidize after harvest, a process that determines their polyphenol makeup and caffeine content. Longer oxidation creates more caffeine and blunts the amount of polyphenols. Black tea, for instance, is the most highly caffeinated of the teas but has fewer polyphenols; with 40 to 60 milligrams of caffeine per 8-ounce (240 ml) cup, it contains about half the caffeine as a cup of coffee. Green tea has half the caffeine as black and twice the polyphenols, thanks to a shorter oxidation process. White and oolong teas fall somewhere between black and green. Processing not only tweaks the phytonutrients in tea, it alters its taste, bringing out a huge spectrum of flavors from bold and woodsy to delicate and floral.

The caffeine in tea and other foods is both a phytonutrient with beneficial brain actions and a stimulant (see the Caffeine sidebar on page 347).

Green tea deserves special mention as a particularly good brain-healthy beverage. While all teas are rich in polyphenols, green tea has more than twice

HERBAL "TEA"

Herbal teas come from steeping flowers, herbs, spices, and fruit in water; basically any plant can be turned into an herbal tea. Their brain health virtue comes from being able to hydrate you on par with plain water plus offering whatever phytonutrients come from their particular plant. Hibiscus flowers, for example, make a bittersweet infusion that can lower blood pressure to the same degree as medication (see the Science Bite on page 353). Chamomile tea is thought to have calming properties, making it a good choice for drinking before bed. Other teas made from plants with brain health nutrients include peppermint, rooibos, passionflower, ginger, and sage.

Herbal teas can be a welcome addition to your brain-healthy dietary pattern. Just don't confuse them with real tea—those made from the *Camellia sinensis* plant and known to possess particularly brain-beneficial nutrients.

as much epigallocatechin-3-gallate (EGCG), one of the most neuroprotective types. EGCG's brain benefit is amplified by the way your body metabolizes it. It first exerts a direct anti-inflammatory and antiamyloid action in the brain. Then it is metabolized in the gut, where your friendly microbiota create even more anti-inflammatory substances that make their way back to the brain. This powerful EGCG two-for-one mechanism may explain why green tea drinkers enjoy lower rates of age-related cognitive decline when compared to drinkers of other types of tea. With 25 to 35 milligrams of caffeine per 8-ounce (240 ml) cup, green tea is mildly caffeinated.

Green tea is the brain-friendliest tea, with matcha being the top of the line within green teas. That's because matcha is made by grinding up whole green tea leaves, not just infusing them in water. The tea is shade grown to optimize the development of its signature grassy flavor as well as its concentration of polyphenols, especially EGCG.

You'll find matcha in two general grades: the highest-quality ceremonial grade (good for drinking straight up as tea) to the less-expensive culinary grade (good for lattes and baking). Avoid matcha that includes added sugar and stabilizers, which are often included to keep the powder from clumping.

Whatever tea you like to drink, do so often. Studies show that the more tea you drink, especially green tea, the lower your risk of Alzheimer's and other dementias.

COFFEE

Coffee contains more than two hundred bioactive substances, many of which are neuroprotective. As a group, coffee drinkers worldwide have been extensively studied with regard to cancer, mortality, and heart and brain health. Drinking three or more cups of coffee per day is associated with a 21 percent lower risk of dying from heart disease and an 18 percent lower risk of dying from any cause. Most of these studies were done with brewed (drip) coffee, but espresso is also thought to be a beneficial way to drink coffee.

Drinking coffee can help you fend off Alzheimer's and other types of dementia, especially Parkinson's disease. Studies show that the risk of cognitive decline goes down with each cup of coffee consumed each day, with a maximum benefit at about four cups. When researchers looked at coffee

BRAIN-HEALTHY TIPS FOR ENJOYING COFFEE

GO FRESH. Seek out freshly roasted coffee beans with a roast date stamped on the label; store in an airtight container and use within about four weeks. Coffee becomes stale with age, losing its bright flavors and much of its antioxidant power. Choose organic to minimize your pesticide exposure, especially if you are a frequent coffee drinker. Other stamps of approval—Fair Trade, Bird Friendly, and Rainforest Alliance—indicate the coffee grower follows ethical treatment of laborers and planet-friendly practices. Avoid any burnt-tasting coffee, which may have spent too much time in the roaster, a process that can rack up AGEs.

DRINK IT BLACK AND UNSWEETENED. These studies mostly look at the impact of drinking black coffee; adding sugar and creamers would confound the results. Dairy products may deactivate the antioxidants in coffee, while sugar turns it into a brain-harming beverage. Enjoy your coffee black or with just a splash of plant-based milk, and wean off sweeteners. (The recipe for Cashew Coffee on page 349 is designed for just that.)

DRINK MINDFULLY. Many studies on coffee's benefits were done in countries where coffee drinking is a social activity. It's difficult to tease out the impact of the actual coffee from the beneficial effect of gathering with friends daily or pausing to enjoy a cup solo. Make your coffee routine a practice in mindfulness rather than gulp it from a to-go cup as you dash off to work. Whenever possible, enjoy coffee in the company of others.

USE A FILTER. How you brew your coffee may have an impact on harmful blood cholesterol. Unfiltered coffee contains dipterans, compounds that can raise cholesterol and possibly attenuate long-term health benefits. Use a filter to brew your coffee, and reserve French press or Turkish unfiltered coffee for rare occasions. Espresso impacts cholesterol somewhere between filtered and unfiltered; because it's made so quickly, the beans aren't in contact with the water long enough to accumulate high levels of dipterans.

BOOST IT. Adding anti-inflammatory spices to your coffee can boost both flavor and nutrition. Add half a teaspoon of ground turmeric, cardamom, cinnamon, or nutmeg to coffee grounds before brewing. Or grind three whole cardamom pods with the beans. Skip the trend of adding butter and/or MCT oil (a supplement that contains medium-chain triglycerides) to coffee; both contain high amounts of saturated fat.

DON'T WASTE IT. Don't toss what's left in the pot—tremendous planetary resources go into growing high-quality coffee. As soon as it's cool, store in an airtight container in the fridge for up to one day or the freezer for up to three months. Use leftover coffee to make the Coffee Berry Smoothie on page 79 or the Coffee, Date, and Oat Bars on page 277. Or make coffee "nice cream" by blending with frozen ripe bananas and cacao powder.

drinkers' brains with high-tech brain scans to measure the amyloid deposition, they found a linear relationship: starting at two more cups of coffee per day, less amyloid was detected in the brain over time. Caffeine has been shown to have antiamyloid action, but one of the flavonoids—quercetin—may be the primary player. Studies suggest that decaffeinated coffee is also neuroprotective. Drink more than six cups a day, though, and one study showed a reduction in brain volume over time.

Even though coffee is mostly water, it won't hydrate you like water. Caffeine has a mild diuretic effect, meaning it acts on the kidneys to excrete more water. Take a tip from the Italians, who always serve espresso with a small glass of sparkling water. They drink the espresso in two or three swallows, then chase it with the water all in one gulp.

JUICE

A daily juice habit may seem like a good way to get an extra dose of vitamins, but in reality, most juices contain too much sugar to be good for your brain.

CAFFEINE

Caffeine wakes you up because it tricks the brain into thinking you are out of adenosine, a brain chemical that calms you down and makes you feel sleepy. By blocking adenosine receptors, caffeine opens the door for other brain-sparking neurotransmitters to flow freely, giving you a surge of energy. Caffeine consumption is proven to increase mental agility, like the ability to do well on a memory test. But does this mean it protects memory long term? Studies are mixed; some show that regular caffeine drinkers have a reduced risk of age-related cognitive decline while others don't. Caffeine's most important role may be to amplify the action of polyphenols in coffee and tea, helping them act as even more effective antioxidants for brain health protection.

Caffeinated beverages are not for everyone. Each person possesses a genetically determined ability to metabolize caffeine slowly or rapidly. Slow metabolizers may be more sensitive to the effects of caffeine, leading to sleep disruption, heart palpitations, irritability, and anxiety. Decaffeinated coffee and tea is just as good for you; taking out the caffeine doesn't reduce the beneficial polyphenols.

Juicing fruits and sugary vegetables (like carrots and beets) removes almost all their fiber. The natural sugars are concentrated in liquid form and, without a fiber matrix to slow absorption, create a blood sugar surge. The juice does retain many beneficial phytonutrients, but these become deactivated quickly.

Studies show that drinking fruit juice (such as apple, orange, and grapefruit) can be just as detrimental to your brain as other sugary drinks. When a population of healthy, middle-aged men and women were studied, a daily fruit juice habit was associated with smaller total brain volume, poorer episodic memory, and smaller hippocampal volume. Researchers estimate that drinking juice on a regular basis adds between three and thirteen years of age to the brain's episodic memory.

Vegetable juices like celery and spinach are lower in sugar and can be a good source of phytonutrients if freshly pressed. Without fiber, however, these nutrients are less bioavailable, so juice doesn't count as a serving of vegetables.

If you enjoy drinking juice, stick to small servings (about 5 ounces/150 ml up to three times a week) of freshly squeezed or pressed juice. Avoid juice in bottles and cans. Combining juice with food will lessen its impact on blood sugar levels and may help you absorb more of its phytonutrients, minerals, and vitamins. Vegetable juices are wonderful to cook with, as in the carrot juice used like a stock in the Creamy Carrot Farrotto (page 259).

BRAIN-HARMING DRINKS

There's no controversy whatsoever about the role of sweet drinks on both short- and long-term brain health: the more sugar-sweetened and artificially sweetened drinks you consume, the greater your risk of stroke and dementia. This includes soda pop, diet soda, sugar-flavored water, energy drinks, sweet tea, lemonade, juice drinks, sports drinks, sweetened milks, and the list goes on and on. Kombucha—a fermented tea with live microorganisms—can be a brain-healthy choice, but some are loaded with added sugar. Approach all drinks marketed to be brain-healthy with a high degree of skepticism (see page 342). As always, go straight to the ingredient list and the nutrition label. A low-sugar drink should have no added sugar and contain less than 5 percent of the daily value (DV) of total sugars.

CREAMY CASHEW COFFEE

SERVES 2

¼ cup (40 g) raw, unsalted cashews

2 cups (480 ml) hot freshly brewed coffee

1 teaspoon honey (optional)

Pinch of kosher salt (optional)

For those who love a splash of cream in their coffee, adding dairy can be a difficult habit to quit. Enter this cashew-based take on a café au lait, which substitutes the nuts for creamer. (Bonus: Cashews last a lot longer than a jug of milk!) The key is a high-powered blender, which whizzes the cashews and coffee into a silky drink.

Combine the cashews, coffee, honey (if using), and salt (if using) in a blender and blend on high speed until completely smooth and frothy, 1 to 2 minutes. Enjoy hot or pour into a glass jar and chill in the refrigerator; shake well before serving over ice.

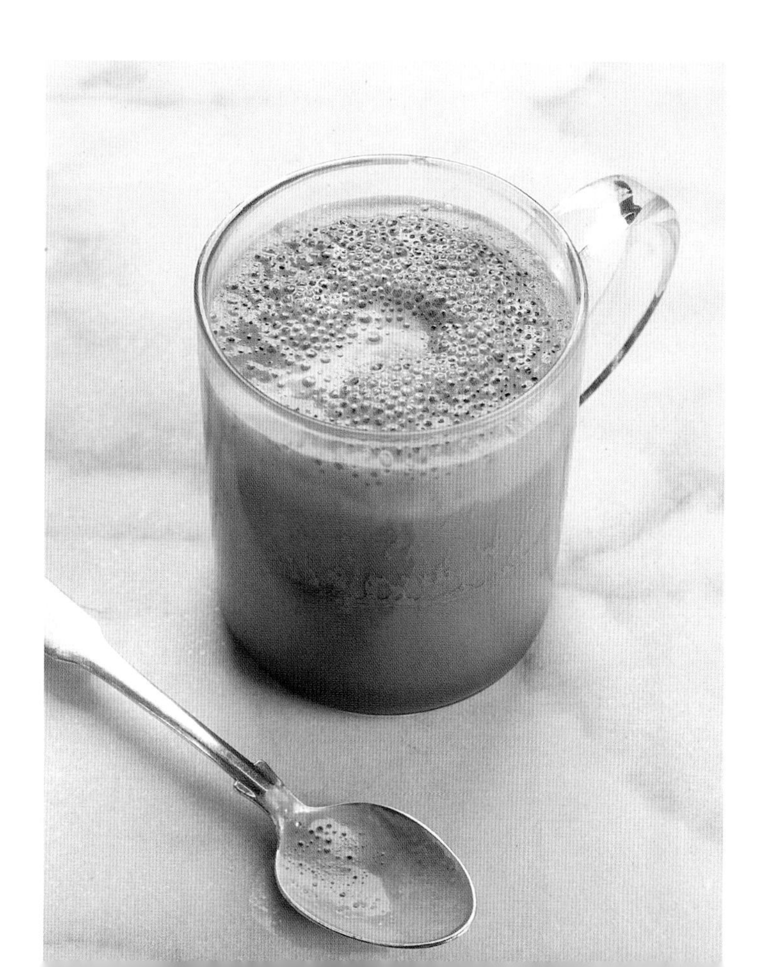

ICED OAT MILK AND MATCHA LATTE

SERVES 2

1 cup (140 g) fresh or frozen blackberries, plus a few for serving

½ cup (120 ml) cold water

½ teaspoon ground cardamom

¼ cup (60 ml) boiling water

1 teaspoon culinary-grade matcha green tea powder

Ice

1½ cups (360 ml) oat milk

Matcha tea rightfully has a reputation for being health promoting, but the popular matcha lattes are usually loaded with added sugar. This pretty, layered version is sweetened with a blackberry syrup and swirled with oat milk. While this ice-cold latte is a natural choice in summer when the blackberries are at their sweetest, you can make the syrup with frozen berries or substitute blueberries instead.

Each latte contains about 30 milligrams of caffeine, roughly equivalent to ¼ cup (60 ml) of coffee.

1. To make the blackberry syrup, bring the blackberries and cold water to a boil in a small saucepan over high heat. Reduce to a low simmer, sprinkle with the cardamom, and cook, stirring often, until the berries soften and collapse, 8 to 10 minutes. Smash the berries with the back of a spoon. Cook until you have a thick syrup that coats the spoon, another 5 to 7 minutes. Transfer the syrup into a small jar and chill in the refrigerator until ready to use.

2. To prepare the tea, pour the boiling water into a small bowl and let cool for about 1 minute. (A temperature of 175°F/80°C is optimal for matcha.) Sprinkle with the matcha powder and whisk until no lumps remain, about 30 seconds.

3. Divide the blackberry syrup between two 10-ounce (295 ml) glasses. Top with ice to reach halfway up the glass, then top with the oat milk, dividing evenly. Set a small fine-mesh strainer over one glass and slowly pour half the matcha over top. Repeat with the second glass. Top with a few whole berries and serve right away with long spoons or straws.

TIPS: *If you prefer a smoother syrup, smash the blackberries more thoroughly (breaking up all the drupelets) and strain before chilling.*

Make a double batch of syrup for more lattes later in the week; store in an airtight container in the fridge for up to five days.

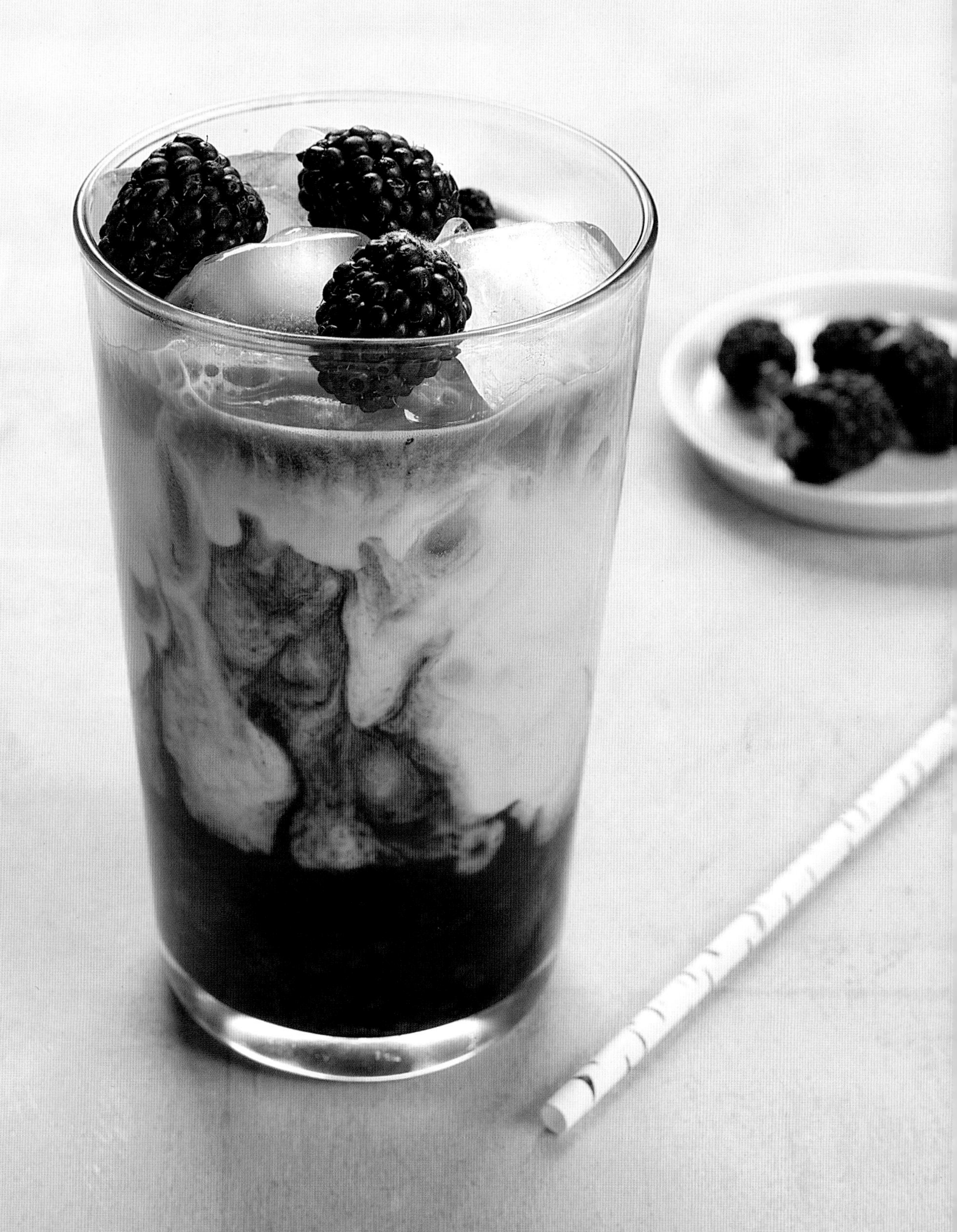

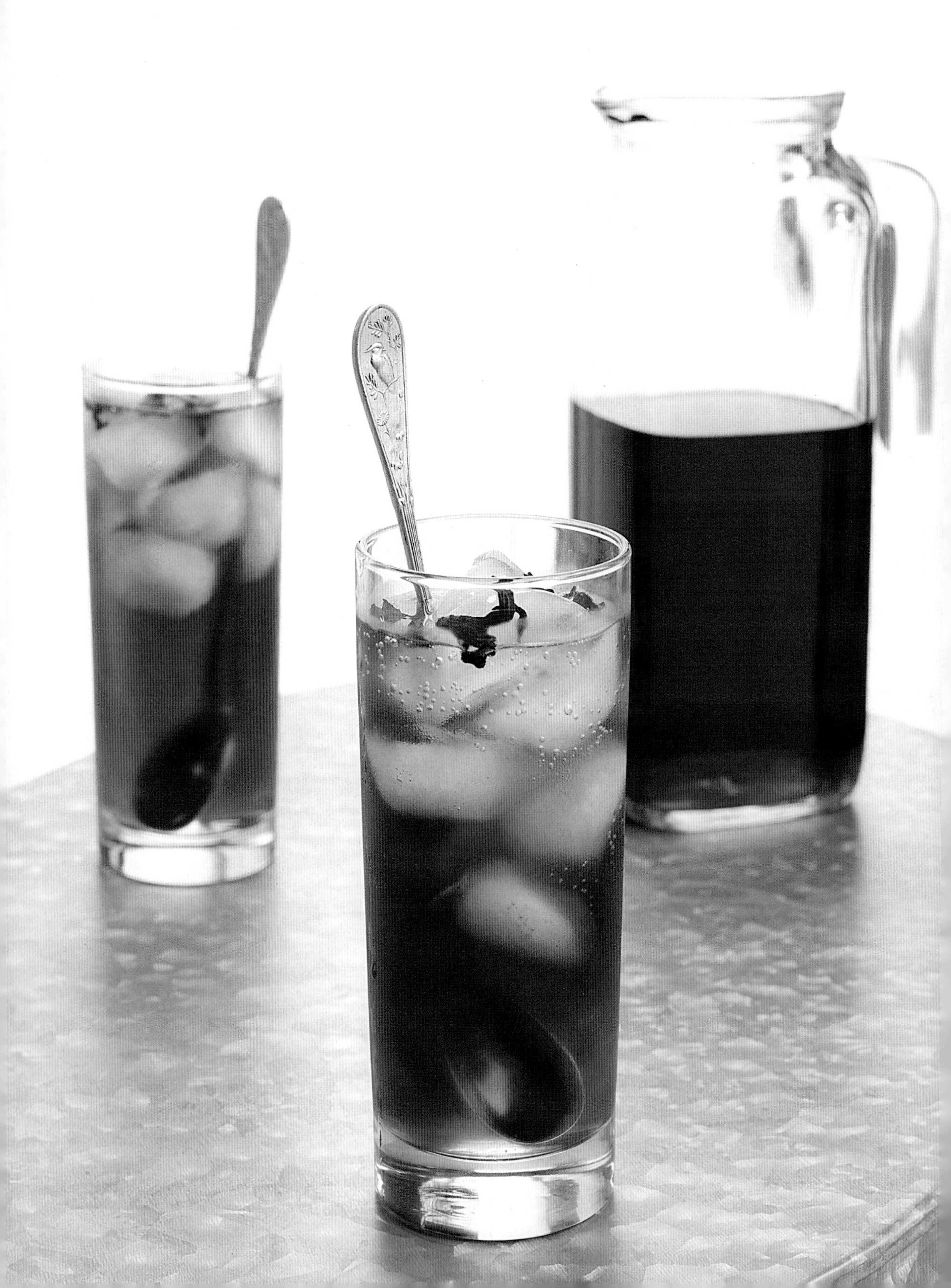

HOT HIBISCUS ICED TEA

SERVES 4

4 cups (1 L) water

2 tablespoons dried hibiscus flowers or 6 hibiscus tea bags

One 2-inch (5 cm) piece fresh ginger, thinly sliced

¼ teaspoon cayenne

Ice

Sparkling water

Everything about this spicy iced tea—from its vibrant red color to its kick from cayenne and ginger—is irresistible. Caffeine-free, it's also a good candidate for a stress-reducing, nonalcoholic beverage.

The phytonutrients in hibiscus have potent blood pressure–lowering properties. If you take blood pressure medication or have naturally low blood pressure, sip slowly and enjoy with food (see the Science Bite).

1. Combine the water, hibiscus, ginger, and cayenne in a small pot and bring to a boil over high heat. Cover and steep away from the heat for about 10 minutes.

2. Place a small fine-mesh strainer over a bowl. Strain the tea infusion into the bowl and discard the rest of the solids. Chill in the refrigerator until ready to use.

3. For each drink, fill a 10-ounce (295 ml) glass halfway with ice and add 1 cup (240 ml) cold tea. Top with sparkling water and gently stir.

TIP: *If using loose-leaf dried hibiscus, set aside a few flowers after straining to garnish the drink.*

SCIENCE BITE:

HIBISCUS TEA LOWERS BLOOD PRESSURE

Keeping blood pressure at a healthy low level prevents Alzheimer's later in life. In a meta-analysis published in the *Journal of Hypertension*, five studies investigating the impact of hibiscus tea on blood pressure underwent scrutiny, confirming that the herb significantly reduces both systolic and diastolic blood pressures. In one study, drinking one cup of hibiscus tea twice a day lowered blood pressure just as well as medication. This antihypertensive effect probably comes from its rich anthocyanin (page 60) content and its ability to form nitrate compounds that make blood vessels more open and pliable.

HERB GARDEN AGUA FRESCA

SERVES 4

2 cups (370 g) cubed pineapple

2 cups (170 g) chopped cucumber

2 cups (480 ml) water

1 cup (20 g) fresh herbs (I like a mix of cilantro, mint, and basil), plus leaves for garnish

¼ cup (60 ml) fresh lime juice

3 pitted Medjool dates (about ¼ cup/50 g), soaked in ½ cup (120 ml) hot water for 30 minutes

¼ teaspoon kosher salt

Ice

This incredibly refreshing drink will keep you feeling sharp by fending off the brain fog that comes from dehydration. Inspired by the sweet fruit drinks served in Mexico and Central America, where *agua fresca* means "cool water," this version is barely sweet from pineapple and dates and includes not just fruit but cucumbers and a mix of any leafy green herbs you like—such as basil, mint, cilantro, and parsley.

This drink is best when enjoyed right away. To save for later, strain it to retain its vibrant green color. Add seltzer for a sparkling refresher, or use your agua fresca as the base for a cocktail.

1. If you plan to strain the agua fresca (see Tip), set a fine-mesh strainer or nut milk bag over a large pitcher.

2. Combine the pineapple, cucumber, water, herbs, lime juice, dates and their soaking water, and salt in a blender. Blend on high speed until frothy and uniformly light green, about 2 minutes. If straining, pour through the strainer, pressing on the solids with the back of a spoon to squeeze out all the juice. Otherwise, pour directly into a pitcher.

3. Serve right away over ice, garnished with a few herb leaves per glass. Or chill in the refrigerator and serve within a few hours.

TIP: *If straining, freeze the pulp to add to your next smoothie.*

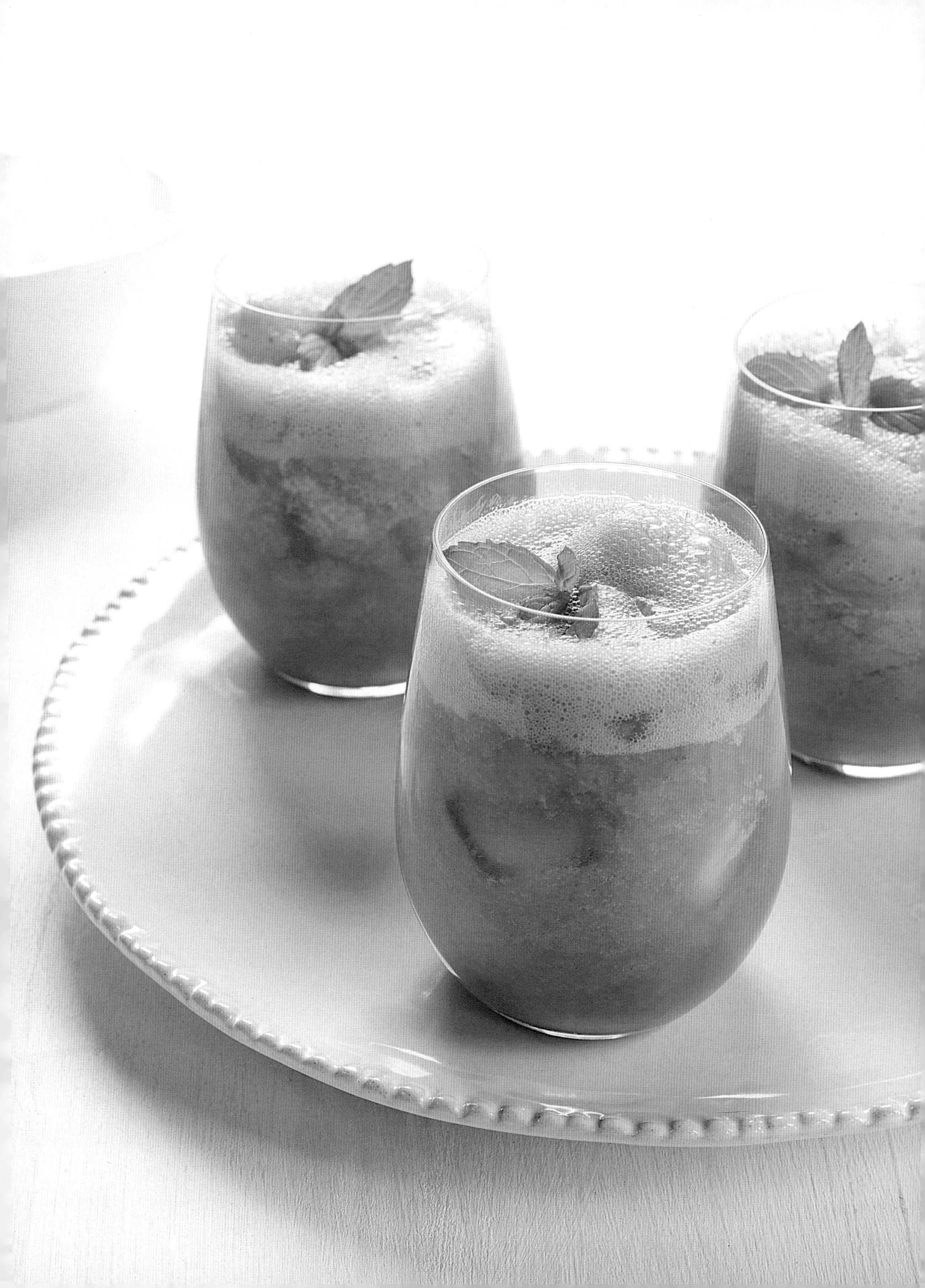

ALCOHOL AND THE BRAIN

You've probably heard that drinking alcohol, specifically red wine, may have brain health benefits. And yet you may also know that alcohol is a depressant, a huge source of addiction and disability, and can be neurotoxic in large quantities. All true! How can one substance be both good and bad for the brain? Like most drugs, dosage is paramount when understanding how alcohol impacts the brain.

Even though red wine is the most studied, it is now thought that all types of alcoholic beverages have a similar impact on the brain. Whether you drink wine, beer, or spirits, what matters most is the quantity of alcohol consumed; in other words—your drinking pattern.

Just like you follow a dietary pattern, if you consume alcoholic beverages, you have a drinking pattern. The Centers for Disease Control and Prevention defines drinking as:

- Light drinking: One to six drinks per week
- Moderate drinking: Seven drinks a week for women, up to fourteen for men
- Heavy drinking: Three or more drinks in one day or more than seven per week for women; more than four drinks in one day or more than fourteen per week for men
- Alcohol use disorder: Inability to stop or control alcohol consumption

Many people are surprised to learn what counts as a drink. A standard glass of wine, for example, is 5 fluid ounces (150 ml). This is equivalent, in actual alcohol content, to 12 ounces (355 ml) of beer and 1.5 ounces (45 ml) of distilled spirits (such as rum, gin, tequila, vodka, or whiskey).

So, how much alcohol is safe to drink? Studies consistently show that heavy drinking is bad for the brain with lower brain volumes and higher rates of Alzheimer's. Historically, many (but not all) studies support that light to moderate drinking has a mild protective effect on the brain.

Now, in the largest brain imaging studies to date with more than 36,000 healthy participants in the UK Biobank, researchers report that even light drinking may be harmful. They found a linear relationship between alcohol intake and brain shrinkage. In other words, the more one drinks, the more the brain shrinks over time, even in light drinkers.

While the study of alcohol and Alzheimer's is complex and not all studies are consistent, most agree on the following:

- Heavy drinking increases the risk of cognitive decline. Light to moderate drinking may not be as brain-protective as was previously thought. Even lower levels of alcohol consumption have been associated with brain shrinkage (a strong marker for cognitive decline).
- If light drinking does confer some brain health benefit, it may be most powerful between the ages of forty-five and sixty-five.
- Women and men metabolize alcohol differently, and men may reap more of the cardiovascular benefits. Women at high risk for breast cancer should limit alcohol consumption.
- The brain health benefits of an alcoholic drink may have more to do with the conviviality of a shared social experience than the actual contents of the drink.

If you choose to include alcohol in your brain-protective lifestyle, do so with caution. Drink mindfully, not moderately. Keep your intake within the guidelines for light drinking. Be strategic about your intake to make sure you aren't tipping over the fine line between light drinking and moderate to heavy. Based on recent studies about how alcohol affects the brain, the difference between brain protection and brain damage can be measured in just a few drinks per week. When the drinking pattern consistently drifts into the heavy category, the brain loses white matter (the myelin-sheath extensions of neurons crucial for communication within the brain) and has a total lower brain volume, both findings consistent with age-related cognitive decline.

Even light drinking may not serve your brain-healthy lifestyle. Women are drinking more than in previous decades, a fact that may contribute to an already higher Alzheimer's risk in coming years. Small amounts of alcohol may be detrimental to the brain if you also have high blood pressure, are overweight, or carry one or two copies of the ApoE4 risk gene for Alzheimer's. If you have a family history of alcohol dependency, proceed with caution.

If you feel like you need to cut back on your drinking, make your stress-reducing end-of-the-day beverage one of the mocktails in this chapter, or stick to sparkling water with lots of fresh lime.

WATERMELON AND BASIL SHRUB

SERVES 4 TO 6

FOR THE SHRUB

Makes 3 cups (710 ml)

1½ pounds (680 g) watermelon, cut into 1-inch (2.5 cm) pieces (about 4 cups)

2 teaspoons raw honey

¼ teaspoon kosher salt

½ cup (120 ml) apple cider vinegar

TO MAKE ONE DRINK

¼ cup (5 g) fresh basil leaves

½ cup (120 ml) watermelon shrub

Ice

Sparkling water

Shrubs—a centuries-old type of fermented drink with roots in Victorian England and Persian cuisine—are a delicious, refreshing treat. This quick, lower-sugar version isn't fermented but has a similar flavor profile thanks to ripe watermelon and apple cider vinegar. Blending the whole fruit means you get more of watermelon's inherent brain-healthy nutrients, like lycopene (page 120) and vitamin C. The shrub comes together in minutes and keeps in the fridge for up to a week.

1. To make the shrub, combine the watermelon, honey, and salt in a blender and blend on high speed until completely smooth, about 1 minute. Pour into a quart (1 L) jar with the vinegar, cover tightly, and shake to combine. Chill in the fridge until ready to use.

2. To make one drink, set aside a few basil leaves for garnish and combine the rest in a 10-ounce (295 ml) glass with ½ cup (120 ml) shrub. Using a muddler or the back of a spoon, gently crush the basil until fragrant. Fill the glass with ice, top with sparkling water, and stir gently. Finish with a few whole basil leaves.

3. To store, refrigerate the watermelon shrub for up to 1 week. Separation is normal; shake well before using.

TO MAKE A BIG BATCH

Muddle 1½ cups (30 g) fresh basil with 3 cups (710 ml) shrub in the bottom of a large measuring cup. Chill thoroughly. To serve, pour into a punch bowl or medium pot over a jumbo-size ice cube. (Look for extra-large ice cube trays online, or simply fill a pint plastic container three-quarters full of water, freeze until solid, and slide out the giant ice cube.) Serve as above; makes about 6 drinks.

TIPS: *For a light cocktail, top with sparkling white wine instead of water.*

For a less-tart drink, use unseasoned rice vinegar instead of apple cider vinegar.

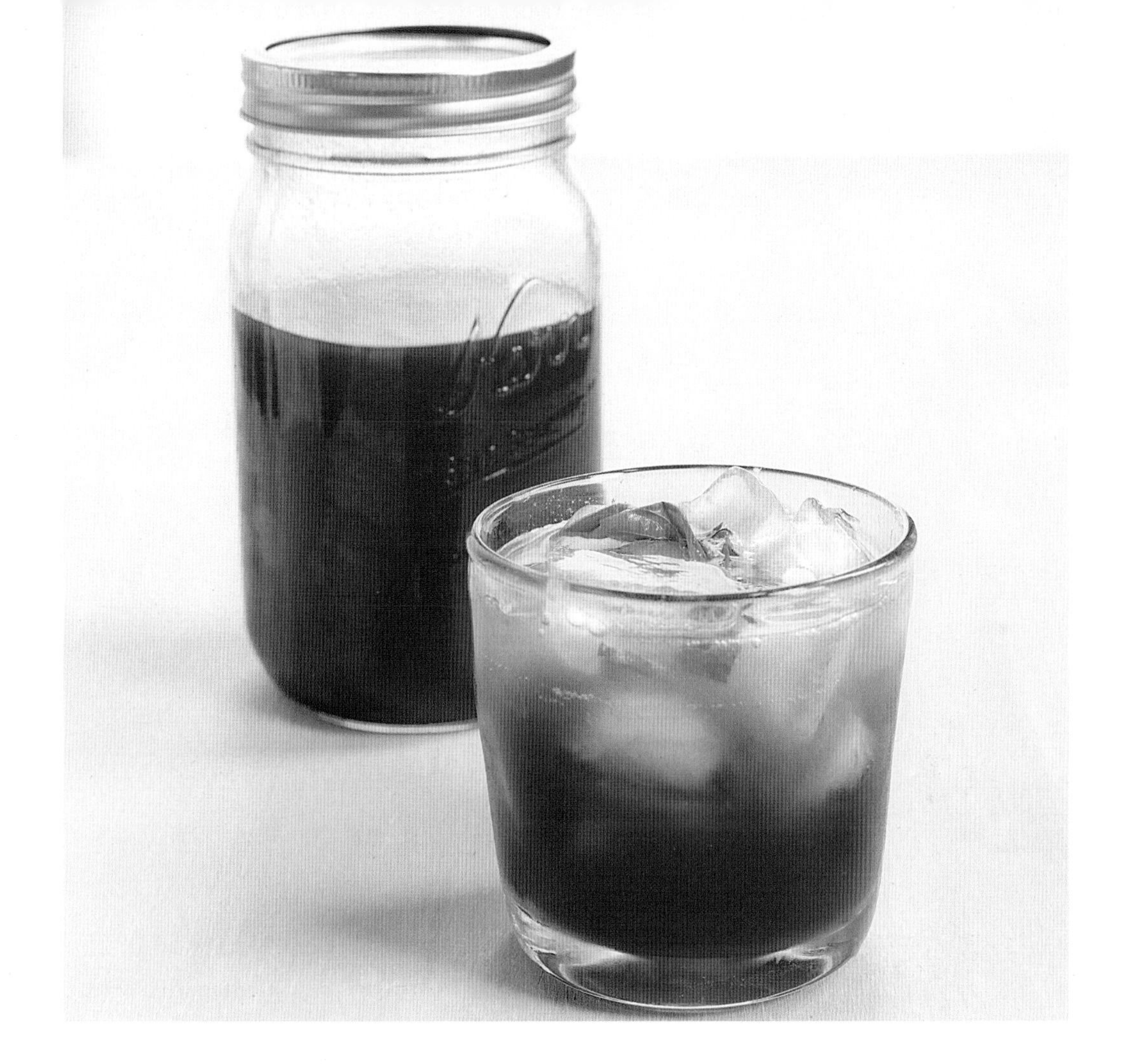

SCIENCE BITE:

APPLE CIDER VINEGAR

Apple cider vinegar may stabilize blood sugar levels after a meal. A recent meta-analysis of studies concluded that consuming vinegar (1 to 2 tablespoons diluted in water) after a carbohydrate-rich meal helps keep blood sugar levels stable, especially in those with type 2 diabetes or insulin resistance. And it held true not just for apple cider but for any vinegar with 5 percent acetic acid. This probably works because it slows digestion after a meal, allowing blood sugar to be absorbed more slowly. (Never drink vinegar straight up; it could damage tooth enamel and disrupt the gut microbiome.)

Choose a bottle with a cloudy collection of sediment at the bottom—called the mother—and you have a fermented food that also provides antioxidants, beneficial bacteria, and potassium.

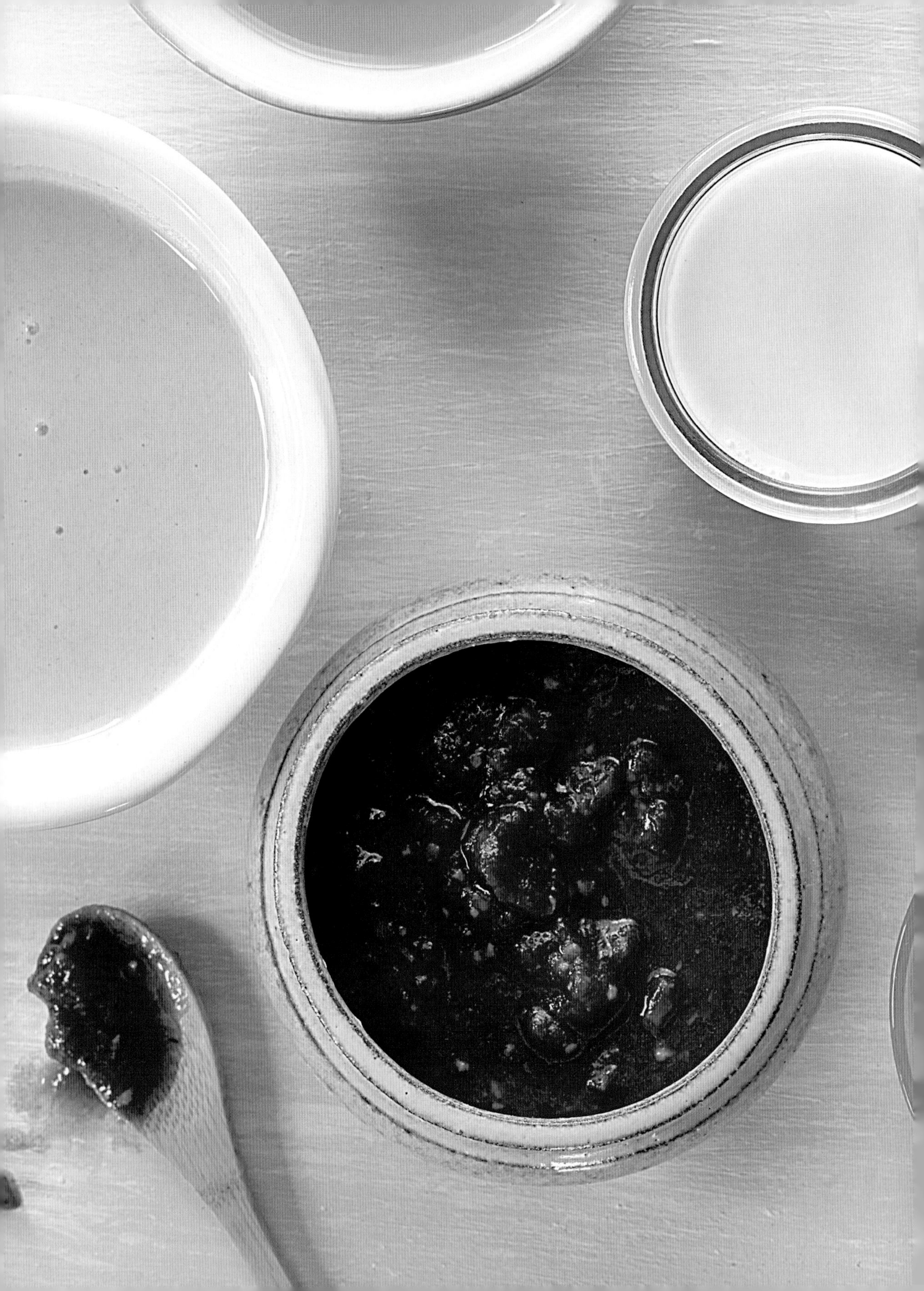

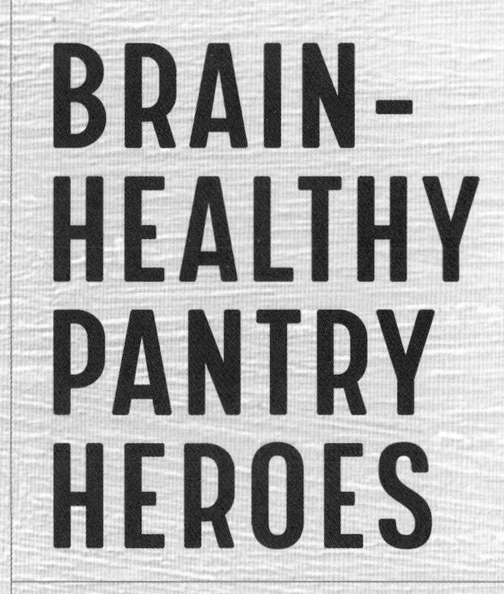

BRAIN-HEALTHY PANTRY HEROES

Your pantry is more than just ingredients. It's also the sauces, dressings, pestos, and core recipes that give your meals depth, personality, and an extra boost of brain health nutrition. Think of the recipes in this chapter as your pantry heroes that provide shortcuts to a delicious meal.

The nut-based milks, creams, and cheeses in this chapter are truly the secret to making dishes that have a pleasing texture and satisfying richness without saturated fat. The Almost Instant Cashew Cream (page 370), for instance, can replace the whipped cream on a bowl of berries or a slice of pie. Because it is nutrient-dense and full of brain-friendly fats, a little goes a long way. Or it can become a savory sour cream spiked with lime to dollop on tacos and beans. Likewise, cashew ricotta can play many roles in your cooking: as a better-for-you sandwich spread; in a garlic and chive dip; or as modern, more brain-healthy way to make your favorite Italian foods—manicotti, stuffed shells, lasagna—light and satisfying. Walnut "Parm" (page 184)—a crumbly nut topping that tastes like Parmesan cheese—could become your go-to flourish for pasta, salads, roasted vegetables, and, well, anywhere you'd use "real" Parmesan.

Some of these pantry hero recipes, like the nut milks, stocks, and marinara, can be store-bought. However, once you discover how easy they are to make, and how fresh they taste, I hope you'll decide to keep your pantry stocked with these homemade versions. If you are accustomed to putting cream (and/or sugar) in your coffee, the coffee creamer (page 365) can be an especially useful recipe to catapult your dietary pattern into a more brain-healthy one.

BASIC NUT MILK

MAKES 5 CUPS (1.2 L)

- **1½ cups raw, unsalted almonds (210 g), cashews (210 g), hazelnuts (195 g), pecans (150 g), pistachios (195 g), or walnuts (150 g)**
- **4 cups (1 L) water, plus more for soaking**
- **1 teaspoon pure vanilla extract or the scraped beans from half a vanilla bean**
- **1 teaspoon honey or 1 pitted Medjool date (optional)**
- **¼ teaspoon kosher salt**

The first time I tasted freshly made almond milk was on the streets of Sicily, where it's a traditional drink served from a kiosk on the street. Up until then, I had only tasted almond milk from a carton and had never considered making it myself. The taste won me over—as fresh as can be with the grassy, almost floral aroma of a just-cracked almond. So did the simplicity of turning almonds—or any other nut—into a nutrient-dense milky drink.

One of the perks of making nut milk at home: you get to control how many nuts go into each batch. This recipe for nut milk is a little thicker than store-bought because it contains a full day's serving (about ¼ cup/30 g) of nuts per cup of milk. If you use almonds or hazelnuts—especially high in the most potent form of vitamin E (d-alpha-tocopherol)—you also get a full day's supply of vitamin E. For a thinner milk (and to stretch your precious nut supply), use 1 cup (about 150 g) of nuts instead.

This recipe gives you the flexibility to make nut milk with a variety of nuts and even add seeds, if you like. You'll need a nut milk bag (see Resources, page 390) or a double layer of cheesecloth to strain the milk if making it from almonds, hazelnuts, or pistachios. Straining is optional with softer nuts, like cashews and pecans.

1. Place the nuts in a deep bowl and cover with water. For almonds, soak at room temperature for 8 to 12 hours. For softer nuts, like cashews, pecans, and walnuts, soak at room temperature for at least 2 hours and up to overnight. Rinse in a colander, discarding the soaking water.

2. Set a nut milk bag over a large bowl. Alternatively, line a colander with a double thickness of cheesecloth and place over a large bowl.

continued

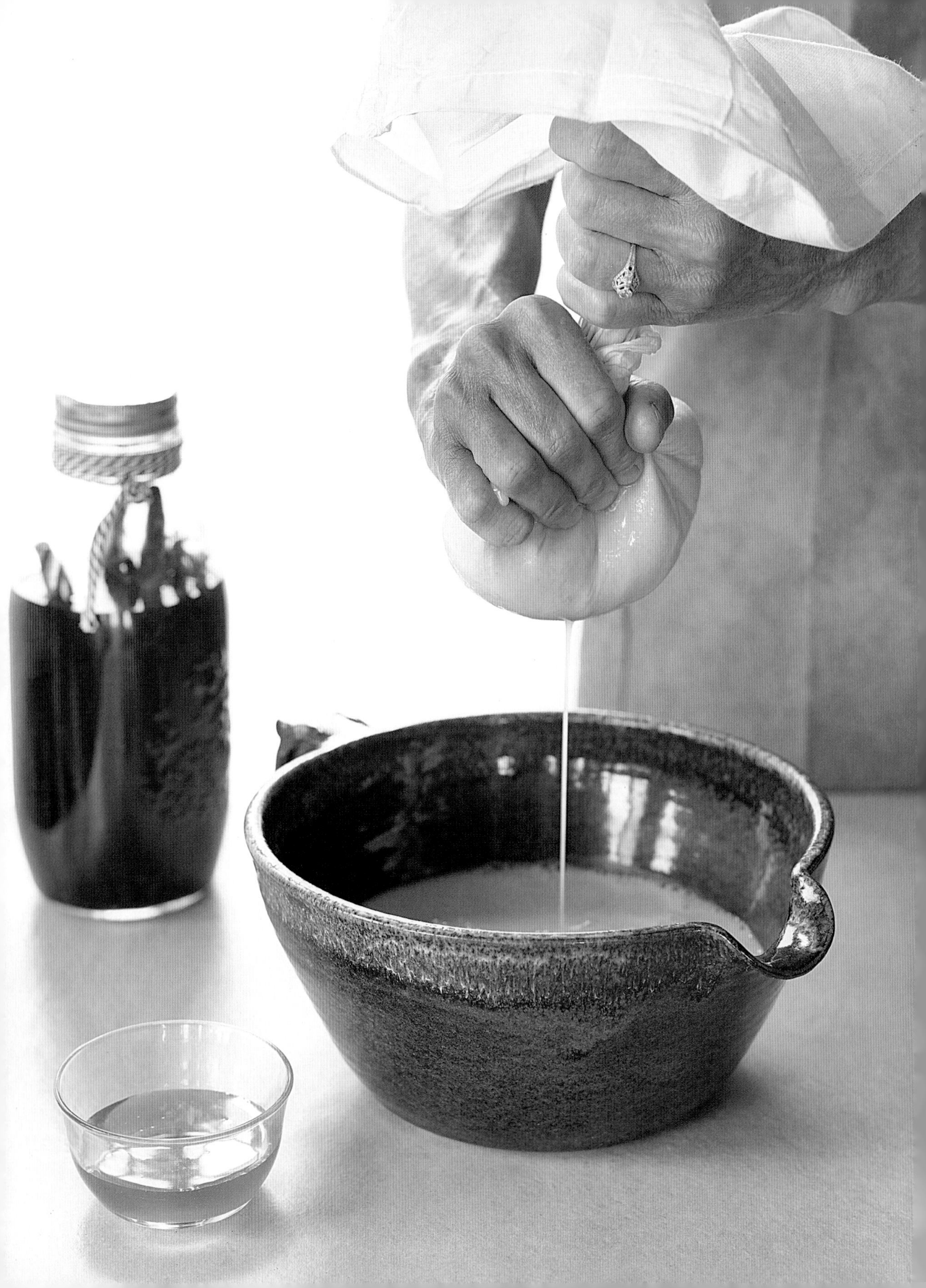

3. Combine the soaked nuts, water, vanilla, honey (if using), and salt in a blender. Blend on high speed until the mixture is frothy and smooth, about 2 minutes. If straining, pour the milk into the nut milk bag and squeeze to extract all of the milk from the pulp. If using a lined colander, press firmly on the pulp with the back of a spoon to extract the milk. Set aside the nut milk meal for another use (see page 367 for ideas).

4. Pour the milk into a glass jar with a tight-fitting lid. Store in the refrigerator for up to 4 days. Shake well before serving.

VARIATIONS

CINNAMON WALNUT MILK

MAKES 5 CUPS (1.2 L)

Make 1 batch basic nut milk using walnuts and 2 teaspoons ground cinnamon. Straining is optional.

CHOCOLATE DATE MILK

MAKES 5 CUPS (1.2 L)

Make 1 batch basic nut milk using hazelnuts, 2 dates, and 3 tablespoons natural cacao powder. Strain.

COFFEE CREAMER

MAKES 3¼ CUPS (770 ML)

Make 1 batch basic nut milk using almonds, 2¼ cups (530 ml) water instead of 4 cups (1 L), and just a pinch of salt. For a flavored creamer, add ¼ teaspoon ground cardamom, cinnamon, or nutmeg. Strain.

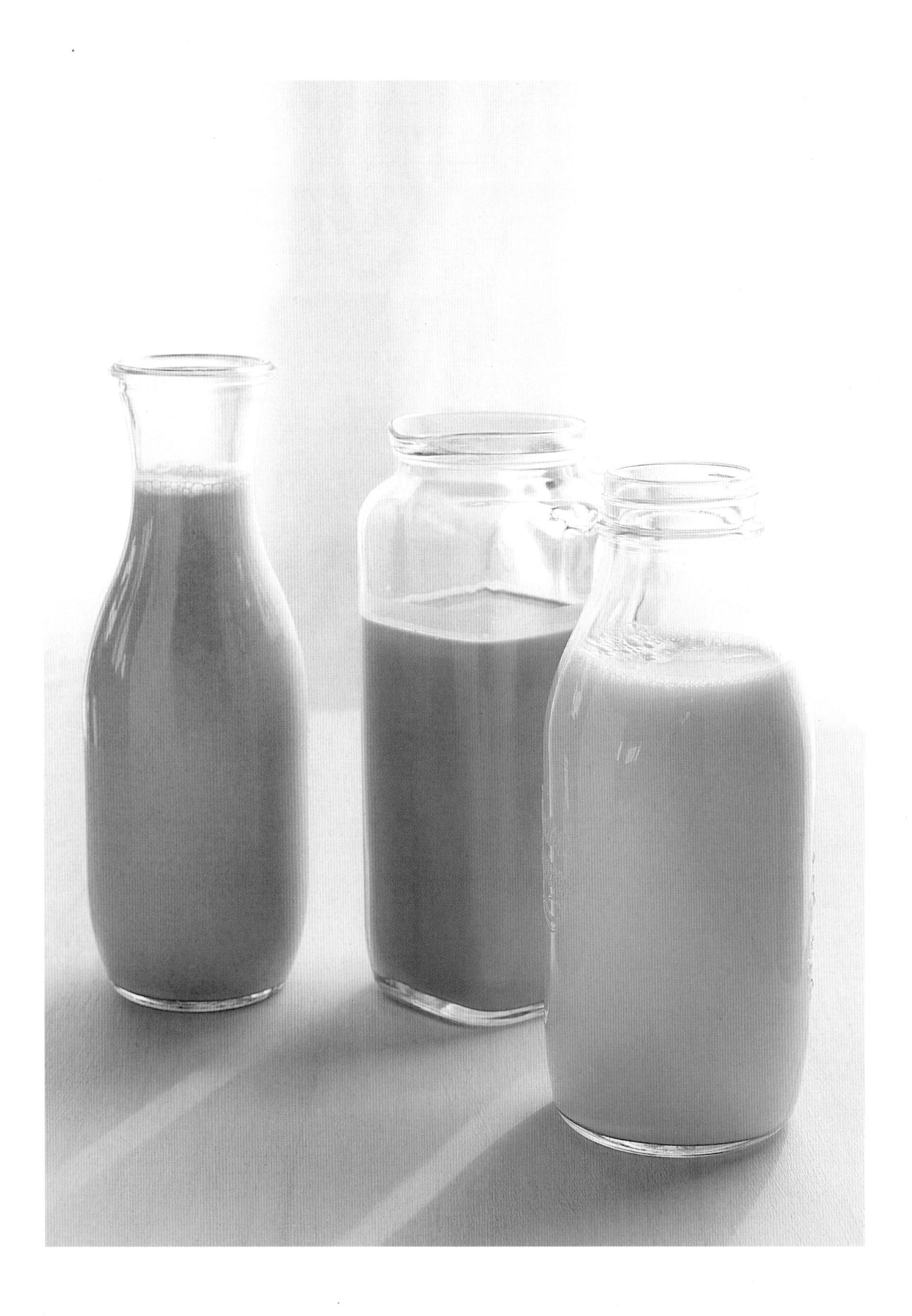

SHORTCUTS, TIPS, AND WHAT TO DO WITH THE PULP

- Straining is optional with soft nuts like pecans and cashews but will result in a smoother milk suitable for sipping. Plan to use your nut milk in a smoothie? Skip the straining step.
- For plain, unsweetened nut milk to use in cooking, omit the sweetener and vanilla.
- To make instant nut milk, use ½ cup (120 ml) nut butter in place of the nuts, blend until completely smooth, and strain.
- Using boiling water to soak softer nuts, such as cashews, pecans, and walnuts, will reduce the soaking time to about one hour. Or even faster, use the "almost instant" method used for making cashew cream (page 370): cover the nuts with water and bring to a boil, then soak, covered, for fifteen minutes. Strain and add fresh water to blend into milk.
- The longer you soak your nuts, the creamier the milk will be. However, after forty-eight hours, the nuts may start to sprout and there is a greater chance of bacterial contamination. Soak nuts at room temperature for up to twelve hours. For longer soaks, change the water every twelve hours and store in the refrigerator.
- For a nut milk that froths well for making a latte, add 2 teaspoons avocado oil to the basic recipe.
- To have soaked nuts on hand for making nut milk, freeze one-and-a-half-cup (see page 363 for weights) portions of soaked and drained nuts in airtight containers for up to three months. Defrost before using.
- For a nut and seed milk, add up to ¼ cup (35 to 40 g) seeds. Hemp seeds don't need to be soaked first. For sunflower, unhulled sesame, or hulled pumpkin seeds (pepitas), soak for ten to twelve hours. If you are also soaking nuts, this can be done in the same bowl.
- Refrigerate leftover nut meal in an airtight container for up to three days. To freeze, spoon into ice cube trays, freeze until solid, and transfer to an airtight container for up to three months. Add nut meal to oatmeal, granola, and smoothies. For DIY almond meal to use in baking, spread almond nut meal on a parchment paper–lined baking sheet, then bake at 250°F (120°C) for one to two hours until dry and easily crumbled. Break into pieces and pulse in a food processor until it is the consistency of flour.

SCIENCE BITE:

COW'S MILK VS. PLANT-BASED MILK

Plant-based milks seem to be taking over the dairy case at the grocery store. Are these so-called milks really better for you than cow's milk? Before going into the pros and cons, it's important to remember that a brain-healthy diet doesn't have to include any type of milk, whether dairy or plant based.

Traditional full-fat cow's milk is a major source of saturated fat in the standard American diet as well as an important source of protein and essential nutrients, such as vitamins A and D, niacin, riboflavin, phosphorus, and calcium. Reduced fat milk (2 percent, 1 percent, and skim) gets rid of most of the saturated fat, but the milk loses nutrients in the process. These get added back in, thanks to the practice of fortification, according to the US Food and Drug Administration's guidelines. Even so, in the absence of fat, these fat-soluble nutrients may not be properly absorbed.

Hence the catch-22 with dairy milk: full-fat cow's milk is too high in saturated fat to be a regular fixture in your brain-healthy dietary pattern, but the low-fat varieties lack nutrient density. Plant-based milks, however, such as nut, soy, seed, and oat milks, offer a variety of brain health advantages. First, unlike low-fat dairy products, they are full of brain-healthy fats. These monounsaturated fats are not only anti-inflammatory in their own right, they also lower harmful blood cholesterol.

Store-bought plant-based milks are undeniably convenient. Most processed nut milks, however, contain only about 2 percent nuts; the remaining 98 percent is water, flavorings, and additives. You'd have to drink an entire half gallon (nearly a liter) of processed nut milk to get the same nutrients in a handful of nuts. And be aware that processed oat milk may raise blood sugar.

If you like to drink plant-based milk, use it to add flavor and body to your cooking. But be sure to shop strategically. Avoid any milk with added sugars, additives like guar gum and carrageenan (which may be disruptive to your gut microbiota), unhealthy oils (like grapeseed and sunflower), and artificial flavors. See Resources (page 390) for recommended brands.

Making nut milk at home in small batches means you get to have it all—nutrient density, fresh nutty flavor, and no unhealthy ingredients. All milks—whether from cows, nuts, or another type of plant—soak up considerable planetary resources to produce, especially water. Drink in small quantities.

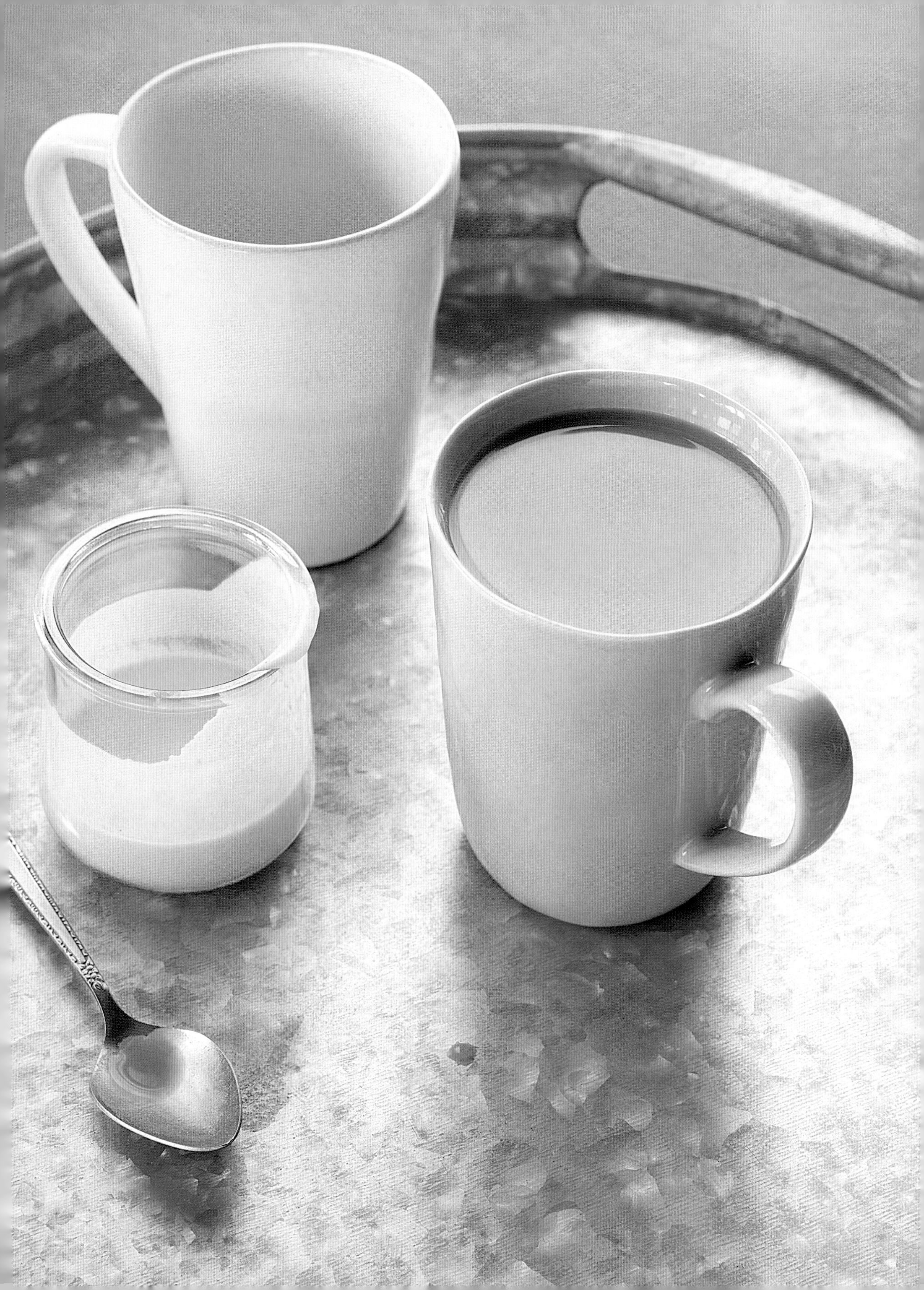

ALMOST INSTANT CASHEW CREAM

MAKES 1¼ CUPS (295 ML)

1½ cups (210 g) raw, unsalted cashews

1 cup (240 ml) fresh water, plus up to ¼ cup (60 ml) more, if needed

¼ teaspoon kosher salt

Cashew cream is a delicious swap for any dish that calls for full-fat cream. Cashews provide mostly brain-friendly monounsaturated fats, but with just enough of the saturated ones to blend up rich and creamy. With my "almost instant" method, making cream from cashews is also quick. Most nut creams call for a long soak before blending, but this version requires only fifteen minutes after bringing the nuts and water to a boil.

Cashew cream is a true secret weapon in your brain-healthy cooking. Add savory ingredients, like garlic and herbs, for a pasta sauce or the base for a cheese-less pizza. Dollop on soups and grain bowls and spread on sandwiches. Or, as an alternative to sweetened whipped cream, fold in vanilla and pure maple syrup instead. Add tahini and it becomes an easy dip for fruit or a stand-in for frangipane in a pear or apple tart.

A powerful blender yields the creamiest result. You can still get good results with a food processor or a standard blender by adding a few minutes to the blending time.

TIP: *If you want to soak the cashews instead of boiling them, combine them in a bowl with enough water to cover for at least 2 hours and up to 12 hours. Discard the soaking water and proceed with the recipe using fresh, room-temperature water.*

1. Place the cashews in a small saucepan, add enough water to cover the nuts, and bring to a boil. Turn off the heat, cover, and let sit for 15 minutes. Drain, discarding the soaking water.

2. Transfer the cashews to a blender with the 1 cup (240 ml) fresh water and salt. Blend on low speed to make a thick paste. With the blender on medium speed, add more water 1 tablespoon at a time until the cashew mixture is the consistency of heavy cream. Increase the power to high and blend until very creamy, about 1 minute.

3. Transfer the cashew cream to a bowl and cover tightly. To store, refrigerate in an airtight container for up to 5 days or freeze for up to 1 month.

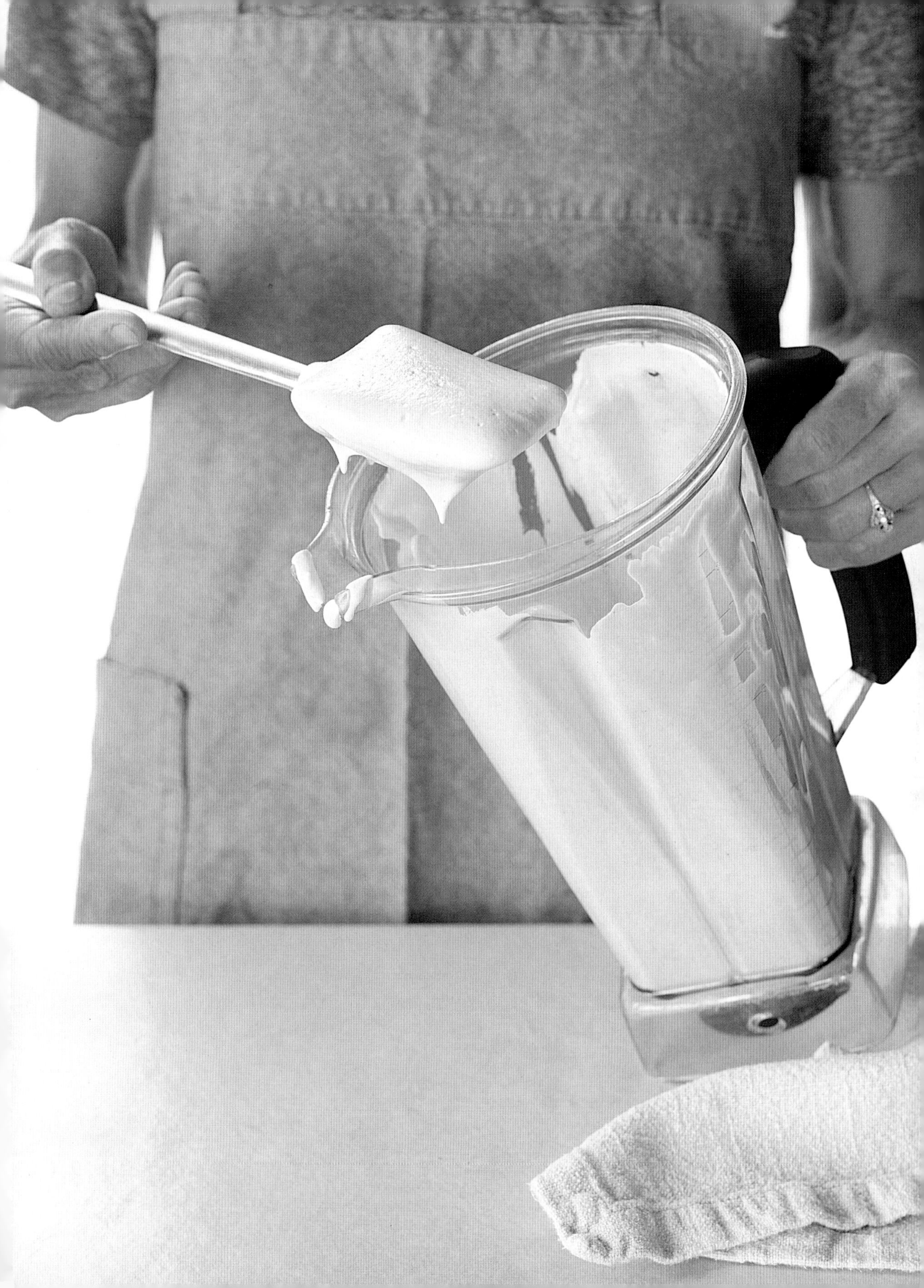

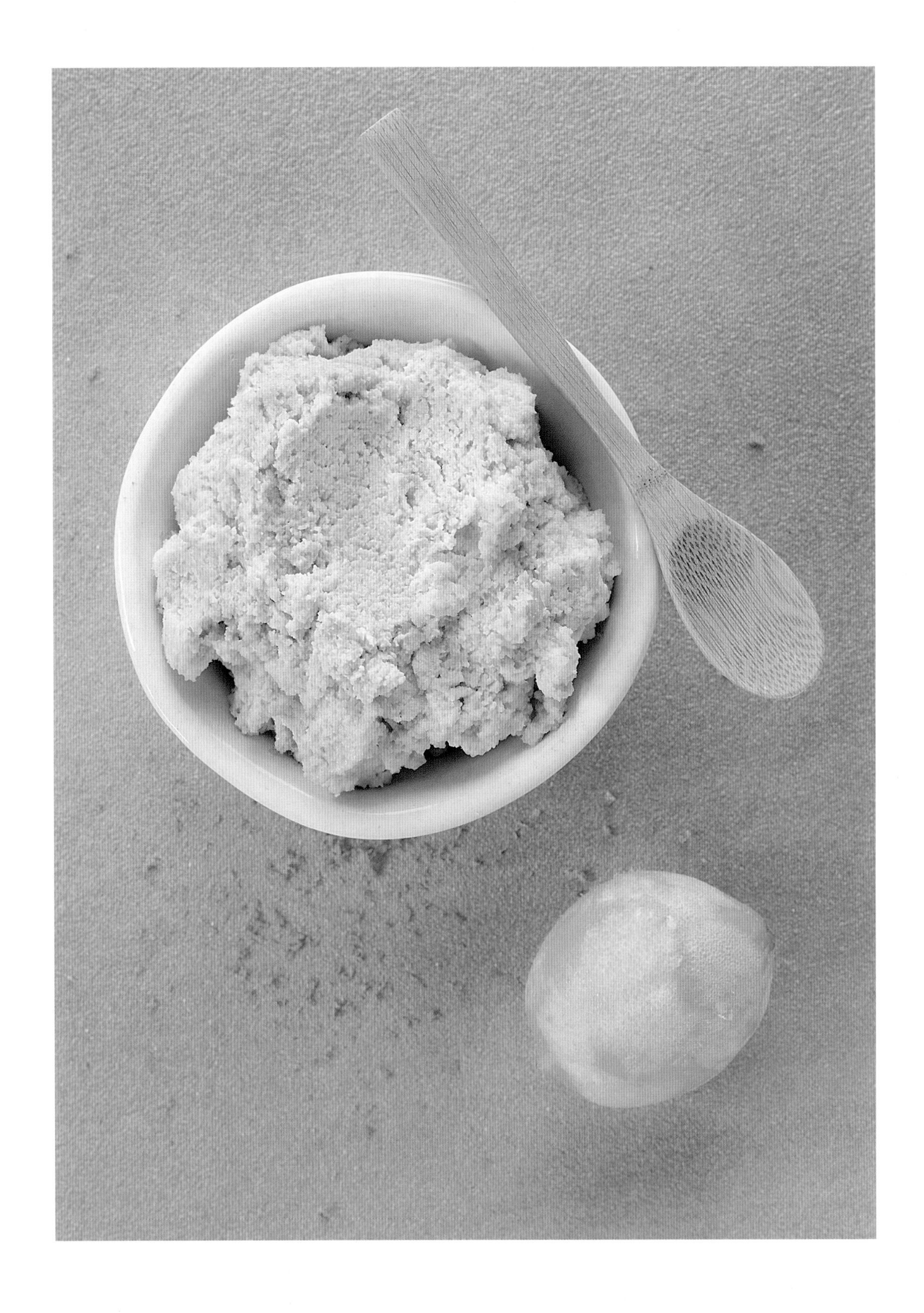

LEMONY CASHEW RICOTTA

MAKES 1½ CUPS (300 G)

1½ cups (210 g) raw, unsalted cashews

Zest of 1 lemon (about 2 teaspoons)

¼ cup (60 ml) fresh lemon juice

½ teaspoon kosher salt

Up to ¼ cup (60 ml) fresh water

One of the key tenets of brain-healthy eating is to reduce saturated fat. Cutting out all dairy might not be in the cards for you, but making selective plant-based swaps is a great strategy. In the case of this cashew-based ricotta, you'll get a delicious alternative for ricotta cheese, which can be used in many traditional dishes like lasagna, manicotti, and stuffed shells. It's extremely versatile, too. By adding a few simple ingredients, such as garlic and chives, this Lemony Cashew Ricotta becomes a dip for crudités, a schmear for your whole-grain bagel, or a much brain-healthier-than-mayo sandwich spread. For a creamy pasta sauce, toss this ricotta with hot pasta and a ladle of the cooking water.

Use the ricotta right away as a dip or spread. For a firmer cheese, place in a nut milk bag or double thickness of cheesecloth and let drain over a bowl in the refrigerator for up to twenty-four hours.

TIP: *To soak the cashews instead, cover with water and soak for at least 2 hours or up to 12 hours; drain before using in the recipe.*

1. Place the cashews in a small saucepan, add enough water to cover the nuts, and bring to a boil. Turn off the heat, cover, and let sit for 15 minutes. Drain, discarding the soaking water.

2. Transfer the cashews to the bowl of a food processor and add the lemon zest, lemon juice, and salt. Pulse about 20 times, or until the cashews take on the consistency of cottage cheese, with curd-like clumps. Scrape down the sides of the bowl and pulse again, adding 1 tablespoon of water at a time, until the mixture has the texture of a moist ricotta.

3. Use right away as a dip or spread. For a firmer cheese, set a nut milk bag or a double thickness of cheesecloth over a bowl. Scrape the cashew ricotta into the nut milk bag or cheesecloth, gather into a bundle, and place over a bowl to catch any water that seeps out. Refrigerate for 24 hours.

GOLDEN STOCKS

Brain-healthy cooking means more meals made from scratch, which comes with a big perk: a treasure trove of scraps for making stock. Homemade stock (whether chicken or vegetable) infuses dishes with deep flavor while also providing health-supporting phytonutrients. Keep a gallon zip-top bag in your freezer to collect scraps and bones. Once it's full, you're ready to make a batch using the recipes below. Of course, you can chop up a few carrots and celery stalks to make a pot off the cuff.

For a stock that's versatile enough to fulfill many uses in your cooking, avoid strongly flavored vegetables and herbs, such as asparagus, broccoli, cabbage, cauliflower, kale, mint, peppers, potatoes, rosemary, and sage. Avoid purple vegetables—such as eggplant and purple carrots and potatoes—that will muddy the stock with an off-putting, murky color.

These stocks are unsalted to build flavor in dishes without added salt. If you like to sip on your stock, salt to taste. The peppercorns here do more than flavor the stock—they add the same type of brain-healthy polyphenols found in green tea and red wine.

GOLDEN VEGETABLE STOCK

MAKES 8 TO 10 CUPS (2 TO 2.4 L)

8 cups (about 910 g) vegetable scraps, such as equal amounts of alliums (onion, leeks, scallion greens, garlic), carrots, celery, fennel, herbs (parsley, thyme), and mushrooms

One 6-inch (15 cm) strip kombu

8 black peppercorns

1 bay leaf

Up to 5 quarts (4.7 L) cold water

This vegetable stock is more flavorful than most, thanks to the addition of kombu, a type of dried seaweed, which adds both umami and a sea saltiness that reduces the need for added salt.

STOVETOP METHOD

1. Combine the vegetable scraps, kombu, peppercorns, bay leaf, and 4 quarts (about 4 L) water in a large pot. Bring to a boil over high heat and reduce the heat to a low simmer. Cover, with the lid slightly ajar, and cook for 1 to 2 hours, or until reduced by about half, adding up to 1 quart (1 L) water as needed to keep the vegetables covered.

2. Set a large-mesh strainer over a 5-quart (4.7 L) or larger bowl or pot. Set the stock aside away from the heat to cool

slightly, then strain into the bowl. Discard the solids and divide the stock between 1-quart (1 L) containers, leaving about ½-inch (1.25 cm) headspace if you plan to freeze them.

3. To store, keep tightly covered in the refrigerator for up to 4 days or the freezer for up to 3 months.

INSTANT POT METHOD

1. Combine the vegetable scraps, kombu, peppercorns, and bay leaf in the bowl of a multicooker. Fill with water to just below the Max line. Lock the lid and cook on high pressure for 40 minutes, then release the pressure naturally.

2. Add up to 1 quart (1 L) water to bring the water level up to where it was.

3. Strain and store as for the stovetop method.

SLOW COOKER METHOD

1. Combine the vegetable scraps, kombu, peppercorns, bay leaf, and 5 quarts (4.7 L) water in a 6-quart (5.7 L) or larger slow cooker. Cook on low for 2 hours.

2. Strain and store as for the stovetop method.

GOLDEN CHICKEN STOCK

MAKES 4 QUARTS (ABOUT 4 L)

1 pound (455 g) chicken bones (raw or leftover from cooked chicken) or other meat bones

6 cups (500 g) vegetable scraps, such as equal amounts of alliums (onion, leeks, scallion greens, garlic), carrots, celery, fennel, herbs (parsley, thyme), mushrooms, parsnips, and zucchini

8 black peppercorns

1 bay leaf

5 quarts (4.7 L) cold water, plus more if needed

This stock makes excellent use of a leftover roasted chicken or other poultry bones, cooked or raw. For bone broth, replace the chicken bones with 1 pound (455 g) beef, bison, lamb, or pork bones, with or without meat.

Seek out the highest-quality bones for your stock, preferably from ethically raised and harvested animals. Good-quality bones are rich in amino acids and collagen, which add body and substance to your stock. Bones with marrow also provide omega-3 fatty acids, like the conjugated alpha-linolenic acid (ALA) found in butter and walnuts.

STOVETOP METHOD

1. Combine the bones, vegetable scraps, peppercorns, bay leaf, and water in a large pot. Bring to a simmer over high heat, but not a full boil, and reduce the heat until the liquid is gently bubbling. Cook, uncovered, for 30 minutes, using a small fine-mesh strainer to skim off any foam that rises to the surface. Cover, with the lid slightly ajar, and adjust the heat so the liquid is gently bubbling. Add more water, if needed, to keep the contents covered, and simmer for another 3 to 4 hours. The stock is done when it has some body and a deep golden color.

2. Set a large fine-mesh strainer over a 5-quart (4.7 L) or larger bowl or pot. Set the stock aside away from the heat to cool slightly, then strain into the bowl. Discard the solids and divide the stock between 1-quart (1 L) containers. Chill thoroughly and scrape off and discard any fat that solidifies on the top of the stock.

3. To store, keep tightly covered in the refrigerator for up to 4 days or the freezer for up to 3 months.

TIP: *For a clear stock, maintain a gently bubbling liquid throughout, avoiding a full boil, and skim off whatever foam (fat and water-soluble proteins) rises to the top.*

continued

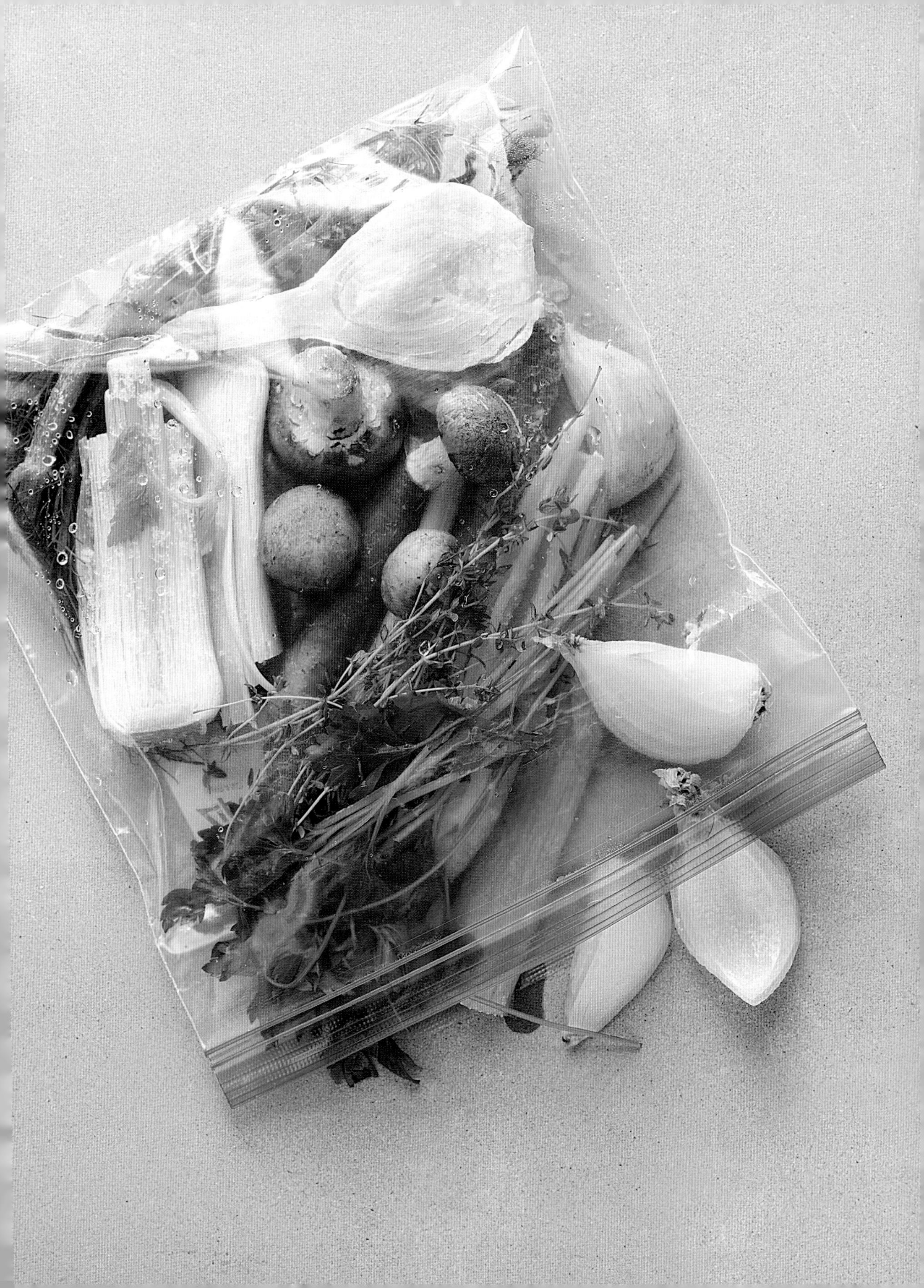

INSTANT POT METHOD

Your yield will vary depending on the size of your multicooker: 3¾ quarts (3.5 L) stock for a 6-quart model, and 4 quarts (3.8 L) for an 8-quart one.

1. Combine the bones, vegetable scraps, peppercorns, and bay leaf in the multicooker. Fill with water to just below the Max line. Cover, lock the lid, then turn the vent knob to the lock position. Select the Manual mode and cook under high pressure for 40 minutes.
2. When the time is up, let the pressure release naturally. Use a small fine-mesh strainer to skim off any foam that has risen to the top. Add the salt, if using, and stir to dissolve.
3. Strain and store as for the stovetop method.

SLOW COOKER METHOD

1. Combine the bones, vegetable scraps, peppercorns, and bay leaf in a 6-qt (5.7 L) or larger slow cooker. Cover and cook on low for 8 hours, using a small fine-mesh strainer to skim off any foam that rises to the surface after the first hour. Add the salt, if using, and stir to dissolve.
2. Strain and store as for the stovetop method.

MARINARA SAUCE

MAKES 6 CUPS (1.4 L)

¼ cup (60 ml) extra-virgin olive oil

8 large garlic cloves, roughly chopped (about 2 tablespoons)

Two 28-ounce (795 g) cans whole peeled tomatoes (preferably San Marzano)

1½ cups (360 ml) water

1 teaspoon dried oregano

1 teaspoon kosher salt

¼ teaspoon crushed red pepper flakes

Your own homemade marinara is a brain health upgrade to most store-bought sauces, which are often laden with sugar, unhealthy oils, and artificial ingredients. Requiring just a few pantry staples—canned tomatoes, extra-virgin olive oil, garlic, and spices—and a quick simmer on the stove, homemade marinara tastes brighter, too.

For this recipe, I've updated my grandmother's marinara method—a messy process of hand-crushing the tomatoes to remove the seeds and core—for one that's less labor intensive and more nutrient-dense. All you do is gently break up the tomatoes with the back of a spoon while still in the pot after they've simmered into a loose sauce. This creates a partly smooth, partly chunky sauce that is well suited for the recipes in this book—it clings nicely to the spicy mussels (page 173), provides a flavorful base for the zucchini lasagna (page 139), and adds pizzazz to Cranberry Bean and Sausage Stew (page 229). And, importantly, you'll include all the fiber from the tomato as well as the seeds and gel, which are rich in vitamin C, lycopene, polyphenols, and the plant-based omega-3—alpha-linolenic acid (ALA).

1. Warm the oil in a large heavy saucepan over medium heat. Add the garlic and cook, stirring often, until translucent but not turning brown, about 1 minute. Pour in the tomatoes (with their sauce), water, oregano, salt, and red pepper flakes. Bring to a boil, then reduce the heat to a gentle simmer with the lid ajar. Cook, stirring often to make sure nothing sticks to the bottom of the pot, for 45 minutes.

2. Using a long wooden spoon, crush any of the tomatoes that are still whole against the side of the pot. Give the sauce

a stir and continue to simmer until the sauce thickens and is mostly smooth, 20 to 30 minutes.

3. Cool slightly and transfer to airtight containers. Keep in the fridge for up to 7 days or the freezer for up to 6 months.

TIPS: *Canned San Marzano tomatoes from Italy are widely available in most grocery stores and are perfect for making this sauce. They are naturally sweet, have just the right flesh-to-pulp ratio, and contain few bitter seeds. Domestic San Marzanos and other canned plum tomatoes can also be good. Look for whole peeled tomatoes with a short ingredient list: just tomatoes, basil (sometimes), citric acid, and salt.* *(See Resources, page 390, for recommended brands.)*

For a smoother sauce, pulse it in a blender or food processor until it's the consistency you like. Alternatively, use an immersion blender to blend the sauce right in the pot.

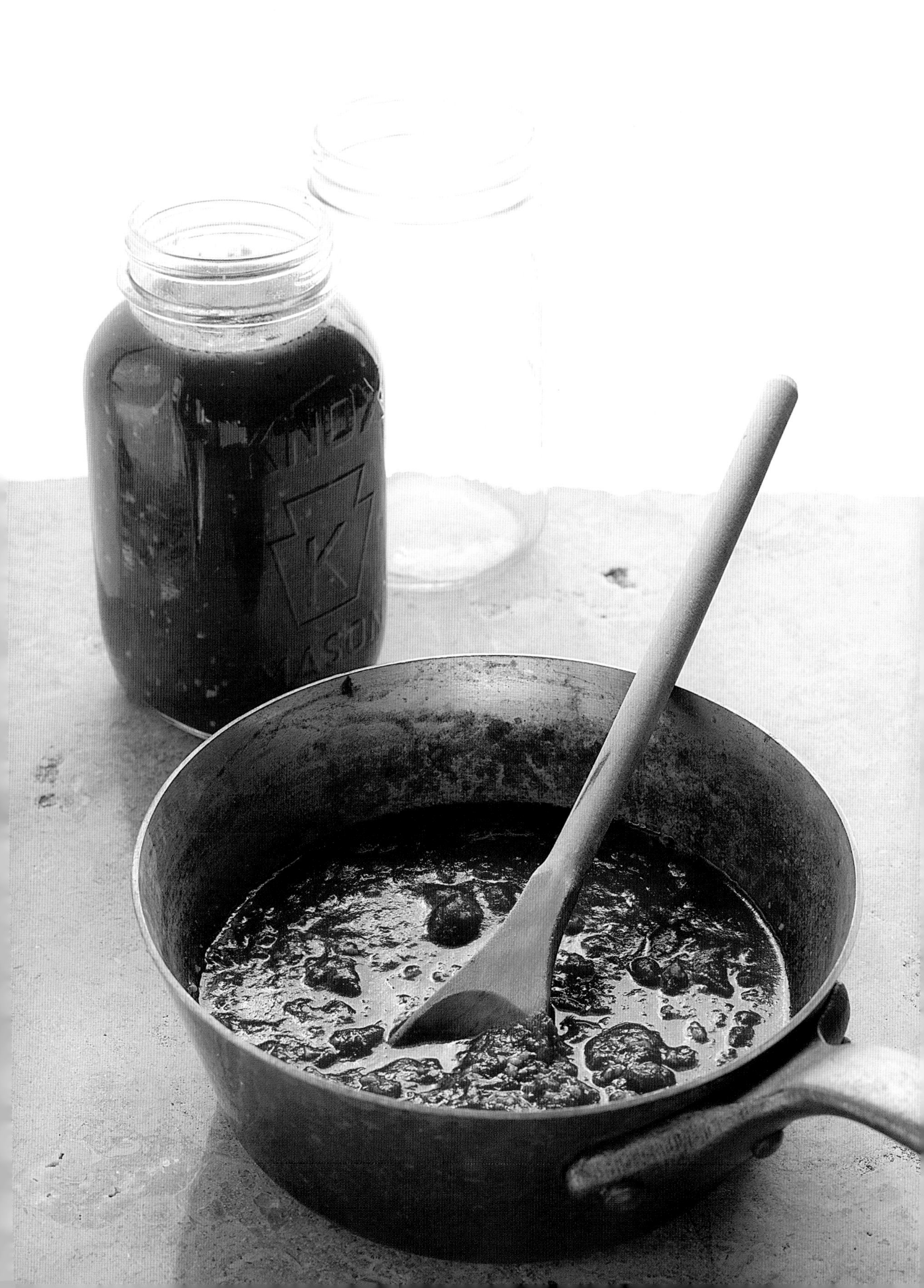

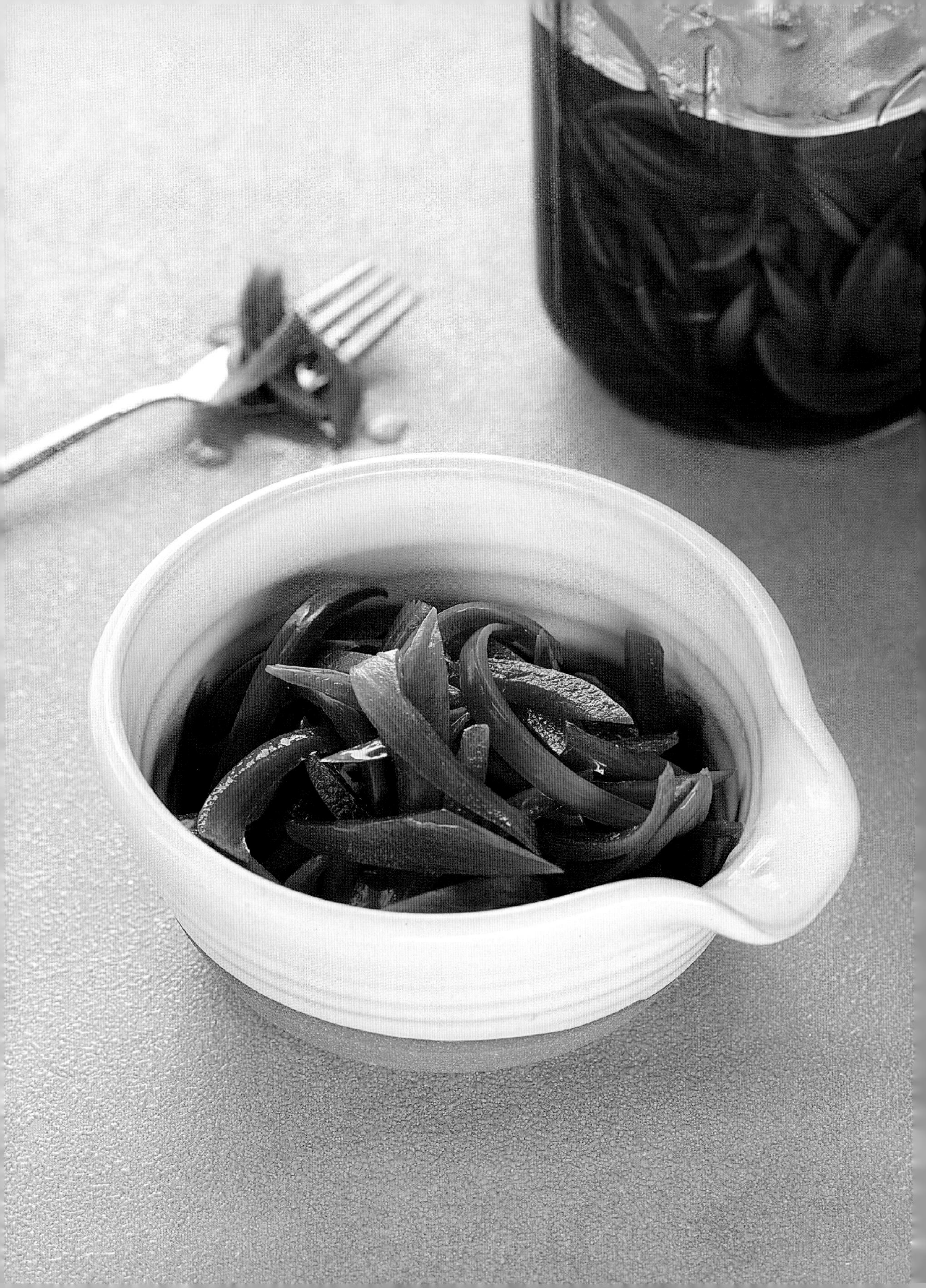

QUICK-PICKLED POMEGRANATE RED ONIONS

MAKES 2 CUPS (480 ML)

1 large red onion (12 ounces/340 g), thinly sliced (about 2 cups)

1 cup (240 ml) white wine vinegar

1 cup (240 ml) pomegranate juice

1 teaspoon kosher salt

Quick pickles typically contain sugar to offset the tartness of the vinegar. Here pomegranate juice replaces the sugar, adding antioxidants and a pretty color to the pickling liquid. Keep a jar of these onions on hand for topping tacos, grain bowls, and salads. Try them on the tuna burgers (page 167), the salsa-poached eggs with black beans (page 311), and the red lentil falafel burgers (page 231). This tart condiment will be welcome wherever you'd like a touch of crisp onion and a pop of color.

TIP: *When the pickled onions are gone, you can reuse the liquid to make another batch. Just pour into a saucepan and bring to a boil before pouring over fresh onions.*

1. Place the onion slices in a large mason jar or other airtight, heatproof container.

2. Combine the vinegar, juice, and salt in a medium saucepan. Bring to a boil over high heat, then carefully pour over the onions. Let sit at room temperature for 2 hours.

3. Cover and store in the refrigerator for up to 2 weeks.

NOTES

PREFACE

9 **if you are an Alzheimer's caregiver** E. B. Dassel et al., "Does Caring for a Spouse with Dementia Accelerate Cognitive Decline? Findings from the Health and Retirement Study," *Gerontologist* 57, no. 2 (April 2017): 319–28, https://pubmed.ncbi.nlm.nih.gov/26582383/.

INTRODUCTION

10 **an estimated fifty million worldwide** Alzheimer's Association, *2022 Alzheimer's Disease Facts and Figures*, https://www.alz.org/media/Documents/alzheimers-facts-and-figures.pdf.

10 **would reduce 40 percent of all cases worldwide** G. Livingston et al., "Dementia Prevention, Intervention, and Care: 2020 Report of the Lancet Commission," *Lancet* 396, no. 10248 (August 8, 2020): 413–46, https://doi.org/10.1016/S0140-6736(20)30367-6.

11 **the number one dementia-reducing behavior** "Healthy Behaviors Independently Linked to Lower Dementia Risk," https://www.practiceupdate.com/C/119032/56?elsca1=emc_enews_topic-alert.

12 **has been shown to reduce Black dementia rates** D. A. Levine et al., "Association between Blood Pressure and Later-Life Cognition among Black and White Individuals," JAMA Neurology 77, no. 7 (July 2020): 810–19, https://pubmed.ncbi.nlm.nih.gov/32282019/.

12 **And while Asian American and Pacific Islander (AAPI) populations** Mehta et al., "Systemic Review of Dementia Prevalence and Incidence in United States Race/Ethnic Populations," *Alzheimer's and Dementia* 13, no. 1 (January 2017): 72–83, https://doi.org/10.1016/j.jalz.2016.06.2360.

14 **Next, I dove into the details of the scientific literature study** M. C. Morris et al., "MIND Diet Associated with Reduced Incidence of Alzheimer's Disease," *Alzheimer's and Dementia* 11, no. 9 (September 2015): 1007–14, https://doi.org/10.1016/j.jalz.2014.11.009.

18 **participants who followed the diet most closely** M. C. Morris et al., "MIND Diet Slows Cognitive Decline with Aging," *Alzheimer's and Dementia* 11, no. 9 (September 2015): 1015–22, https://doi.org/10.1016/j.jalz.2015.04.011

18 **the MIND diet study has been replicated** D. E. Hosking et al., "MIND Not Mediterranean Diet Related to 12-Year Incidence of Cognitive Impairment in an Australian Longitudinal Cohort Study," *Alzheimer's and Dementia* 15, no. 4 (April 2019): 581–89, https://doi.org/10.1016/j.jalz.2018.12.011. Y. A. Metcalfe-Roach et al., "MIND and Mediterranean Diets Associated with Later Onset of Parkinson's Disease," *Movement Disorders* 36, no. 4 (April 2021): 977–84, https://doi.org/10.1002/mds.28464. J. K. Dhana et al., "MIND Diet, Common Brain Pathologies, and Cognition in Community-Dwelling Older Adults," *Journal of Alzheimer's Disease* 83, no. 2 (2021): 683–92, https://doi.org/10.3233/JAD-210107.

18 **Researchers in Israel compared three groups of people** Alon Kaplan et al., "The Effect of a High-Polyphenol Mediterranean Diet (GREEN-MED) Combined with Physical Activity on Age-Related Brain Atrophy: The DIRECT PLUS Randomized Controlled Trial," *American Journal of Clinical Nutrition* (Jan. 11, 2022), nqac001, doi:10.1093/ajcn/nqac001

19 **Buettner (author of *The Blue Zones*)** Dan Buettner, *The Blue Zones: Lessons for Living Longer from the People Who've Lived the Longest* (Washington, DC: National Geographic, 2008).

19 **Campbell (author of *The China Study*)** T. Colin Campbell with Thomas M. Campbell II, *The China Study: The Most Comprehensive Study of Nutrition Ever Conducted and the Startling Implications for Diet, Weight Loss and Long-Term Health* (Dallas: BenBella Books, 2005).

19 **strict vegetarians had half the risk of dementia** Giem et al., "The Incidence of Dementia and Intake of Animal Products: Preliminary Findings from the Adventist Health Study," *Neuroepidemiology* 12 (1993): 28–36, https://doi.org/10.1159/000110296.

19 **updated studies of vegetarian and WFPB diets** T. H. T. Chiu et al., "Vegetarian Diet and Incidence of Total, Ischemic, and Hemorrhagic Stroke in 2 Cohorts in Taiwan," *Neurology* 94, no. 11 (2020): e1112–21, https://doi.org/10.1212/WNL.0000000000009093. M. J. O'Donnell et al. (INTERSTROKE investigators), "Global and Regional Effects of Potentially Modifiable Risk Factors Associated with Acute Stroke in 32 Countries (INTERSTROKE): A Case-Control Study," *Lancet* 388, no. 10046 (August 20, 2016): 761–75, https://doi.org/10.1016/S0140-6736(16)30506-2.

20 **two thousand healthy older adults in Sweden** B. Shakersain et al., "The Nordic Prudent Diet Reduces Risk of Cognitive Decline in the Swedish Older Adults: A Population-Based Cohort Study," *Nutrients* 10, no. 2 (February 17, 2018): 229, https://pubmed.ncbi.nlm.nih.gov/29462973/.

21 **a single night of sleep deprivation** Winer, Joseph R., Kacie D. Deters, Gabriel Kennedy, Meghan Jin, Andrea Goldstein-Piekarski, Kathleen L. Poston, and Elizabeth C. Mormino. "Association of short and long sleep duration with amyloid-ß burden and cognition in aging." *JAMA Neurology* 78, no. 10 (2021): 1187-1196.

24 **Lisa Genova's book *Still Alice*** Lisa Genova, *Still Alice* (New York: Pocket Books, 2009).

25 **the female brain is well equipped** L. Mosconi, R. D. Brinton et al., "Menopause Impacts Human Brain Structure, Connectivity, Energy Metabolism, and Amyloid-Beta Deposition," *Scientific Reports* 11, no. 1 (June 9, 2021): 10867, https://doi.org/10.1038/s41598-021-90084-y.

25 **female ApoE4 carriers have unique** N. G. Norwitz, R. S. Isaacson, et al., "Precision Nutrition for Alzheimer's Prevention in ApoE4 Carriers," *Nutrients* 13, no. 4 (April 19, 2021): 1362, https://doi.org/10.3390/nu13041362.

26 **The decision to take hormones** J. M. Matyi et al., "Lifetime Estrogen Exposure and Cognition in Late Life: The Cache County Study," *Menopause* 26, no. 12

(December 2019): 1366–74, https://doi.org/10.1097/GME.0000000000001405.

27 **Lack of early childhood education** Livingston et al., "Dementia Prevention, Intervention, and Care."

28 **have younger-performing brains** M. C. Morris et al., "Nutrients and Bioactives in Green Leafy Vegetables and Cognitive Decline: Prospective Study," *Neurology* 30, no. 3 (2018): e214–22, https://doi.org/10.1212/WNL.0000000000004815.

29 **clinical trial of a nasal vaccine against Alzheimer's** Brigham and Women's Hospital, "Brigham and Women's Hospital Launches Clinical Trial of Nasal Vaccine for Alzheimer's Disease," press release, November 16, 2021, https://www.brighamandwomens.org/about-bwh/newsroom/press-releases-detail?id=4029.

29 **A blood test now being used** "Early Clinical Data of a Blood Biomarker Test in the Evaluation of Patients with Cognitive Impairment" (poster presentation, Gerontological Society of America 2021 Annual Scientific Meeting, online November 10–13, 2021).

36 **the amount in a few spoonfuls of honey** Lisa Mosconi, *Brain Food: The Surprising Science of Eating for Cognitive Power* (New York: Avery, 2018), 87.

36 **readings that are consistently high** P. Crane et al., "Glucose Levels and Risk of Dementia," *New England Journal of Medicine* 369, no. 6 (October 10, 2013): 540–48, https://doi.org/10.1056/NEJMoa1215740.

37 **overall rates of death from any cause** Guasch-Ferré M, Li Y, Willett WC, et al. Consumption of Olive Oil and Risk of Total and Cause-Specific Mortality Among U.S. Adults. J Am Coll Cardiol. 2022;79(2):101-112. doi:10.1016/j.jacc.2021.10.041

BRAIN HEALTH BEGINS IN THE KITCHEN

32 **if berries are enjoyed daily** R. Krikorian et al., "Blueberry Supplementation Improves Memory in Older Adults. *Journal of Agricultural and Food Chemistry* 58, no. 7 (April 14, 2010): 3996–4000, https://doi.org/10.1021/jf9029332. E. L. Boespflug et al., "Enhanced Neural Activation with Blueberry Supplementation in Mild Cognitive Impairment," *Nutritional Neuroscience* 21, no. 4 (2018): 297–305, https://doi.org/10.1080/1028415X.2017.1287833.

35 **avoid foods with long ingredient lists** A. Rico-Campà et al., "Association between Consumption of Ultra-Processed Foods and All Cause Mortality: SUN Prospective Cohort Study," *BMJ* 365 (May 29, 2019): l1949, https://doi.org/10.1136/bmj.l1949.

39 **certain flavonoid-containing foods** T. M. Holland et al., "Dietary Flavonols and Risk of Alzheimer Dementia," *Neurology* 94, no. 16 (April 21, 2020): e1749–56, https://doi.org/10.1212/WNL.0000000000008981.

LEAFY GREENS

83 **up to forty times more potent** Choe et al., "The Science behind Microgreens as an Exciting New Food for the 21st Century," *Journal of Agricultural and Food Chemistry* 66, no. 44 (November 7, 2018): 11519–30, https://doi.org/10.1021/acs.jafc.8b03096.

86 **build resilient brain cell membranes** G. Ferland, "Vitamin K and the Nervous System: An Overview of Its Actions," *Advances in Nutrition* 3, no. 2 (March 1, 2012): 204–12, https://doi.org/10.3945/an.111.001784.

86 **cognitively healthy, age-matched adults** N. Presse et al., "Low Vitamin K Intakes in Community-Dwelling Elders at an Early Stage of Alzheimer's Disease," *Journal of the American Dietetic Association* 108, no. 12 (December 2008): 2095–99, https://doi.org/10.1016/j.jada.2008.09.013.

94 **That's because parsley** Le Zhao et al, "Neuroprotective, Anti-Amyloidogenic and Neurotrophic Effects of Apigenin in an Alzheimer's Disease Mouse Model," *Molecules* 18, no. 8 (2013): 9949–65. Kalivarathan et al., "Apigenin Attenuates Hippocampal Oxidative Events, Inflammation and Pathological Alterations in Rats Fed High Fat, Fructose Diet," *Biomedicine & Pharmacotherapy* 89 (2017): 323–31.

100 **First, the vitamin C in citrus** J. D. Cook et al., "Effect of Ascorbic Acid Intake on Nonheme-Iron Absorption from a Complete Diet," *American Journal of Clinical Nutrition* 73, no. 1 (January 2001): 93–98, https://doi.org/10.1093/ajcn/73.1.93.

100 **higher scores on cognitive testing** B. L. Tan et al., "Carotenoids: How Effective Are They to Prevent Age-Related Diseases?," *Molecules* 24, no. 9 (May 9, 2019): 1801, https://doi.org/10.3390/molecules24091801.

100 **counting backward, recalling words, and speaking fluently** E. Kesse-Guyot et al., "Carotenoid-Rich Dietary Patterns during Midlife and Subsequent Cognitive Function," *British Journal of Nutrition* 111, no. 5 (March 14, 2014): 915–23, https://doi.org/10.1017/S0007114513003188.

103 **Getting lutein and zeaxanthin from food** B. Eisenhauer et al., "Lutein and Zeaxanthin-Food Sources, Bioavailability and Dietary Variety in Age-Related Macular Degeneration Protection," *Nutrients* 9, no. 2 (February 9, 2017): 120, https://doi.org/10.3390/nu9020120.

VEGETABLES

117 **detrimental effect of bombarding brain cells** E. E. Nwanna et al., "Eggplant (Solanum spp.) Supplemented Fruits Diet Modulated the Activities of Ectonucleoside Triphosphate Diphosphohydrolase (ENTPdase), Monoamine Oxidase (MAO), and Cholinesterases (AChE/BChE) in the Brain of Diabetic Wistar Male Rats," *Journal of Food Biochemistry* 43, no. 8 (August 2019): e12910, https://doi.org/10.1111/jfbc.12910.

FISH AND SEAFOOD

163 **based on MRI studies** Z. S. Tan, W. S. Harris, et al., "Red Blood Cell Omega-3 Fatty Acid Levels and Markers of Accelerated Brain Aging," *Neurology* 78, no. 9 (February 28, 2012): 658–64, https://doi.org/10.1212/WNL.0b013e318249f6a9.

163 **A recent study** Arellanes, Isabella C et al. "Brain delivery of supplemental docosahexaenoic acid (DHA): A randomized placebo-controlled clinical trial." *EBioMedicine* vol. 59 (2020): 102883. doi:10.1016/j.ebiom.2020.102883.

164 **PCBs (polychlorinated biphenyls) and pesticides** "Monterey Bay Aquarium Seafood Watch," accessed July 30, 2021, https://www.seafoodwatch.org/.

164 **Marine Stewardship Council stamp of approval** "Marine Stewardship Council," accessed July 30, 2021, https://www.msc.org/en-us/.

165 **Animal studies have documented** Taksima et al., "Effects of Astaxanthin from Shrimp Shell on Oxidative Stress and Behavior in Animal Model of Alzheimer's Disease," *Marine Drugs* 17, no. 11 (November 4, 2019): 628, https://doi .org/10.3390/md17110628.

168 **A 2015 study** Morris et al., "Association of Seafood Consumption, Brain Mercury Level, and APOE e4 Status with Brain Neuropathology in Older Adults," *JAMA* 315, no. 5 (February 2, 2016): 489–97, https://doi.org/10.1001/jama.2015.19451.

NUTS AND SEEDS

180 **Snacking on nuts** R. Estruch et al., "Primary Prevention of Cardiovascular Disease with a Mediterranean Diet Supplemented with Extra-Virgin Olive Oil or Nuts," *New England Journal of Medicine* 378, no. 25 (June 21, 2018): e34, https://www.nejm.org/doi/metrics/10.1056/NEJMoa1800389.

180 **In numerous large-scale, prospective studies** O'Brien et al., "Long-Term Intake of Nuts in Relation to Cognitive Function in Older Women," *Journal of Nutrition, Health, and Aging* 18, no. 5 (May 2014): 496–502, https://pubmed.ncbi.nlm.nih.gov/24886736/. Koyama et al., "Evaluation of a Self-Administered Computerized Cognitive Battery in an Older Population," *Neuroepidemiology* 45, no. 4 (2015): 264–72, https://doi.org/10.1159/439592. L. Arab et al., "A Cross Sectional Study of the Association between Walnut Consumption and Cognitive Function among Adult US Populations Represented in NHANES," *Journal of Nutrition, Health and Aging* 19, no. 3 (March 2015): 284–90, https://link.springer.com/article/10.1007/s12603-014-0569-2.

184 **Now a study of older adults** M. Petrie et al., "Beet Root Juice: An Ergogenic Aid for Exercise and the Aging Brain," *Journals of Gerontology, Series A, Biological Sciences and Medical Sciences* 72, no. 9 (September 2017): 1284–89, https://doi.org/10.1093/gerona/glw219.

BEANS AND LENTILS

223 **And oregano,** Zotti et al., "Carvacrol: From Ancient Flavoring to Neuromodulatory Agent," *Molecules* 18, no. 6 (May 24, 2013): 6161–72.

223 **Carvacrol has also been found** Raeni et al., "Carvacrol Suppresses Learning and Memory Dysfunction and Hippocampal Damages Caused by Chronic Cerebral Hypoperfusion," *Nauyn-Schmiedeberg's Archives of Pharmacology* 393, no. 4 (April 2020): 581–89.

225 **When you eat a legume-rich meal** I. Darmadi-Blackberry et al., "Legumes: The Most Important Dietary Predictor of Survival in Older People of Different Ethnicities," *Asia Pacific Journal of Clinical Nutrition* 13, no. 2 (2004): 217–20, https://pubmed.ncbi.nlm.nih.gov/15228991/.

230 **in elderly Japanese women** M. Nakamoto et al., "Soy Food and Isoflavone Intake Reduces the Risk of Cognitive Impairment in Elderly Japanese Women," *European Journal of Clinical Nutrition* 72, no. 10 (2018): 1458–62, https://www.nature.com/articles/s41430-017-0061-2.

230 **to combat aging** Y. Lu et al., "Dietary Soybean Isoflavones in Alzheimer's Disease Prevention," *Asia Pacific Journal of Clinical Nutrition* 27, no. 5 (2018): 946–54, http://apjcn.nhri.org.tw/server/APJCN/27/5/946.pdf.

WHOLE GRAINS

244 **Rolled oats, for example, are rich in avenanthramides** L. Nie et al., "Avenanthramide, a Polyphenol from Oats, Inhibits Vascular Smooth Muscle Cell Proliferation and Enhances Nitric Oxide Production," *Atherosclerosis* 186, no. 2 (June 2006): 260–66, https://doi.org/10.1016/j.atherosclerosis.2005.07.027.

245 **More than fifty-seven studies** G. Zong et al., "Whole Grain Intake and Mortality from All Causes, Cardiovascular Disease, and Cancer: A Meta-Analysis of Prospective Cohort Studies," *Circulation* 133, no. 24 (June 14, 2016): 2370–80. E. Yu et al., "Diet, Lifestyle, Biomarkers, Genetic Factors, and Risk of Cardiovascular Disease in the Nurses' Health Studies," *American Journal of Public Health* 106, no. 9 (September 2016): 1616–23, https://www.ncbi.nlm.nih.gov/pmc/articles/PMC4981798/.

245 **PREDIMED, the same study** R. Casas et al., "Long-Term Immunomodulatory Effects of a Mediterranean Diet in Adults at High Risk of Cardiovascular Disease in the PREvención con DIeta MEDiterránea (PREDIMED) Randomized Controlled Trial," *Journal of Nutrition* 146, no. 9 (September 2016): 1684–93, https://doi.org/10.3945/jn.115.229476.

246 **a formula you can easily do in your head** R. S. Mozaffarian et al., "Identifying Whole Grain Foods: A Comparison of Different Approaches for Selecting More Healthful Whole Grain Products," *Public Health Nutrition* 16, no. 12 (December 2013): 2255–64, https://doi.org/10.1017/S1368980012005447.

258 **Alzheimer's drug donazepil** Adalier et al., "Vitamin E, Turmeric and Saffron in Treatment of Alzheimer's Disease," *Antioxidants* 5, no. 4 (October 25, 2016): 40, https://doi.org/10.3390/antiox5040040.

264 **quell inflammation in the brain by turning off FOXO3** B. Morris et al., "FOXO3: A Major Gene for Human Longevity—A Mini-Review," *Gerontology* 61, no. 6 (2015): 515–25, https://doi.org/10.1159/000375235.

264 **Other Okinawan dietary staples** D. Wilcox et al., "Healthy Aging Diets Other Than the Mediterranean: A Focus on the Okinawan Diet," *Mechanisms of Ageing and Development* 136–137 (March–April 2014): 148–62, https://doi.org/10.1159/000375235.

267 **A recent meta-analysis** Whitehead et al., "Cholesterol-Lowering Effects of Oat b-glycan: A Meta-Analysis of Randomized Controlled Trials," *American Journal of Clinical Nutrition* 100, no. 6 (December 2014): 1413–21, https://academic.oup.com/ajcn/article/10Ju0/6/1413/4576477.

274 **It's one of the richest food sources** Lin et al., "Quinoa Secondary Metabolites and Their Biological Activities or Functions," *Molecules* 24, no. 13 (July 2019): 2512, https://doi.org/10.3390/molecules24132512.

MEAT, POULTRY, AND EGGS

280 **the plants also act as a buffer** J. Uribarri, et al., "Advanced Glycation End Products in Foods and a Practical Guide to Their Reduction in the Diet," *Journal of the American Dietary Association* 110, no. 6 (June 2010): 911–16.e12, https://doi.org/10.1016/j.jada.2010.03.018.

282 **an analysis of more than fifty studies** J. S. Carson et al., "Dietary Cholesterol and Cardiovascular

Risk: A Science Advisory from the American Heart Association," *Circulation* 141, no. 3 (January 21, 2020): e39–53, https://doi.org/10.1161/CIR.0000000000000743.

282 **The fats from the yolk** J. E. Kim et al., "Effects of Egg Consumption on Carotenoid Absorption from Co-consumed, Raw Vegetables," *American Journal of Clinical Nutrition* 102, no. 4 (October 2015): 981, https://doi.org/10.3945/ajcn.115.111062.

283 **promising reports that dietary sources of niacin** M. C. Morris et al., "Dietary Niacin and the Risk of Incident Alzheimer's Disease and of Cognitive Decline," *Journal of Neurology, Neurosurgery, and Psychiatry* 75, no. 8 (2004): 1093–99, https://doi.org/10.1136/jnnp.2003.025858.

283 **In a recent review of twenty-nine scientific studies** H. Zhang et al., "Meat Consumption, Cognitive Function and Disorders: A Systematic Review with Narrative Synthesis and Meta-Analysis," *Nutrients* 12, no. 5 (May 24, 2020): 1528, https://doi.org/10.3390/nu12051528.

283 **participants had better blood lipid tests** J. A. Fleming,et al., "Effect of Varying Quantities of Lean Beef as Part of a Mediterranean-Style Dietary Pattern on Lipids and Lipoproteins: A Randomized Crossover Controlled Feeding Trial," *American Journal of Clinical Nutrition* 113, no. 5 (May 8, 2021): 1126–36, https://doi.org/10.1093/ajcn/nqaa375.

283 **Participants who ate unprocessed meat** H. Zhang et al., "Meat Consumption and Risk of Incident Dementia: Cohort Study of 493,888 UK Biobank Participants," *American Journal of Clinical Nutrition* 114, no. 1 (July 1, 2021): 175–84, https://doi.org/10.1093/ajcn/nqab028.

285 **The World Health Organization's definition** World Health Organization, "Cancer: Carcinogenicity of the Consumption of Red Meat and Processed Meat," October 26, 2015, https://www.who.int/news-room/questions-and-answers/item/cancer-carcinogenicity-of-the-consumption-of-red-meat-and-processed-meat.

307 **In a study from Tufts University** T. Boumenna et al., "Folate, Vitamin B-12, and Cognitive Function in the Boston Puerto Rican Health Study," *American Journal of Clinical Nutrition* 113, no. 1 (November 12, 2020): 179–86, https://doi.org/10.1093/ajcn/nqaa293.

307 **When asparagus is metabolized by the body** P. Kashyap et al., "Sarsasapogenin: A Steroidal Saponin from Asparagus racemosus as Multi Target Directed Ligand in Alzheimer's Disease," *Steroids* 153 (January 2020): 108529, https://www.sciencedirect.com/science/article/abs/pii/S0039128X19302193?via%3Dihub.

OLIVES AND OLIVE OIL

314 **Homer called it "liquid gold."** Clodoveo et al., "In the Ancient World, Virgin Olive Oil was Called 'Liquid Gold' by Homer and 'the Great Healer' by Hippocrates. Why Has This Mythic Image Been Forgotten?," *Food Research International* 62 (2014): 1062–68, https://doi.org/10.1016/j.foodres.2014.05.034.

314 **Athletes in ancient Greece** Nomikos et al., "The Use of Deep Friction Massage with Olive Oil as a Means of Prevention and Treatment of Sports Injuries in Ancient Times," *Archives of Medical Science* 6, no. 5 (2010): 642–45. https://doi.org/10.5114/aoms.2010.17074.

314 **olive oil may blunt the insulin response** R. Estruch et al., "Primary Prevention of Cardiovascular Disease with a Mediterranean Diet," *New England Journal of Medicine* 368, no. 14 (April 4, 2013): 1279–90, https://www.nejm.org/doi/full/10.1056/NEJMoa1200303.

314 **serve to drive down harmful blood cholesterol** Guasch-Ferré et al., "Olive Oil Consumption and Cardiovascular Risk in US Adults," *Journal of the American College of Cardiology* 75, no. 15 (2020): 1729–39, https://www.jacc.org/doi/full/10.1016/j.jacc.2020.02.036.

328 **the Spanish PREDIMED study showed** Estruch, "Primary Prevention of Cardiovascular Disease."

328 **in a similar U.S. study, Harvard researchers** Guasch-Ferré, "Olive Oil Consumption."

328 **The latest study (of more than 90,000 participants over 28 years)** Marta Guasch-Ferré et al., "Consumption of Olive Oil and Risk of Total and Cause-Specific Mortality Among U.S. Adults," *Journal of the American College of Cardiology* 79, no. 2 (2022): 101–112, doi:10.1016/j.jacc.2021.10.041

339 **In one randomized, controlled trial from Greece** M. Tsolaki et al., "A Randomized Clinical Trial of Greek High Phenolic Early Harvest Extra Virgin Olive Oil in Mild Cognitive Impairment: The MICOIL Pilot Study," *Journal of Alzheimer's Disease* 78, no. 2 (2020): 801–17, https://doi.org/10.3233/JAD-200405.

COFFEE, TEA, AND OTHER DRINKS

333 **These phytonutrients specifically protect the brain** X. Li et al., "Neuroprotective and Anti-Amyloid ? Effect and Main Chemical Profiles of White Tea: Comparison against Green, Oolong, and Black Tea," *Molecules* 24, no. 10 (May 2019): 1926, https://doi.org/10.3390/molecules24101926.

345 **Studies show that the more tea you drink** X Liu et al., "Association between Tea Consumption and Risk of Cognitive Disorders: A Dose-Response Meta-Analysis of Observational Studies," *Oncotarget* 8, no. 26 (June 27, 2017): 43306–21, https://doi.org/10.18632/oncotarget.17429.

345 **Drinking three or more cups of coffee** A. Crippa et al., "Coffee Consumption and Mortality from All Causes, Cardiovascular Disease, and Cancer: A Dose-Response Meta-Analysis," *American Journal of Epidemiology* 180, no. 8 (October 15, 2014): 763–75, https://doi.org/10.1093/aje/kwu194.

345 **Drink more than six cups a day** Pham et al., "High Coffee Consumption, Brain Volume, and Risk of Dementia and Stroke," *Nutritional Neuroscience* 1–12 (June 24, 2021), https://doi.org/10.1080/1028415X.2021.1945858.

346 **Unfiltered coffee contains dipterans** Y. Fukumoto, "Filtered, Not Unfiltered, Coffee in Cardiovascular Disease," *European Journal of Preventive Cardiology* 27, no. 18 (December 1, 2020): 1983–85, https://doi.org/10.1177/2047487320920415.

348 **a daily fruit juice habit** Pase et al., "Sugary Beverage Intake and Preclinical Alzheimer's Disease in the Community," *Alzheimer's and Dementia* 13, no. 9 (2017): 955–64, https://doi.org/10.1016/j.jalz.2017.01.024.

348 **There's no controversy whatsoever** M. P. Pase et al., "Sugar- and Artificially Sweetened Beverages and the

Risks of Incident Stroke and Dementia: A Prospective Cohort Study," *Stroke* 48, no. 5 (May 2017): 1139–46, https://doi.org/10.1161/strokeaha.116.016027.

353 **In one study, patients with high blood pressure** M. Jalalyazdi et al., "Effect of Hibiscus sabdariffa on Blood Pressure in Patients with Stage 1 Hypertension," *Journal of Advanced Pharmaceutical Technology and Research* 10, no. 3 (2019): 107–111, https://doi.org/10.4103/japtr.JAPTR_402_18.

353 **five studies investigating the impact of hibiscus tea** C. Serban et al., "Effect of Sour Tea (Hibiscus sabdariffa L.) on Arterial Hypertension," *Journal of Hypertension* 33, no. 6 (June 2015): 1119–27, https://doi.org/10.1097/HJH.0000000000000585.

356 **Whether you drink wine, beer, or spirits,** E. T. Reas et al., "Moderate, Regular Alcohol Consumption Is Associated with Higher Cognitive Function in Older Community-Dwelling Adults," *Journal of Prevention of Alzheimer's Disease* 3, no. 2 (September 2016): 105–13, https://doi.org/10.14283/jpad.2016.89. A. Ruitenberg et al., "Alcohol Consumption and Risk of Dementia: The Rotterdam Study," *Lancet* 359, no. 9303 (January 26, 2002): 281–86, https://doi.org/10.1016/s0140-6736(02)07493-7.

357 **the risk of cognitive decline goes down** L. S. Ran et al., "Alcohol, Coffee and Tea Intake and the Risk of Cognitive Deficits: A Dose-Response Meta-Analysis," *Epidemiology and Psychiatric Sciences* 30 (February 11, 2021): e13, https://doi.org/10.1017/S2045796020001183.

357 **If light drinking does confer** S. Sabia et al., "Alcohol Consumption and Risk of Dementia: 23 Year Follow-up of Whitehall II Cohort Study," *BMJ* 362 (August 1, 2018): k2927, https://doi.org/10.1136/bmj.k2927.

357 **When the drinking pattern consistently drifts** Topiwala et al., "No Safe Level of Alcohol Consumption for Brain Health: Observational Cohort Study of 25,378 UK Biobank Participants." Publication pending, https://doi.org/10.1101/2021.05.10.21256931.

357 **one or two copies of the ApoE4 risk gene** Norwitz, "Precision Nutrition for Alzheimer's Prevention in ApoE4 Carriers."

359 **A recent meta-analysis of studies concluded** Shishehbor et al., "Vinegar Consumption Can Attenuate Postprandial Glucose and Insulin Responses; A Systematic Review and Meta-Analysis of Clinical Trials," *Diabetes Research and Clinical Practice* 127 (May 2017): 1–9, https://doi.org/10.1016/j.diabres.2017.01.021.

ACKNOWLEDGMENTS

When my mother was diagnosed with Alzheimer's, little did I know it would lead to meeting some of the best people of my life.

First, to my book coach (and so much more), Lindsay Maitland Hunt: Thank you for your incredible support from proposal to finished book; for always bringing out my voice and best recipe ideas; and for infusing our work with your professionalism, smarts, and patented Lindsay humor.

To my agent, Sarah Smith, at David Black Agency: Thank you for believing in this book and for helping me find my home at Artisan. Thank you for your ever-patient answers to my questions and all the questions I don't know to ask.

Thank you, Judy Pray, my editor at Artisan Books, for taking the time to see the vision of this book through my eyes, and then for guiding me through every step of the process. You bring out the best in my writing. Thank you to Suet Chong, Zach Greenwald, Nina Simoneaux, Sibylle Kazeroid, Karen Tongish, Ivy McFadden, and Rachel Markowitz for making the book both gorgeous and useful. Thank you, Allison McGeehon, for getting the word out about the book.

Thank you to photographer Alexandra Grablewski, for capturing my food in perfect light, for your meticulous attention to detail, and for always having just the right prop. To Cyd McDowell: Thank you for putting all of your heart into each dish, for drizzling, splattering, and sprinkling the food with your magic. To Christine Buckley: Thank you for lovingly stamping each recipe with your immense artistic talent. Thank you Brooke Mockler for on-set beautification. Thank you dear friends who lent props for the shoot: Lisa Wan, Peggy Davenport, and Julie Walker.

To my physician friends: Thank you Andrew Budson, for your unbelievable support at every stage of the book; John Tew, for being a trailblazer and true friend; Jeanne Rosner and Angie Neison, for being my soul sisters in culinary medicine; Drew Ramsey, for your friendship and brain food love.

Thank you to my partners in Alzheimer's prevention: Stacy Fisher, Elizabeth Humphreys, Lisa Mosconi, Ed Park, Matthew Zuraw, everyone at HFC, especially Bonnie Wattles and Alexandra Villano, and everyone at the Women's Alzheimer's Movement, especially Maria Shriver and Sandy Gleysteen. For Dan Jaworsky, carpe diem to you, friend. Thank you to my friends in the book world: Ted Kerasote and Becky Benenate, for bolstering my earliest ideas about the book; Sheryl Flug, for always-spot-on gut checking; Ina Garten, for specific and meaningful encouragement; and Dianne Jacob, for early input on the proposal.

To my tribe, the luminous, talented, and heartful group of women who constantly shower me with unconditional love: Carrie, Casey, Catherine, Chris, Dana, Erika, Frances, Gina, Jamie, Jodi, Julie, Laely, Lisa, Margaret, Mary Kate, Nanette, Nicole, Patty, Peggy, Robin, Sheryl, Susan, Veronica. Thank you for being my Hucklebetties.

Thank you Linda Carroll for keeping me sane; Jim Shaw for pecan oil and hilarious emails; and Mark Caraluzzi for beans, turnips, and more.

For everyone in the Brain Health Kitchen community—former patients, cooking students, newsletter subscribers, and Instagram pals: Thank you for reading, commenting, posting photos of my recipes, and keeping in touch. Special thanks to one of my first students, Chaco Sorenson, who gave me the mantra for my mission when you said: "You're not just giving us recipes, Annie, you are giving us hope."

To my recipe testers, your stellar work in the kitchen is the secret sauce that makes each recipe the best it can be. I can't thank you enough: Lettie, Susan, Meredith, Catherine, Jennifer, Mark, Grace, Julie, Carter, Robin, Caryn, Lisa, Nicole, Elly, Maria, Liz, Laura, Carrie, Hayden, Lannie, Erika, Terri, Patty, Patti, Trina, Frances, Susan, Cynthia, Elizabeth, Margaret, Andrea, Jeanne, Lexi, Nikki, Veronica, Kathleen, Karen, Julie, Susan, Christine, Mary, Emily, and Temple.

For my brothers, John and Peter Barranco, and my mom, Diana: Thank you for a lifetime of love and support.

For my boys, Jack and Nick: Thank you for being my favorite people to cook for. Special thanks to Nick for coming up with the idea for a Coffee Berry Smoothie.

Finally, thank you to my husband, Jon, for providing the love and scaffolding for pursuing my dreams. As this book increasingly consumed my life, thank you for being there with coffee (just the way I like it) every day at 6.

RESOURCES

ALZHEIMER'S EDUCATION AND CAREGIVER SUPPORT

Alzheimer's Association
Nonprofit organization that educates and funds research to drive early detection, risk reduction, and care and support for people with Alzheimer's.
https://www.alz.org/

Alzheimer's Research and Prevention Foundation
Nonprofit organization that funds research about the impact of lifestyle on Alzheimer's disease and trains allied health professionals with their Brain Longevity Therapy Training program.
https://alzheimersprevention.org/

HFC
Nonprofit organization that supports families impacted by Alzheimer's disease, activates the next generation of Alzheimer's advocates, and is a leader in brain health research and education.
https://wearehfc.org/

Mind What Matters
Nonprofit organization that supports Alzheimer's caregivers with its Caregiver Relief Fund and raises awareness about memory disorders through the *Mind What Matters* podcast.
https://www.weremindwhatmatters.org/

Women's Alzheimer's Movement
Nonprofit organization that funds women-based Alzheimer's research, supports those impacted by the disease, and educates about brain health and Alzheimer's prevention.
https://thewomensalzheimersmovement.org/

BOOKS

Books about Alzheimer's, Dementia, and Brain Health

Brain Food: The Surprising Science of Eating for Cognitive Power by Lisa Mosconi, PhD (Avery, 2018).

Diet for the MIND: The Latest Science on What to Eat to Prevent Alzheimer's and Cognitive Decline—From the Creator of the MIND Diet by Martha Clare Morris, PhD (Little, Brown Spark, 2017).

Seven Steps to Managing Your Memory: What's Normal, What's Not, and What to Do about It by Andrew Budson, MD, with Maureen K. O'Connor, PsyD (Oxford University Press, 2017).

Six Steps to Managing Alzheimer's: A Guide for Families by Andrew Budson, MD, with Maureen K. O'Connor, PsyD (Oxford University Press, 2021).

The 30-Day Alzheimer's Solution: The Definitive Food and Lifestyle Guide to Preventing Cognitive Decline by Dean Sherzai, MD, PhD, and Ayesha Sherzai, MD, MAS (HarperOne, 2021).

The XX Brain: The Groundbreaking Science Empowering Women to Maximize Cognitive Health and Prevent Alzheimer's Disease by Lisa Mosconi, PhD (Avery, 2020).

Books about Food and Mental Health

Eat to Beat Anxiety and Depression: Nourish Your Way to Better Mental Health in Six Weeks by Drew Ramsey, MD (Harper Wave, 2021).

This Is Your Brain on Food: An Indispensable Guide to the Surprising Foods That Fight Depression, Anxiety, PTSD, OCD, ADHD, and More by Uma Naidoo, MD (Little, Brown Spark, 2020).

Books about Healthy Aging

The New Rules of Aging Well: A Simple Program for Immune Resilience, Strength, and Vitality by Frank Lipman, MD, and Danielle Claro (Artisan, 2020).

Cookbooks

The Blue Zones Kitchen: 100 Recipes to Live to 100 by Dan Buettner (National Geographic, 2019).

The Complete Mediterranean Diet Cookbook: 500 Vibrant, Kitchen-Tested Recipes for Living and Eating Well Every Day by the editors at America's Test Kitchen (America's Test Kitchen, 2016).

Cool Beans: The Ultimate Guide to Cooking with the World's Most Versatile Plant-Based Protein, with 125 Recipes by Joe Yonan (Ten Speed Press, 2020).

Grains for Every Season: Rethinking Our Way with Grains by Joshua McFadden (Artisan, 2021).

More with Less: Whole Food Cooking Made Irresistibly Simple by Jodi Moreno (Roost Books, 2018).

Whole Food Cooking Every Day: Transform the Way You Eat with 250 Vegetarian Recipes Free of Gluten, Dairy, and Refined Sugar by Amy Chaplin (Artisan, 2019).

FOOD ADVOCACY

Marine Stewardship Council
Global nonprofit organization working to avoid overfishing and help consumers make sustainable fish and seafood choices.
https://www.msc.org/en-us/

Monterey Bay Aquarium Seafood Watch
Shopper's guide for purchasing the most environmentally friendly and healthful fish and seafood ranked from Most Sustainable to Avoid, updated frequently.
https://www.seafoodwatch.org/

Oldways Whole Grains Council
Nonprofit consumer advocacy organization that educates about choosing whole-grain foods.
https://wholegrainscouncil.org/

DIETARY PATTERN SCORING SYSTEMS

Mediterranean Diet Score
A questionnaire used in research settings to quantify adherence to a Mediterranean diet. Numerous variations exist; this Med Diet Score was developed for consumers by the Mediterranean Food Alliance in partnership with Oldways.org, creator of the most widely used Mediterranean Diet Pyramid.
https://oldwayspt.org/system/files/atoms/files/RateYourMedDietScore.pdf

MIND Diet Score
A scoring system used to quantify adherence to the MIND (Mediterranean-DASH Intervention for Neurodegenerative Delay) diet in the MIND diet study published in 2015. A slightly modified version of the scoring system is being used in the ongoing MIND Diet Trial (publication pending): cheese was increased from one to two servings per week, and red wine was eliminated as a brain-healthy food group.

INGREDIENTS

BEANS AND LEGUMES

Eden Foods
Organic canned beans in phthalate-free cans
https://store.edenfoods.com/

Rancho Gordo
Heirloom beans
https://www.ranchogordo.com/

365 by Whole Foods Market
Cooked beans and lentils in BPA-free boxes
https://www.wholefoodsmarket.com/

Thrive Market
Dry and cooked beans and lentils in BPA-free pouches
https://thrivemarket.com/

Zursun Beans
Heirloom beans
https://www.zursunbeans.com/

CANNED AND JARRED INGREDIENTS

Available at most grocery stores

ENCHILADA SAUCE

Frontera Red and Green Enchilada Sauce (consider reducing the salt in a dish when using this)

Hatch Green Chile Enchilada Sauce (consider reducing the salt in a dish when using this)
Simply Organic Red Enchilada Sauce

CANNED TOMATOES

Bianco di Napoli San Marzano tomatoes
Cento Organic tomatoes
Mutti crushed tomatoes
REGA San Marzano tomatoes
San Marzano tomatoes

MARINARA SAUCE

Classico Riserva Marinara
Newman's Own Organics Marinara
Rao's Homemade Marinara

COOKING OILS

California Olive Ranch
100 percent California extra-virgin olive oil and avocado oil blend for everyday use
https://californiaoliveranch.com/

Fresh-Pressed Olive Oil Club
Subscription service for high-end extra-virgin olive oils from around the world
https://freshpressedoliveoil.com/home/

Kinloch Plantation Products
Virgin pecan oil for everyday, high-heat cooking
https://pecanoil.com/

Nutiva
Organic avocado oil for everyday cooking
https://www.nutiva.com/

Podere Ricavo
High-end extra-virgin olive oil from Tuscany, Italy
https://ricavo.it/

FISH AND SEAFOOD

Tinned and Jarred Seafood
High-quality, sustainable anchovies, sardines, mussels, and tuna
Conservasortiz.com
Patagoniaprovisions.com
Wildplanetfoods.com
Vitalchoice.com

Wild For Salmon
Wild-caught, sustainable, traceable salmon from Alaska
https://www.wildforsalmon.com/

FLOUR AND OTHER BAKING INGREDIENTS

Anson Mills
Buckwheat, stone-ground cornmeal, and whole-wheat flour
https://ansonmills.com/

Bob's Red Mill
Almond, buckwheat, chickpea, hazelnut, oat, quinoa, spelt, and whole-grain flours and meals; ground flaxseed
https://www.bobsredmill.com/

Hayden Flour Mills
Buckwheat, chickpea, oat, spelt, stone-ground cornmeal, and whole-grain flours
https://www.haydenflourmills.com/

Jovial Foods
Whole-wheat flour
https://jovialfoods.com/

EXTRACTS

Nielsen-Massey Orange Blossom Water
nielsenmassey.com

King Arthur Baking Company Pure Orange Oil
https://www.kingarthurbaking.com/

Simply Organic Orange Flavor
simplyorganic.com

GRAINS AND PASTA

Anson Mills
Farro, oats, polenta, rice, and oats
https://ansonmills.com/

Barilla
Whole-grain pasta
https://www.barilla.com/en-us

Bob's Red Mill
Amaranth, barley, farro, oats, millet, quinoa, teff
https://www.bobsredmill.com/

DeLallo
Whole-wheat pasta
https://www.delallo.com/

Jovial Foods
Gluten-free pasta
https://jovialfoods.com/

Lundberg Family Farms
Wide variety of organic rice
https://www.lundberg.com/

Lotus Foods
Organic Forbidden black rice, rice noodles, and brown and black rice noodles
https://www.lotusfoods.com/

Sfoglini
Whole-grain pasta
https://www.sfoglini.com/

365 by Whole Foods Market
Amaranth, barley, farro, freekeh, and wild rice
https://www.wholefoodsmarket.com/

Thrive Market Organic Biodynamic
Whole-wheat pasta
https://thrivemarket.com/

MEAT, POULTRY, AND DAIRY-FREE MILK AND CHEESE

Belcampo
Grass-fed beef
https://belcampo.com/collections/beef

Butcher Box
Grass-fed beef, organic chicken, and sustainable meats
https://www.butcherbox.com/

Califia Farms
Unsweetened almond and oat milk
https://www.califiafarms.com/

Jackson Hole Buffalo Meat Company
Grass-fed bison
https://jhbuffalomeat.com/

Kite Hill
Almond ricotta cheese
https://www.kite-hill.com/

Lockhart Cattle Company
Grass-fed beef
https://lockhartcattle.com/

Three Trees Organics
Unsweetened almond, pistachio, oat, and seed milks
https://www.threetrees.com/

NUTS AND SEEDS

Nuts.com
Organic and conventional nuts and seeds
https://nuts.com/

Kirkland
Organic almonds, cashews, pecans, and walnuts available in bulk online or at Costco retail stores
https://www.costco.com

Soom Foods
Organic tahini
https://soomfoods.com/

365 by Whole Foods Market
Organic tahini
https://www.wholefoodsmarket.com/

Thrive Market
Organic almonds, cashews, walnuts, pecans, pine nuts, and pistachios; organic chia, hemp, and pumpkin seeds; cloth nut milk bags
https://thrivemarket.com/

OLIVES

Divina
https://divinamarket.com/

Mediterranean Organic
https://www.mediterraneanorganic.com/

SEASONINGS AND CONDIMENTS

Diaspora Co.
Turmeric, chiles, pepper, saffron, sumac, and other spices
https://www.diasporaco.com/

Eden Foods
Lower-sodium shiro white miso paste
https://store.edenfoods.com/

The Ginger People
Organic pickled sushi ginger
https://gingerpeople.com/

Maldon Salt Company
Flaky sea salt
https://maldonsalt.com/

Mina
Harissa paste, preserved lemons
https://mina.co/

Miso Master Organic
Organic red, chickpea, and white miso paste
https://great-eastern-sun.com/

Mother-In-Law's
Gochujang (without corn syrup or MSG), kimchi
https://milkimchi.com/

New York Shuk
Harissa, preserved lemons, sumac, za'atar
https://www.nyshuk.com/

SUPPLEMENTS

Nordic Naturals Algae Omega
Vegan source of DHA and EPA from algae
https://www.nordic.com/

Relevate
Brain-supporting nutrients, including DHA and EPA from fish roe
https://neuroreserve.com/

Index

Page numbers in italic refer to photos and figures.